MCP HAHNEMANN UNIVERSITY
D0870025

HANDBOOK OF Clinical Ophthalmology FOR Eyecare Professionals

Edited by:

Janice K. Ledford, COMT
EyeWrite Productions
Franklin, North Carolina

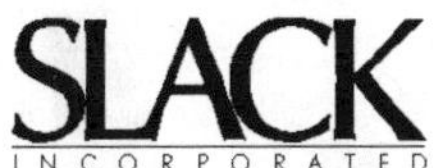

an innovative information, education, and management company

6900 Grove Road • Thorofare, NJ 08086

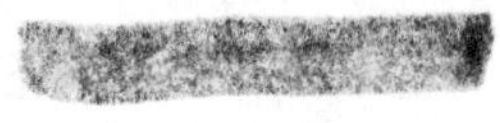

WW
39
H2356
2000

Publisher: John H. Bond
Editorial Director: Amy E. Drummond
Editorial Assistant: April C. Johnson

Copyright © 2001 by SLACK Incorporated

All rights reserved. No part of this book may be reproduced, stored in a retrieval system or transmitted in any form or by any means, electronic, mechanical, photocopying, recording or otherwise, without written permission from the publisher, except for brief quotations embodied in critical articles and reviews.

The author, editor, and publisher cannot accept responsibility for errors or exclusions or for the outcome of the application of the material presented herein. There is no expressed or implied warranty of this book or information imparted by it.

Care has been taken to ensure that drug selection, dosages, and treatments are in accordance with currently accepted/recommended practice. Due to continuing research, changes in government policy and regulations, and various effects of drug reactions and interactions, it is recommended that the reader review all materials and literature provided for each drug use, especially those that are new or not frequently used.

Handbook of clinical ophthalmology for eyecare professionals/ Jan K. Ledford, editor.
p. ; cm.
Includes index.
ISBN 1-55642-464-7 (alk. paper)
1. Ophthalmology--Handbook, manuals, etc. I. Ledford, Janice K.
[DNLM: 1. Eye Diseases--Handbooks. 2. Ophthalmology--Handbooks. WW 39 H2356 2000]
RE48.9 .H364 2000
617.7--dc21

00-057412

Printed in the United States of America.

Published by: SLACK Incorporated
6900 Grove Road
Thorofare, NJ 08086-9447 USA
Telephone: 856-848-1000
Fax: 856-853-5991
www.slackbooks.com

Contact SLACK Incorporated for more information about other books in this field or about the availability of our books from distributors outside the United States.

Authorization to photocopy items for internal or personal use, or the internal or personal use of specific clients, is granted by SLACK Incorporated, provided that the appropriate fee is paid directly to Copyright Clearance Center, 222 Rosewood Drive, Danvers, MA 01923 USA, 978-750-8400. Prior to photocopying items for educational classroom use, please contact the CCC at the address above. Please reference Account Number 9106324 for SLACK Incorporated's Professional Book Division.

For further information on CCC, check CCC Online at the following address: http://www.copyright.com.

Last digit is print number: 10 9 8 7 6 5 4 3 2 1

Dedication

This book is dedicated to the memory of William "Bill" Borover—master optician, author, lecturer, consultant, and friend.

D10060107
1-4-01 Rittenhouse $28.05

Contents

Acknowledgments

My first debt of thanks goes to SLACK Incorporated and its wonderful staff. In the field of eyecare, they have been part of making my every book publishing dream come true. No author or editor could ask for better. The exciting thing is that we are not through yet! Many thanks to John Bond, Amy Drummond, Debra Toulson, Vikki Kristiansson, April Johnson, Michele McDonnell, and Lauren Plummer. There are other behind-the-scenes folks who have also worked hard, whether it is answering the switchboard, reading proofs, handling computers, or what have you. I appreciate your contributions as well.

Next are a number of folks I have been privileged to meet during my career in eyecare, especially since I have been the Series Editor of the *Basic Bookshelf*. Ken Woodworth and Todd Hostetter did not have time to write (believe me, I begged them!), but were glad to give other assistance on many occasions. Ruth Bahr, Donna Leef, Cindy Dean, Jeff Freund, Seglinda Freed, Marsha Price, and Peggy Yamada also deserve a thank you. Those who kindly gave permission to use material and illustrations from their textbooks in this handbook include Norma Garber, Mark Greenwald, Sheila Nemeth, and Carolyn Shea. (If those lists sound like a Who's Who in ophthalmology, it is with good reason. These people are movers and shakers!) I must also express my appreciation for Bob Campbell, who is the ophthalmic editor for the *Bookshelf*, and thus inherited the job of editing *my* writing!

Now that the *Bookshelf* is nearly complete (we think!), I find that I have not only gained experience but new friends and special memories. For some, writing a book is a dream come true, and it was neat to be a part of that. Denise Cunningham was able to use her manuscript as part of earning a master's degree. Gretchen Van Boemel invited me to share her room at Academy. (I will never forget running about New Orleans with her! She has 10 times my energy!) One and all, there is no doubt that the authors and coauthors of the *Bookshelf* are experts in their field. They were willing to give extraordinary amounts of time and effort to share their knowledge with others. That is a tremendous gift that many benefit from, and I thank them all. On a sad note, we lost Bill Borover soon after the book he co-authored was published.

I would be remiss if I did not thank my family as well. Jim, TJ, Collin: you are the very best. No wife or mom could ask for more.

I have been truly blessed because of each one of you.

Jan Ledford, COMT
EyeWrite Productions
Franklin, North Carolina

About the Editor

It has been a long journey from Janice (Jan) Ledford's beginnings as an ophthalmic assistant to Series Editor of the *Basic Bookshelf for Eyecare Professionals.*

The journey began in 1982 when Dr. George Hubbard in Columbus, GA hired Jan. She became certified first as an assistant (1983) and then as a technician (1984) under his tutelage. Her interest in teaching others began to surface, and she was named Continuing Education Coordinator for the practice.

The Ledfords returned to their hometown of Warner Robins, GA in 1985. Jan began working for Eyesight Associates of Middle Georgia, an eyecare empire created and run by Dr. Johnny Gayton. The idea of becoming certified as a ophthalmic medical technologist began to surface during the next 2 years. By 1988 she had made it a reality.

In this practice, other talents began to emerge as well. By the time SLACK Incorporated began looking for an editor for a new series, she had already published several books in the field. She had also broken into professional journals with articles, case studies, and research reports. (Journals include the *Journal of Ophthalmic Nursing and Technology, Ophthalmic Surgery, Ophthalmic Plastic and Reconstructive Surgery, Annals of Ophthalmology*, and *Contact Lens Spectrum.*) In 1993, Alcon Surgical awarded her its Achievement in Ophthalmology for coauthorship of the side approach cataract technique. In 1994, she was named to the *International Who's Who in Medicine.* Her editing experience included a seat on the editorial board of the *Professional Medical Assistant* journal.

When she heard that SLACK was doing a new series, she asked if they had chosen an editor yet. Next thing she knew, she was interviewing for the job. "Amy Drummond, SLACK's acquisition editor at that time, was in Atlanta for a meeting and suggested that we get together," Jan remembers. "We met at the Whistle Stop Café (where the movie "Fried Green Tomatoes" was filmed) and talked over a plate of fried green tomatoes. She must have liked them... I got the job!"

Jan, her husband, Jim, their two boys (TJ and Collin), and four cats have since moved to the mountains of Franklin, NC. She works part-time with Dr. Charles Kirby and Western North Carolina Eyecare Associates. Her writing talents have expanded to include a published novel and numerous awards for both fiction and nonfiction. She is a member of the National League of American Pen Women (Atlanta Branch), as well as the editorial board of the *Journal of Ophthalmic Nursing and Technology.*

Preface

There's been an explosion!

You didn't hear it. But if you're reading this book, I'll bet you're a part of it. The field of eyecare has not just grown or expanded. It has erupted with a big bang of technology.

Eyecare has got to be one of the most exciting of all medical fields. The eye is the only organ of the body that can be looked into without incision or intubation. This unique feature, in and of itself, is responsible for so much that has become possible in ophthalmology, optometry, and opticianry.

Now, with the advent of instruments such as the microendolaser, we can see even more. I stood in an operating room a few years ago and watched a video screen in awe as the back side of the iris came into focus. Only a year or two prior, no one had ever seen the back of the iris in a living eye. It was my mother's eye.

The truth is, besides the desire to offer the best patient care possible, we all have a personal interest in eyecare. How many of you are nearsighted like me? Chances are your grandparents have cataracts. Your teenagers wear contacts. We're not just talking about "the public." We're talking family.

Education has become more critical than ever because of this explosion (both in technology and in the population). That is the contribution that the *Basic Bookshelf for Eyecare Professionals* wants to make. We series authors want to teach you everything you need to know about the eye, ocular procedures and devices, patient care, even about your own career.

Before we ever started, before the first word went on paper or screen, we talked to a lot of you and we listened.

You want to perform your job not just adequately but fantastically. You want to learn what you need for the task at hand without a lot of history lessons, weighty theory, or research notes. When you spend time studying, you want it to count for something, so the details you need have to be right there. You demand information that you can use where you live… in the exam lane, dispensary, or operating room.

Job performance isn't your only goal. You want to grow professionally. Taking certifying examinations is an important part of that growth. You need to know where to start and what to study. You want the material to be available without having to dig through tons of print.

We heard you, and we did our best to make the *Bookshelf* meet those needs.

Now, with this handbook, we have put the finishing touch on our work. We have put the tools at your fingertips. You'll be equipped to do your best, and because of that, the world of eyecare will be a better place.

Janice K. Ledford

Introduction

It was very difficult to determine exactly what should go into this handbook. After all, we've already devoted a complete book to each topic. The *Basic Bookshelf for Eyecare Professionals* has been well received. What sense does it make to offer a condensed version?

It makes a lot of sense in fact, unless you want to put your 24 *Bookshelf* books on a rolling cart to take them into the exam room with you. While each book is necessary for the background and details on each topic, we decided to put out one more text… a handbook small enough to fit into your lab coat pocket. Something you *could* take into the exam room.

As I said, compiling this handbook wasn't easy, especially regarding the clinical aspects of eyecare. For those topics, the bottom line became "what information might a tech need during the exam?" Thus, we filled the handbook with useful tables, charts, and how-to's. The more academic subjects are highlighted by key text and notes.

We've done our best with each *Bookshelf* text to make sure our information is accurate and current, even down to the spelling. In some cases, however, controversy exists. For example, is it Grave, Grave's, or Graves' ophthalmopathy? Even when I consulted a long list of experts, the answers varied. The best we could do was to go with the most popular answer and strive to be consistent in this particular volume.

If these efforts enable you to provide even better patient care, then we have achieved our goal.

Janice K. Ledford

CHAPTER 1

Ocular Anatomy and Physiology

Embryology (Table 1-1)

- The eyes begin to develop during the second week of pregnancy.
- The process of ocular formation is largely a product of different growth rates of various cells, in addition to cellular specialization as development takes place.
- The eye begins as a thickened area called the optic primordium, becomes the optic grove, then invaginates (folds in) to form the optic vesicle. The optic vesicle is later pushed outward, forming the optic cup, from which will develop the individual structures of the eye.
- The optic cup predetermines the size and shape of the orbit. Postnatal growth of the orbit coincides with the growth of the globe.
- Eyelids are fused together at first, then separate during months 5 through 7.
- Most babies are hyperopic at birth.

A newborn baby can see light and closes his or her eyes to bright light. Most newborns will exhibit a jerky following response to a target (a human face is preferred). There is poorly controlled eye movement, and intermittent eye deviations may be present. These conditions usually phase out around the fourth month of life, and fixation becomes increasingly sharper. The visual acuity of a 2-month-old is estimated to be around 20/400. This rises to 20/100 at 6 months, 20/50 at 1 year, and 20/20 by 3 years of age.

The Bony Orbit (Figure 1-1)

- The bony orbit contains the globe, fat, fascia (supportive tissues), blood vessels, and extraocular muscles.
- The orbit serves as a protective housing for the globe and a framework for the attachments of the extraocular muscles.
- The seven bones that comprise the orbit are the frontal, sphenoid, zygomatic, maxilla, ethmoid, lacrimal, and palatine bones.

Table 1-1.
Gestational Development of Ocular Structures

Gestation Month(s)	Embryologic Occurrence
0 to 1	Formation of optic pit, optic stalk, optic vesicle, and optic cup Lens begins forming Primary vitreous is present
1 to 2	Lens separates from optic cup Cornea forms: epithelium and endothelium Sclera begins forming anteriorly Iris tissues fuse Orbit begins forming Anterior chamber begins forming Pupils form Secondary vitreous is present Eyelids form and fuse Eyebrows form Extraocular muscles begin to form Nasolacrimal drainage system begins to form Optic nerve fibers present in stalk
3	Eyes positioned in center of face Lens is 2 mm in diameter Descemet's membrane forms Sclera surrounds optic nerve Optic cup pushes forward Tertiary vitreous is present
4	Ciliary muscle begins to form Precursors of photoreceptors present Primitive retinal vasculature present Vitreous fully formed Zonules begin to form Schlemm's canal forms
5	Pupillary membrane disappears Bowman's membrane forms Corneal nerve endings present Sphincter muscle begins to form Macula begins to differentiate Lids begin to separate
6	Dilator muscle forms Retinal layers fully formed Aqueous begins to form

(continued)

Table 1-1. (continued)

Gestational Development of Ocular Structures

Gestation Month(s)	Embryologic Occurrence
7	Lids fully separate Eyelashes present
8	Lens is 6 mm in diameter Hyaloid artery degenerates Nasolacrimal cord hollows out Pupillary membrane atrophies

Reprinted with permission from Lens A, Langley T, Nemeth SC, Shea C. Ocular Anatomy and Physiology. *Thorofare, NJ: SLACK Incorporated; 1999.*

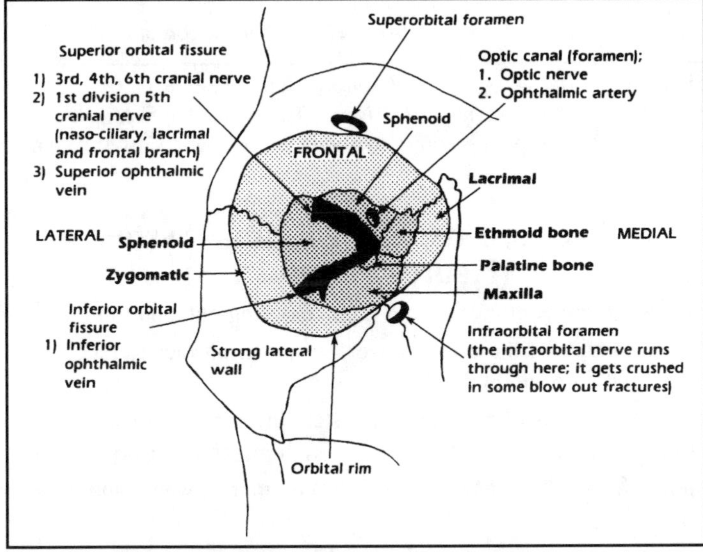

Figure 1-1. Bones and openings in the orbit (reprinted from Nemeth SC, Shea CA. *Medical Sciences for the Ophthalmic Assistant.* Thorofare, NJ: SLACK Incorporated; 1988, with permission from Sheila Nemeth and Carolyn Shea).

- The orbit has a roof, a floor, and a lateral and medial wall. The floor of the orbit is comprised mostly of the thin maxillary bone, which is commonly broken from the pressure of blunt trauma in a blow-out fracture.
- The thinness of the ethmoid bone, located in the medial orbital wall, makes it susceptible to erosion from sinusitis originating from the ethmoid sinuses. Infections from the ethmoid sinuses, on occasion, can enter the orbital cavity and move into the brain via the orbital veins.

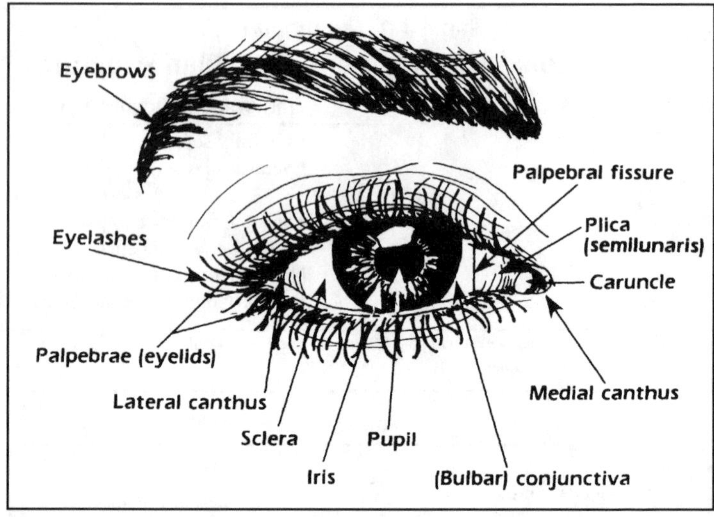

Figure 1-2. External eye (reprinted from Nemeth SC, Shea CA. *Medical Sciences for the Ophthalmic Assistant.* Thorofare, NJ: SLACK Incorporated; 1988, with permission from Sheila Nemeth and Carolyn Shea).

Brows, Lids, and Lacrimal System (Figures 1-2 and 1-3)

- The eyelids protect the eye from trauma, drying out, and too much light.
- The appearance of the external eye can vary from race to race and is simply a variation of normal.
- The two divisions of the lacrimal system are the secretory system for the delivery of the tears and the excretory system, which disposes of the tears.
- A normal tear film consists of three layers: mucin, water, and oil.

The Globe

(For information on the extraocular muscles, see Chapter 12.)

- Each globe is located in the anterior portion of the orbit, nearer to the roof and lateral wall.
- The globe occupies only one-fifth of the orbital cavity.
- The globe is least protected on the lateral side.
- The globe is not spherical but is made up of two modified spheres fused together with their junction at the limbus (Figure 1-4). The anterior cornea is the smaller "sphere" with a radius of 7.8 mm, and the larger posterior "sphere" has a radius of 17 mm.

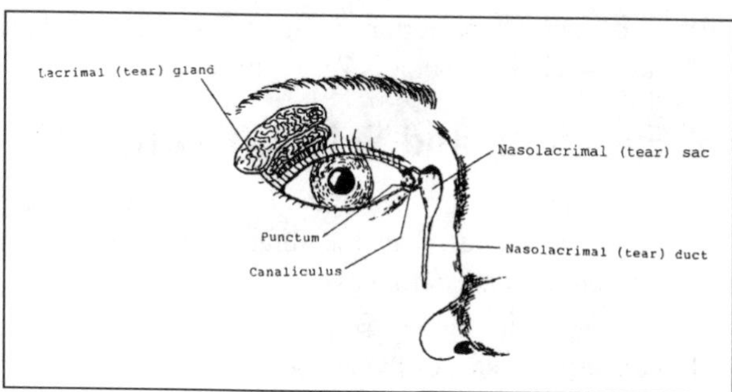

Figure 1-3. The lacrimal system (drawing by Holly Hess. Reprinted with permission-from Gayton JL, Ledford JK. *The Crystal Clear Guide to Sight for Life*. Lancaster, Pa: Starburst Publishers, 1996).

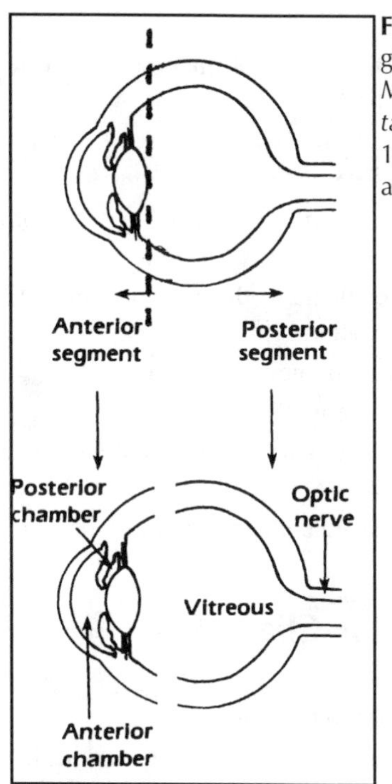

Figure 1-4. Segments and chambers of the globe (reprinted from Nemeth SC, Shea CA. *Medical Sciences for the Ophthalmic Assistant.* Thorofare, NJ: SLACK Incorporated; 1988, with permission from Sheila Nemeth and Carolyn Shea).

- The globe is widest at the anterior posterior diameter (24 mm) and flatter vertically (23 mm). Its horizontal diameter is 23.5 mm (Figure 1-5).

Conjunctiva, Episclera, and Sclera (Figure 1-6)

- The conjunctiva is the vascular mucous membrane that covers the anterior globe and inner surface of the eyelids. This membrane plays a role in the immunologic defense system of the external eye.
- The bulbar conjunctiva covers the globe itself, while the palpebral conjunctiva is attached to the tarsal plates of the eyelids.
- The episclera is the outermost layer of the sclera and has an extensive blood supply from the anterior ciliary arteries. Inflammation makes these vessels much more visible (when viewed with a slit lamp), as they sit posterior to the bulbar conjunctiva.
- The sclera, composed of dense collagen fibers, is the firm, protective white housing for the inner contents of the globe.

The Cornea

- The cornea is the strongest refractive entity within our visual system, contributing two-thirds of the refractive power of the eye.
- The cornea is made up of five layers: epithelium, Bowman's membrane, stroma, Descemet's membrane, and endothelium (Figure 1-7).
- The epithelium is one of the fastest healing tissues of the body.
- The stroma makes up 90% of the cornea's structure.
- The endothelium functions as a water pump to maintain proper tissue hydration.
- The anatomy and physiology of the cornea are both geared toward one end: corneal clarity.

Anterior and Posterior Chambers

- The anterior segment is the small asymmetric cavity of the globe, which includes the lens and all structures anterior to the lens.
- The anterior segment is made up of the anterior and posterior chambers.
- The anterior chamber lies anterior to the iris and behind the cornea and contains aqueous. The posterior chamber lies posterior to the iris and contains the lens.

The iris can be thought of as a colored muscular shutter attaching peripherally to the ciliary body (Figure 1-8). The central aperture, or opening, is the pupil. The primary function of the iris is to regulate the size of the pupil via the innervation of its muscles. The iris prevents excessive light from entering the system and helps to form clear images on the retina by preventing peripheral rays of light from entering the eye (see Chapter 8 for pupil evaluation).

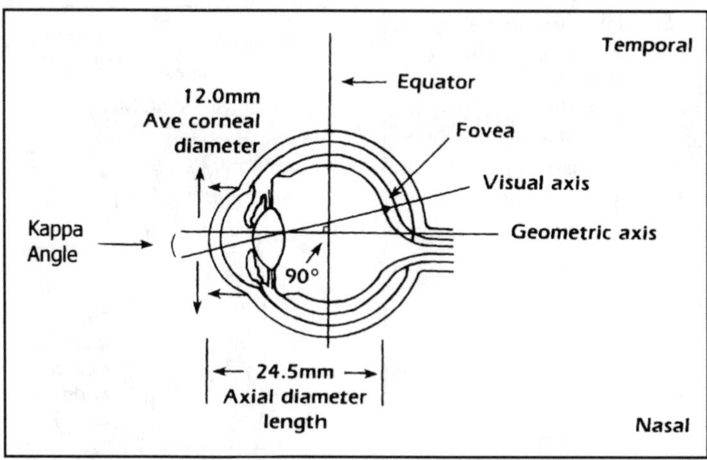

Figure 1-5. Ocular landmarks and dimensions (reprinted from Nemeth SC, Shea CA. *Medical Sciences for the Ophthalmic Assistant*. Thorofare, NJ: SLACK Incorporated; 1988, with permission from Sheila Nemeth and Carolyn Shea).

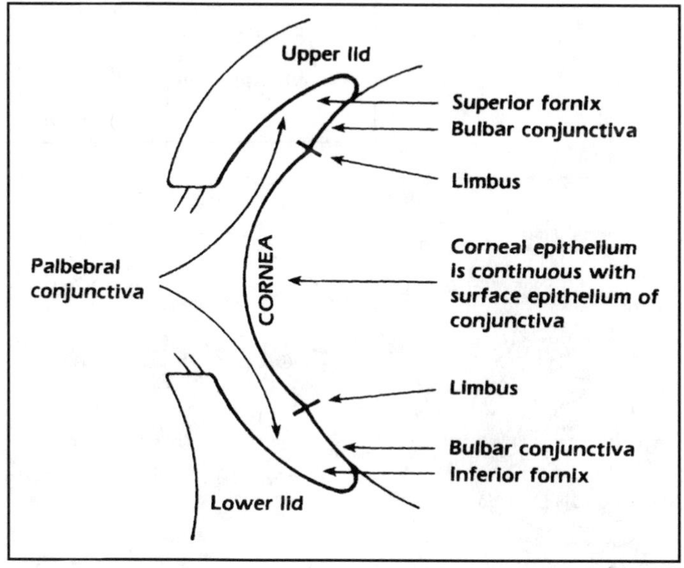

Figure 1-6. Cross-section of conjunctival topography (reprinted from Nemeth SC, Shea CA. *Medical Sciences for the Ophthalmic Assistant.* Thorofare, NJ: SLACK Incorporated; 1988, with permission from Sheila Nemeth and Carolyn Shea).

Figure 1-7. Histological cross-section of the cornea (reprinted from Nemeth SC, Shea CA. *Medical Sciences for the Ophthalmic Assistant*. Thorofare, NJ: SLACK Incorporated; 1988, with permission from Sheila Nemeth and Carolyn Shea).

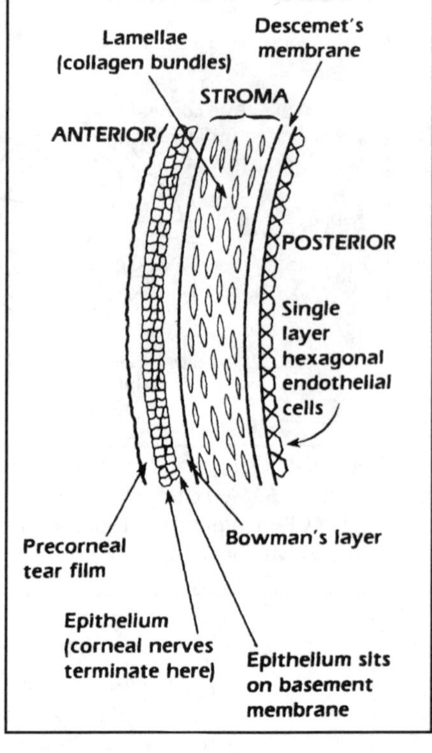

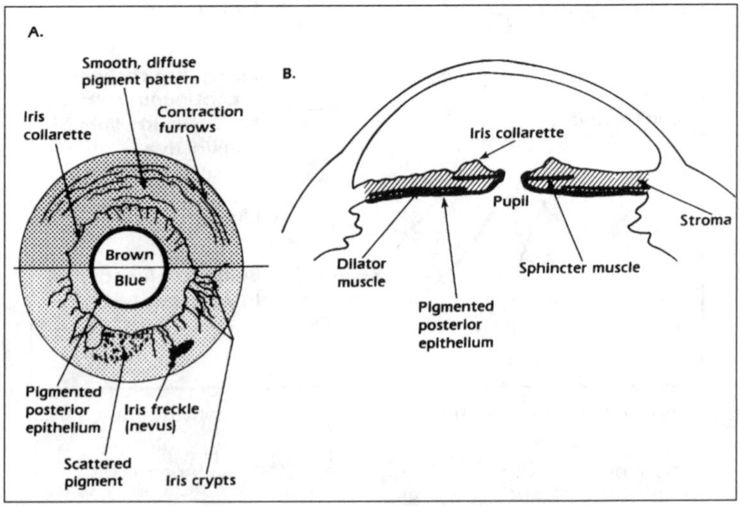

Figure 1-8. A. External view of blue and brown irides. B. Cross-section of iris anatomy (reprinted from Nemeth SC, Shea CA. *Medical Sciences for the Ophthalmic Assistant*. Thorofare, NJ: SLACK Incorporated; 1988, with permission from Sheila Nemeth and Carolyn Shea).

The ciliary body lies between the iris and the choroid. The ciliary body contains pigment and a rich vascular network. It is divided into two sections: the anterior pars plicata and the more posterior pars plana (Figure 1-9).

The aqueous (aqueous humor) is the watery fluid that occupies the anterior and posterior chambers of the eye. In addition to contributing to corneal and lenticular metabolism, the aqueous is a part of the pathway that light must take on its way to the retina. In its normal state, the aqueous is clear. Aqueous is formed in the posterior chamber, then circulates through the pupil into the anterior chamber (Figure 1-10). The aqueous then leaves the eye through the angle. The presence of the aqueous in the eye helps create a certain amount of resistance to sustain a constant shape of the ocular coat. It also creates a pressure, known as intraocular pressure (IOP), within the eye. (For measuring IOP, see Chapter 8.)

The angle is the actual angle created by the root of the iris and the peripheral corneal vault (Figure 1-11). The aqueous leaves the anterior chamber through the trabecular meshwork (TM), a mesh-like band lying just posterior to the peripheral corneal endothelium. If the iris and corneal endothelium have too small a separation, or are "closed" against one another, the aqueous will not have access to the TM.

IOP is created by the dynamics of the production of aqueous at the ciliary processes (termed inflow) and the drainage of aqueous through the TM to Schlemm's canal (termed outflow). There is a normal physiologic balance between these two forces. However, when these dynamics are disturbed and the inflow exceeds the outflow, the result is increased IOP. IOP is measured with a tonometer (see Chapter 8).

The lens is the transparent biconvex intraocular structure that actively participates in the functions of accommodation and refraction. The lens is located directly behind the iris. Fine zonular fibers (or zonulae) originating from the ciliary body (pars plicata portion) attach to the lens, suspending it behind the pupil. Anatomically, it has three distinct parts: the capsule, the epithelium, and the lens substance (the cortex and nucleus).

The Posterior Segment

- The posterior segment includes the vitreous, posterior sclera, choroid, and retina (Figure 1-12).
- The choroid is a dense network of blood vessels sandwiched between the retina and sclera. It provides nourishment to the photoreceptors (rods and cones) and the retinal pigment epithelium (RPE). The choroid is the posterior part of the uvea. (Other uveal tissue is the iris and ciliary body.)
- The retina contains the photochemicals (ie, rhodopsin) and the neurologic connections (rods, cones, and ganglion cells) that process light energy and relay it to our visual cortex for visual perception and integration.

Figure 1-9. Ciliary body and related structures (reprinted from Nemeth SC, Shea CA. *Medical Sciences for the Ophthalmic Assistant*. Thorofare, NJ: SLACK Incorporated; 1988, with permission from Sheila Nemeth and Carolyn Shea).

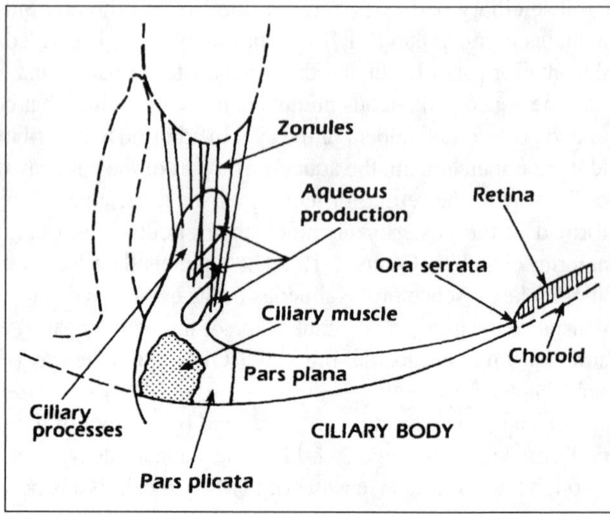

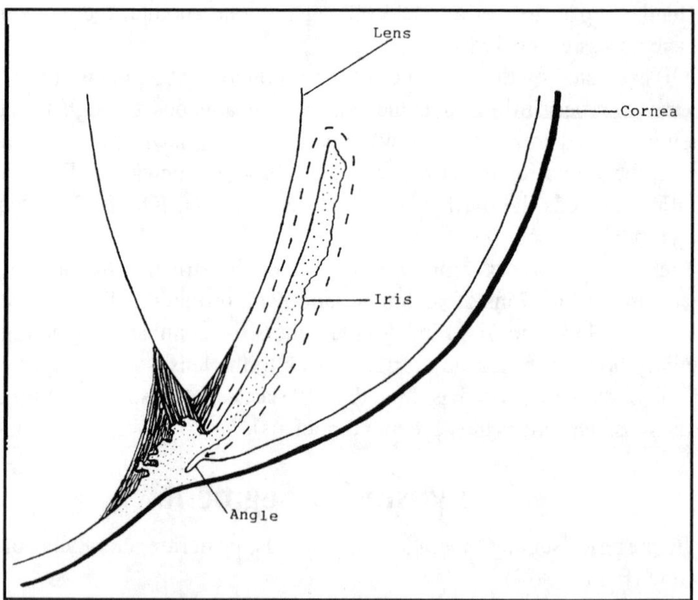

Figure 1-10. Flow of aqueous humor through the anterior chamber and posterior chamber (drawing by Holly Hess. Reprinted from Gayton JL, Ledford JK. *The Crystal Clear Guide to Sight for Life*. Lancaster, Pa: Starburst Publishers; 1996).

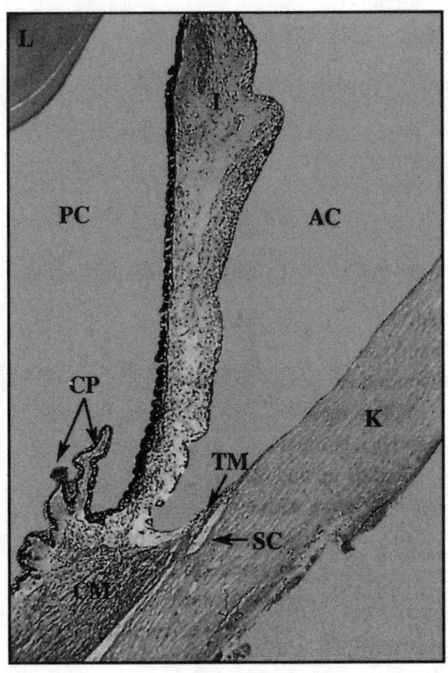

Figure 1-11. Microscopic section of an angle (reprinted with permission from Lens A, Langley T, Nemeth SC, Shea C. *Ocular Anatomy and Physiology.* Thorofare, NJ: SLACK Incorporated; 1999. Photo by Mark Greenwald, University of Tennessee-Memphis).

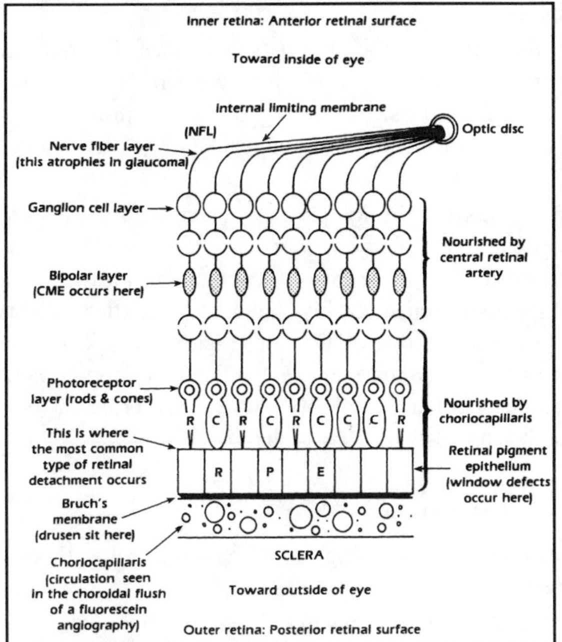

Figure 1-12. Schematic of retinal anatomy (reprinted from Nemeth SC, Shea CA. *Medical Sciences for the Ophthalmic Assistant.* Thorofare, NJ: SLACK Incorporated; 1988, with permission from Sheila Nemeth and Carolyn Shea).

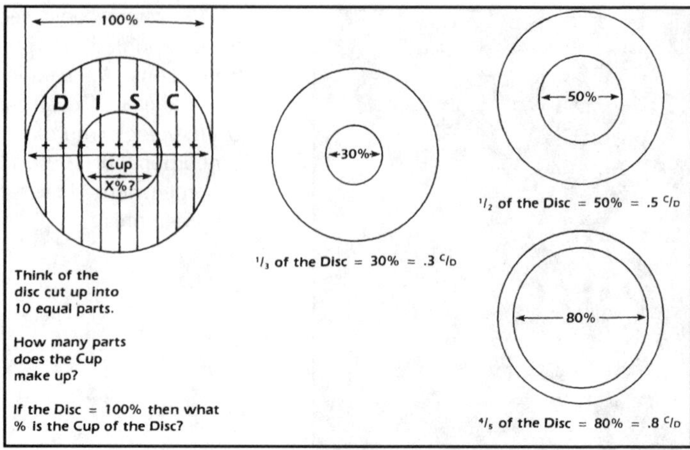

Figure 1-13. Cup-to-disc estimation technique (reprinted from Nemeth SC, Shea CA. *Medical Sciences for the Ophthalmic Assistant*. Thorofare, NJ: SLACK Incorporated; 1988, with permission from Sheila Nemeth and Carolyn Shea).

- The macula is the 1.5 mm of central retina that surrounds the fovea, which is approximately 500 microns in diameter and the site from which our most detailed vision originates.
- The photoreceptor cells of the retina are the rods and cones. The rods, of which there are 130 million, are responsible for peripheral and scotopic (low luminance) vision. The cones, numbering 6 million, provide both color vision and the ability to see detail and fine resolution in higher luminance.

The optic disc develops a normal physiologic cup, or depression, in its center from the recession of fetal tissue. This cup varies greatly in size from one individual to another. The cup size of the disc is an important measurement because various disease processes (most notably, glaucoma) can affect it. This measurement is known as the cup-to-disc (C/D) ratio (Figure 1-13). This ratio is first assessed as a fraction: the disc represents a "10," and the proportion of the cup represents a percentage of that overall "10." As a general rule, the normal C/D ratio is 0.3 (ie, the cup takes up 30% of the total disc).

Visual Pathway

- Understanding the anatomy and physiology of the visual pathway (Figure 1-14) aids in localizing lesions (Figure 1-15).
- Lesions located in front of the chiasm (prechiasm) will affect only one eye; lesions at or behind the chiasm will affect both eyes.

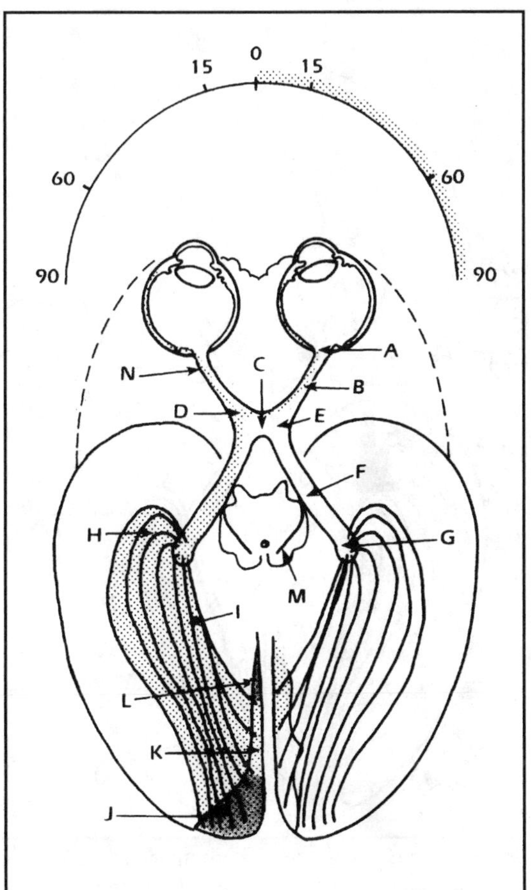

Figure 1-14. Visual pathways. A. The optic nerve. B. The nasal retinal fibers in the optic nerve. C. Nasal fibers crossing at the chiasm. D. Von Willebrandt's knee of the right eye's nasal fibers positioned in the left optic nerve. E. Chiasm or crossing. F. The optic tract. G. The lateral geniculate body. H. Meyer's loop of the temporal radiations. I. Parietal optic radiations. J. Macular area of the calcarine cortex in the occipital lobe. K. Peripheral binocular calcarine cortex. L. Monocular (extreme peripheral) calcarine cortex. M. Afferent fibers to the brainstem, which are comprised of about 10% of the visual sensory information. N. Temporal fibers from the retina traveling on the same side of the head to the same side visual cortex (courtesy of Norma Garber, Productivity Enhancement Group, Inc. Reprinted with permission from Lens A, Langley T, Nemeth SC, Shea C. *Ocular Anatomy and Physiology*. Thorofare, NJ: SLACK Incorporated; 1999).

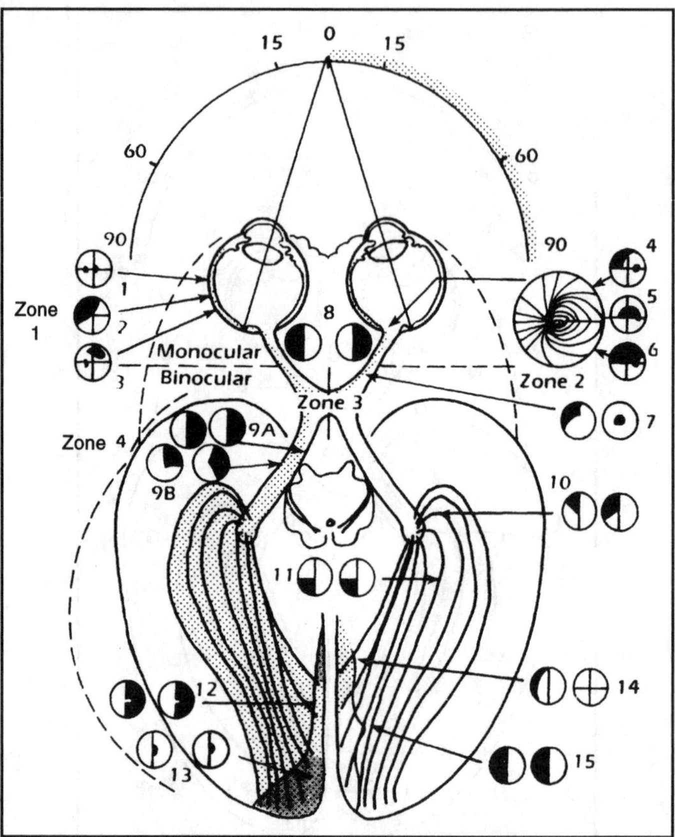

Figure 1-15. Typical field patterns seen with damage along the visual pathways. Zone 1—Retinal: 1. central scotoma; 2. retinal detachment; 3. isolated scotoma. Zone 2—The NFL: 4. nasal step; 5. arcuate scotoma; 6. altitudinal radiating scotoma. Zone 3—The chiasm: 7. prechiasmal anterior junctional scotoma; 8. chiasmal bitemporal hemianopsia. Zone 4—The retrochiasmal regions: 9A. optic tract complete right homonymous hemianopsia; 9B. optic tract incomplete incongruous hemianopsia; 10. temporal lobe left incongruous quandrantanopsia; 11. parietal lobe left congruous quandrantanopsia; 12. macular sparing occipital homonymous hemianopsia; 13. congruous occipital right macular hemianopsia; 14. left temporal crescent damage to deep right occipital cortex; 15. left complete homonymous hemianopsia. Note: Complete homonymous hemianopsias can occur anywhere posterior to the chiasm. If they are incomplete, they are helpful in localizing pathology. As a general rule, the more anterior the pathology, the more unlike or incongruous the field defects. The more posterior the pathology, the more exquisitely congruous the field defects become (courtesy of Norma Garber, Productivity Enhancement Group, Inc. Reprinted with permission from Lens A, Langley T, Nemeth SC, Shea C. *Ocular Anatomy and Physiology*. Thorofare, NJ: SLACK Incorporated; 1999).

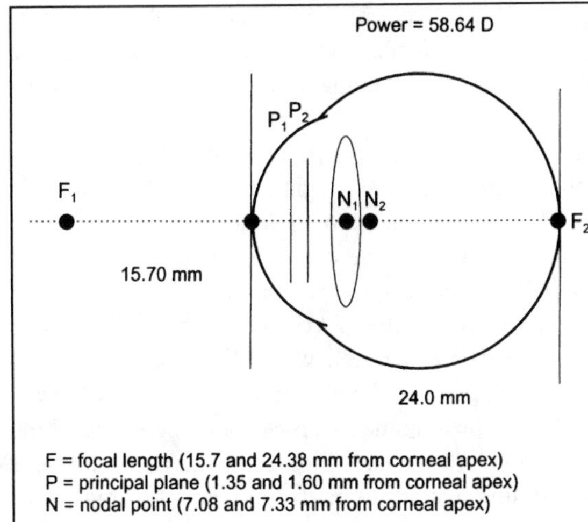

Figure 1-16. Schematic eye (reprinted with permission from Lens A, Langley T, Nemeth SC, Shea C. *Ocular Anatomy and Physiology*. Thorofare, NJ: SLACK Incorporated; 1999).

- The eyes only collect the images we see. The brain is responsible for interpreting what is viewed.
- Various parts of the brain respond to visual stimuli. The responses range from recognizing the image to sending impulses to other parts of the body.
- Important terms to remember when relating to visual field (see also Chapter 11) include:

  Homonymous—relating to the same half of each eye's visual field.
  Bitemporal—pertaining to the temporal visual field in each eye.
  Hemianopsia—defect in the right or left half of the visual field.
  Congruous—similar defect in each eye.

Miscellaneous

The *schematic eye of Gullstrand* (Figure 1-16) is a model that uses average values for the optical system of the eye (see also Chapter 3). The schematic eye is used as a general reference for determining mathematical values. It makes certain assumptions, however, that can lead to inaccuracies if the values in the schematic eye are accepted as true.

Accommodation is stimulated by either the blurred image of a nearby object or an awareness of the object's proximity. About 70 thread-like fibers, known as zonulae, extend from the ciliary muscle to the lens capsule. As the ciliary muscle contracts, it relaxes the tension on the zonulae. This results in increased curvature and power of the crystalline lens. Accommodation also causes the eyes to converge and the pupils to constrict. This chain of events is known as the accommodative triad, or the near response.

Emmetropia is the lack of a refractive error—the state of a "normal" eye. Light from a distant object (20 or more feet away) has essentially parallel light rays. When these light rays enter a relaxed emmetropic eye, they are focused on the retina.

Myopia, or *nearsightedness*, is caused by the power of the refractive structures being too strong for the length of the eye—light comes to a focus in front of the retina (Figure 1-17). This can be related to an eye of normal length, but the power is too strong; more commonly, the eye is too long for its power. Myopia is corrected with minus-powered spherical lenses.

Most humans are born with some degree of *hyperopia*, or *farsightedness*. In normal eyes, emmetropia occurs in the teen years. However, some eyes remain too short for the focusing power of the eye (in its relaxed state), causing hyperopia. In this case, light fails to come to a focus point before reaching the retina (light is focused "behind" the retina) (Figure 1-18). When the eye is young, it is capable of overcoming a small to moderate amount of hyperopia using accommodation. Therefore, hyperopia may not manifest itself until later in life. Hyperopia is corrected with plus-powered spherical lenses.

Astigmatism is a refractive error that is not equal in all meridians. An unequally curved cornea is the usual cause of astigmatism, but it may occur in the lens as well (lenticular astigmatism). In regular astigmatism, the meridians with the greatest and least amount of curvature (or refractive error) are perpendicular (90 degrees) to each other. Instead of light being focused to a point, two focus lines are created perpendicular to each other (one focus line for each primary meridian). This causes the image to be stretched out. Regular astigmatism is corrected with a cylindrical lens. Irregular astigmatism is not entirely correctable.

The types of astigmatism associated with the position of the focal lines are called simple, compound, and mixed astigmatism (Figure 1-19). Simple astigmatism is present when one focal line is on the retina. Simple myopic astigmatism has the second focal line is in front of the retina, and in simple hyperopic astigmatism, the second focal line is behind the retina. Compound astigmatism has both focal lines on the same side of the retina. Compound myopic astigmatism has both focal lines in front of the retina, and compound hyperopic astigmatism has both focal lines behind the retina. Mixed astigmatism is present when one focal line is in front of the retina and the other is behind the retina.

Presbyopia is caused by a decrease in the elasticity of the crystalline lens. When the ciliary muscle contracts, it releases tension on the zonulae that are attached to the capsule of the lens. In a young eye, this allows the lens to assume a more round (and powerful) shape. In an older eye, the lens has lost its ability to change shape, reducing the capacity to accommodate. The ability of the eye to change its focus (accommodate) naturally diminishes each year. Its effects are not usually noticed, however, until age 40 to 45. Presbyopia is corrected using plus-powered spheres placed over whatever correction, if any, is required for clear distance vision.

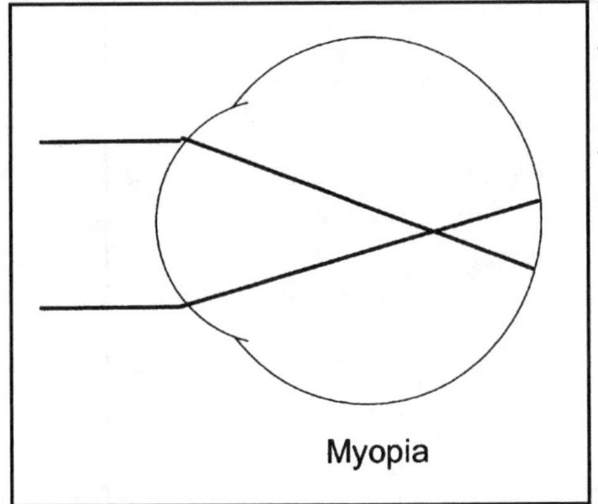

Figure 1-17. Myopia (reprinted with permission from Lens A, Langley T, Nemeth SC, Shea C. *Ocular Anatomy and Physiology*. Thorofare, NJ: SLACK Incorporated; 1999).

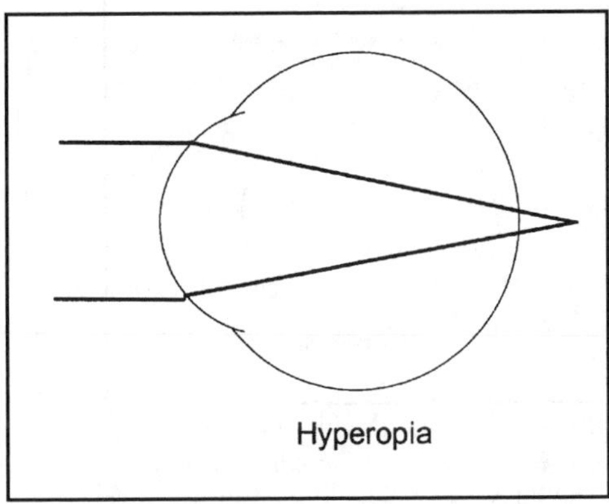

Figure 1-18. Hyperopia (reprinted with permission from Lens A, Langley T, Nemeth SC, Shea C. *Ocular Anatomy and Physiology*. Thorofare, NJ: SLACK Incorporated; 1999).

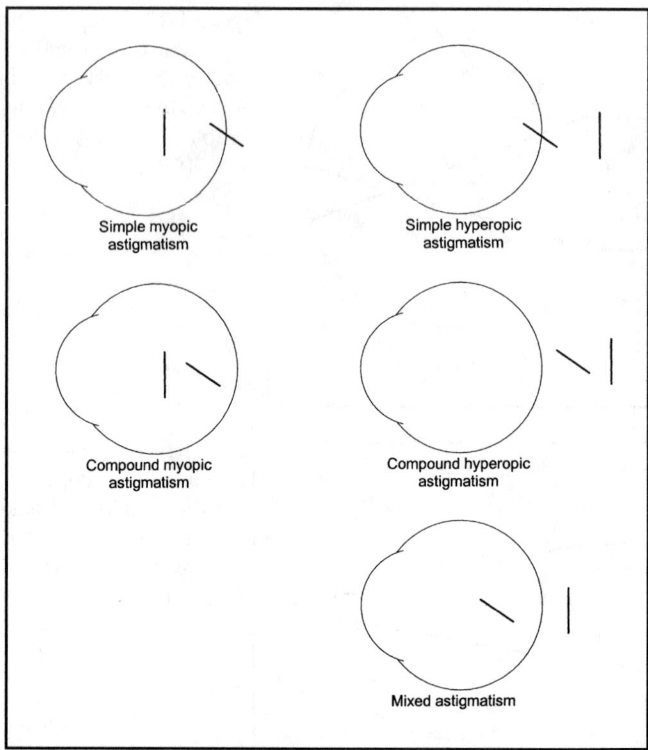

Figure 1-19. Types of astigmatism (reprinted with permission from Lens A, Langley T, Nemeth SC, Shea C. *Ocular Anatomy and Physiology*. Thorofare, NJ: SLACK Incorporated; 1999).

Unless otherwise noted , all text, tables, and figures are adapted or reprinted with permission from Lens A, Langley T, Nemeth SC, Shea C. Ocular Anatomy and Physiology. *Thorofare, NJ: SLACK Incorporated; 1999.*

CHAPTER 2

General Medical Knowledge

Anatomy and Physiology

- The body has four basic parts: cells, tissues, organs, and organ systems.
- The major systems of the body are musculoskeletal, nervous, gastrointestinal, respiratory, cardiovascular, genitourinary, and reproductive.
- The three regions of the body are head and neck, trunk, and limbs.

Like using a compass and a map to take a trip, positional terms give the ability to know position and direction when studying the human body. The *anatomical position* is defined as standing erect, eyes looking forward to the horizon, arms by the side, palms of hands directed forward, thumbs outward, and toes directed forward. The midline is an imaginary line drawn vertically down the middle of the body while in the anatomical position. It separates the body into right and left halves. A number of positional terms are used when describing the body (Table 2-1). All of these are defined relative to the anatomical position.

- Cells and tissues form the basic substance of the human body.
- Organs and the systems they form derive identity and structure from their cell and tissue make-up.
- Cells are the "concrete" from which tissue "building blocks" are made.
- Cells bound together form the "foundation" of the human body.

The body is composed of four types of tissues: nerve, muscle, epithelial, and connective. *Nerve tissue* is the body's postal service. It transmits messages in the form of electrical impulses from one place to another. Nerve tissue is comprised of the brain, the spinal cord, and the myriad of nerve fibers throughout the body. Movement is produced by *muscle tissue*. *Epithelial tissue* performs three functions: protection, absorption, and secretion. Skin is the epithelial tissue with which we are most familiar. *Connective tissue* takes many different forms and is found in many different places in the body. Adipose, or fat, tissue insulates the body and acts as a shock absorber. The connective tissue fills the spaces between

Table 2-1.
Anatomical Positions

Anatomical Positions
Anterior, ventral—Nearer the front surface of the body
Posterior, dorsal—Nearer the back surface of the body
Superior—Nearer the top of the head
Inferior—Nearer the soles of the feet
Medial—Nearer the midline
Lateral—Farther away from the midline
Superficial—Nearer the surface
Deep—Farther away from the surface
Ipsilateral—Same side of the body
Contralateral—Opposite side of the body
Internal—Nearer the center of the body
External—Away from the center of the body
Proximal—Near a specified region
Distal—Farther away from a specified region
Plantar—Sole of the foot
Palmar—Palm of the hand
Left—To the left of the midline of a subject in anatomical position
Right—To the right of the midline of a subject in anatomical position

other tissues and organs. Bone and cartilage are specialized connective tissues that give support to the body. Blood, another specialized connective tissue, is the body's transportation system, carrying nutrients and other products to all parts of the body.

- The heart, blood vessels, and blood make up the cardiovascular system. This system functions as the body's transportation system, carrying life-sustaining nutrients to all parts of the body.
- The respiratory system supplies vital oxygen to cells and expels carbon dioxide (a waste product) from the body.
- Without the ability to adjust to a constantly changing internal and external environment, the body would soon die. Maintaining homeostasis in the face of these forces is a major function of the endocrine system.
- Five glands make up the endocrine system: pituitary, thyroid, parathyroid, pancreas, and adrenal glands.

- The nervous system directs and coordinates most of the body's activities. Directly or indirectly, the nervous system affects every part of the body.
- The nervous system has two parts: the central nervous system (CNS) and the peripheral nervous system. The brain and spinal cord make up the CNS. The peripheral nervous system is composed of nerves that travel to and from the brain (cranial nerves) and spinal cord (spinal nerves).
- Cranial nerves (CN) II through VII are involved in normal eye function (Table 2-2). (See also Chapter 12.)

Disorders

The body is a collection of systems that work together. Any disease or condition that affects the body may also affect the eyes (Table 2-3). In addition, medication taken for any disorder may also have the potential for ocular side effects (Table 2-4).

Diagnostics

- Blood tests that may be indicated in eyecare include complete blood count (CBC), blood glucose level, rheumatoid factor, and sedimentation rate (Table 2-5).
- X-rays are used to image bony structures.
- Computed tomography (CT) uses fanned-out x-rays to create a cross-sectional picture of structures.
- Ultrasound utilizes sound waves to measure or create an image of the eye (see Chapter 10).
- Magnetic resonance imaging (MRI) utilizes a magnetic field to create a picture. It is especially useful in imaging soft tissue.

Table 2-2.
Cranial Nerves

CN #	Nerve Name	Ocular Action
II	Optic	Carries information from the retina to the brain
III	Oculomotor	Controls all EOMs except SO and LR Innervates superior levator palpebrae Functions in pupillary dilation Controls accommodation
IV	Trochlear	Controls SO muscle
V	Trigeminal	
	Branch 1: Ophthalmic	Sensation to lids, eyeball, conjunctiva, lacrimal gland, and other nonocular structures
	Branch 2: Maxillary	Sensation to lower lids and other nonocular areas
VI	Abducens	Controls LR muscle
VII	Facial	Controls muscles of facial expression

Table 2-3.
Systemic Disorders and Their Effects on the Eye

Disorder	Ocular Complications
I. Cardiovascular	
A. Atherosclerosis/ carotid artery disease	Retinal artery obstruction
B. Endocarditis	Conjunctival and retinal hemorrhage (Roth's spot) Infection Artery occlusion
C. Hypertension	Narrowing, twisting, and fibrosis of retinal blood vessels Retinal hemorrhage Papilledema Cotton-wool spots
D. Mitral valve prolapse	Retinal vessel occlusion

(continued)

Table 2-3. (continued)

Systemic Disorders and Their Effects on the Eye

II. Endocrine	
A. Diabetes	Leaking and rupturing of retinal blood vessels Neovascularization of retinal vessels Iris rubeosis Retinal detachment Macular edema Increased incidence of glaucoma and cataract
B. Graves' disease	Inflammation of EOMs Corneal exposure Compression of optic nerve
C. Hypothyroid	Partial loss of eyebrows and eyelashes Keratoconus Cataracts Optic atrophy
D. Pituitary tumor	Visual field loss Optic atrophy Nerve palsy
III. Infections	
A. AIDS	Swelling of retinal vessels Cotton-wool patches Kaposi's sarcoma of lids, conjunctiva, or orbit
B. Chlamydia	Trachoma
C. Herpes simplex 1	Corneal opacity
D. Influenza	Conjunctivitis Dacryoadenitis
E. Lyme disease	Conjunctivitis Periorbital edema Corneal infiltrates Uveitis Endophthalmitis
F. Measles	Conjunctivitis Subconjunctival hemorrhage Superficial keratitis

(continued)

Table 2-3. (continued)

Systemic Disorders and Their Effects on the Eye

G. Shingles (Herpes zoster)	Corneal and lid lesions Inflammation of conjunctiva, sclera, and uvea
H. Syphilis	Eyelid chancre Argyll Robertson pupil Swelling of optic disc Optic atrophy EOM weakness
I. Toxoplasmosis	Chorioretinitis
J. Tuberculosis	Ocular tubercles
IV. Connective tissue disease	
A. Lupus	Scleritis Damage to lacrimal gland Optic neuritis Cotton-wool spots
B. Multiple sclerosis	Optic neuritis Paralysis of EOMs Nystagmus
C. Rheumatoid arthritis	Keratoconjunctivitis sicca Scleritis Episcleritis Uveitis (in juveniles)
D. Temporal arteritis	Ischemic optic neuritis Weakness of EOMs
V. Muscle disorders	
A. Muscular dystrophy	Weakness of EOMs (causing diplopia) Weakness of levator muscle (causing ptosis)
B. Myasthenia gravis	Weakness of EOMs Ptosis
VI. Blood dyscrasias	
A. Anemia	Pale conjunctiva Retinal hemorrhage Cotton-wool spots and hard exudates
B. Leukemia	Optic nerve compression Elevated IOP

(continued)

Table 2-3. (continued)

Systemic Disorders and Their Effects on the Eye

C. Sickle cell disease	Neovascularization Vitreous hemorrhage Retinal detachment
VII. Age-related disorders	
A. Elderly	Cataract Macular degeneration Dry eye Increased incidence of glaucoma Increased incidence of infection Presbyopia (first noticed around age 40) Loss of skin and muscle tone (entropion, ectropion, dermatochalasis, EOM dysfunction)
B. Prematurity	O_2 damage to retina Blocked development of retinal blood vessels Retinal detachment Retinal scarring
VIII. Environmental disorders	
A. Alcoholism	Visual field defects Nerve palsies Optic atrophy Alcohol amblyopia Decreased color vision Cataracts
B. Child abuse	Retinal and vitreal hemorrhage Periorbital bruising and swelling Subconjunctival hemorrhage Orbital fractures Hyphema Dislocated lens Retinal detachment
C. Malnutrition	Night blindness Retinopathy Corneal ulceration/necrosis
D. Smoking	Chronic conjunctivitis Increased risk of nuclear sclerosis Increased risk of macular degeneration Increased optic nerve damage in glaucoma Nystagmus Optic neuropathy

(continued)

Table 2-3. (continued)

Systemic Disorders and Their Effects on the Eye

Disorder	Effects on the Eye
IX. Genetic disorders	
A. Albinism	Blue-gray to pink iris Nystagmus Decreased visual acuity Strabismus Photophobia
B. Down syndrome	Short, slanted palpebral fissures Epicanthal folds Strabismus Nystagmus Myopia Cataracts Keratoconus Brushfield's spots
X. Neoplastic disorders	
A. Cancer	Ocular metastasis (iris most common)
B. Non-Hodgkin's lymphoma	Proptosis Conjunctival growths Diplopia Lacrimal gland infiltration
XI. Other disorders/conditions	
A. Chronic obstructive pulmonary disease	Dilation of retinal vessels Retinal hemorrhage Darkening of blood vessels (conjunctiva and retina)
B. Gout	Conjunctivitis Episcleritis Scleritis Elevated IOP Uric acid crystals (cornea or sclera)
C. Pregnancy	Minor refractive shifts Difficulty with accommodation Drop in IOP Mild ptosis Hyperpigmentation of lids
D. Sarcoidosis	Bilateral anterior uveitis Granulomas Optic neuritis Optic atrophy

Table 2-4.

Ocular Side Effects of Systemic Medications

Drug	Ocular Side Effect
Allopurinol	Cataract
Aminoglycosides	Corneal epithelial breakdown Keratopathy
Amiodarone	Corneal deposits
Amphetamines	Elevated IOP
Anesthetics	EOM paralysis
Antibiotics	Conjunctival inflammation Follicular proliferation
Anticoagulants	Retinal hemorrhage
Barbiturates	Conjunctivitis Stevens-Johnson type syndrome with inflammation of mucous membranes Ptosis Optic atrophy
Busalfan	Cataract
Chlorambucil	Papilledema
Chloramphenicol	Optic atrophy Optic neuritis
Chloroquin	Loss of night vision Progressive deterioration of central visual acuity Corneal deposits Macular degeneration syndromes
Choloral hydrate	Conjunctivitis
Chorpropamide	Corneal deposits Stevens-Johnson type syndrome with inflammation of mucous membranes EOM paralysis
Clofazimine	Corneal deposits Conjunctival deposits
Diazepam	Nystagmus
Disulfiram	Optic neuritis
Ethambutol hydrochloride	Optic neuritis
Glycosides	Macular degeneration syndromes
Gold salts	Corneal deposits Conjunctival deposits Nystagmus Lens deposits
Guanethidine	Conjunctivitis Ptosis
Haloperidol	Cataract

(continued)

Table 2-4. (continued)

Ocular Side Effects of Systemic Medications

Hexamethonium	Changes in retinal vascular patterns
Indomethacin	Corneal deposits
Iodoquinol	Optic atrophy
Isoniazid	Optic neuritis
Ketamine hydrochloride	Nystagmus
Lovastatin	Cataract
Malidixic acid	Papilledema
MAO inhibitors	Optic atrophy
Methyldopa	Conjunctivitis
Methysergide	Conjunctivitis
Morphine	Optic neuritis
Nonsteroidal anti-inflammatory drugs (NSAIDs)	Increased IOP
Oral contraceptives	Corneal swelling
	Nystagmus
	Papilledema
	Retinal edema
	Changes in retinal vascular patterns
Penicillamine	EOM paralysis
	Ptosis
	Optic neuritis
Phenothiazine	Conjunctival deposits
	Corneal deposits
	Lens deposits
	Macular degeneration syndromes
Phenylbutazone	Conjunctivitis
	Retinal hemorrhage
	Keratitis
Phenytoin	Nystagmus
	EOM paralysis
Quinacrine hydrochloride	Conjunctival deposits
Quinine	Changes in retinal vascular patterns
Rifampin	Optic neuritis
Salicylates	Nystagmus
	Retinal hemorrhage
Steroids	Increased IOP
	Posterior subcapsular cataracts
	Optic atrophy
Streptomycin	Optic neuritis
Sulfonamides	Conjunctivitis
	Stevens-Johnson type syndrome with inflammation of mucous membranes
	Retinal hemorrhage

(continued)

Table 2-4. (continued)

Ocular Side Effects of Systemic Medications

Tetracycline	Papilledema
Tricyclic antidepressants	Increased IOP
Vitamin A	Conjunctival deposits Papilledema
Vitamin D	Corneal deposits

Reprinted with permission from Duvall B, Kershner RM. Ophthalmic Medications and Pharmacology. *Thorofare, NJ: SLACK Incorporated; 1998.*

Table 2-5.

Normal Values of Common Blood Tests

1. CBC—Checks the number of red blood cells, white blood cells, and platelets present in a blood sample. Normal values are:
   - White blood cell count: 4300 to 10,800/cu mm
   - Platelet count: 150,000 to 350,000/cu mm
   - Red cell count
     - Male: 4.6 to 6.2 million/cu mm
     - Female: 4.2 to 5.4 million/cu mm
   - Hemoglobin
     - Male: 14 to 17 g/dL
     - Female: 12 to 15 g/dL
   - Hematocrit
     - Male: 41% to 50%
     - Female: 36% to 44%

2. Prothrombin time—Evaluates the blood's ability to clot. A normal value is between 9 and 18 seconds.

3. Blood glucose level—Used to detect the presence of diabetes and to monitor its treatment. Normal fasting blood glucose level is 60 to 100 mg/dL.

4. Rheumatoid factor—A test for rheumatoid arthritis. If the patient does not have rheumatoid arthritis, the test will usually be negative.

5. Erythrocyte sedimentation rate—Indicates the presence and intensity of an inflammatory process such as arthritis or cancer. It is not specific for any one disease. Normal values (Westergren) are:
   - Male: 0 to 13 mm/hour
   - Female: 0 to 20 mm/hour

6. Creatinine and blood urea nitrogen (BUN)—Both creatinine and BUN are tests of kidney function. Normal values are:
   - Creatinine: 0.8 to 1.2 mg/dL
   - BUN: 8 to 25 mg/dL

(continued)

Table 2-5. (continued)

Normal Values of Common Blood Tests

7. Potassium—3.3 to 4.9 mmol/L

8. Sodium—135 to 145 mmol/L

9. Calcium—8.9 to 10.3 mg/dL

Unless otherwise noted, all text, tables, and figures are adapted or reprinted with permission from Bittinger M. General Medical Knowledge for Eyecare Paraprofessionals. *Thorofare, NJ: SLACK Incorporated; 1999.*

CHAPTER 3

Optics, Retinoscopy, and Refractometry

Optics

Optics in ophthalmology can be divided into three components: physical, geometric, and physiologic.

Physical Optics

Physical optics is the study of light itself, including the theories of light travel and the electromagnetic spectrum. The two main theories of light travel are the corpuscular theory and the wave theory. It is uncertain which theory is correct, but it seems that light has both properties. The electromagnetic spectrum encompasses all light energy, ranging from the shortest (cosmic) rays to the longest (radio) waves. Clinical optics includes the visible spectrum (wavelengths 400 to 760 nonometers), which lies between ultraviolet and infrared. White light is a combination of all the colors. The pattern of color in visible light follows a certain order according to its wavelength: red, orange, yellow, green, blue, indigo, and violet.

Geometric Optics

Geometric optics relates to how light rays are affected by various surfaces and media. The speed of light in a vacuum is 186,282 miles per second. This speed changes in different media. Light also travels in a straight line until its path is bent by a medium. (A medium is a substance that light can pass through, such as gases, liquids, and glass.) Bending of light is called refraction. In optics, the media we usually deal with are lenses of some type.

Light emanating from a light source is always divergent (rays spread apart as they travel away from the source). If the source is more than 20 feet (6 meters) away, then the light is considered to have parallel rays (although they are still very slightly divergent). Light traveling through a lens will have its vergence (angle of the rays of light in relation to each other) affected. This effect will depend on the properties of the lens. Parallel light entering a minus-powered lens will become divergent (negative vergence or spreading apart of the light rays). A plus-powered lens causes convergence (positive vergence or coming together of light rays toward a focus) (Figure 3-1). Plus-powered lenses are used to correct hyperopia (farsightedness) and cause magnification of the image. A minus-powered lens causes divergence (negative vergence or spreading apart of light rays). Minus-powered lenses correct myopia (nearsightedness) and cause minification.

Light passing through a lens produces an image. Sometimes this image is real, other times it is virtual. First, one should understand that *object rays* exist only on the incoming side of an optical system, and *image rays* exist only on the outgoing side. (An optical system is a lens [or a combination of more than one lens] and the surrounding media, usually air.) When the image is on the same side as the outgoing rays, it is called a real image. Virtual images appear on the same side of the lens as the incoming rays. Generally speaking, real images can be formed on a screen, whereas virtual images cannot.

A real, inverted image is created on the opposite side of the lens when parallel rays (from 20 or more feet away) enter a plus-powered lens. However, since a minus-powered lens causes light to diverge, its focal point (place where the image is focused) is in front of the lens (on the same side as the object), thereby producing a virtual, upright image. The distance between the center of the lens and the focal point is the focal distance (or focal length).

The power of a lens is measured in diopters. A 1 diopter (D) lens will bend parallel light rays to a focal point that is 1 m from the lens. To put it in a formula, 1 D is equal to the reciprocal of the focal length of the lens (in meters). The formula is $D = 1/f$, where D is the dioptric power of the lens, and f is the focal length of the lens (in meters). The focal length of a lens is related to its power. Lenses with shorter focal lengths have higher powers and vice-versa.

Lenses

Light traveling through a *prism* will be bent toward the base (thickest part) of the prism. The power of a prism (measured in diopters) is determined by the amount of deviation of light (in centimeters) that occurs at 1 m. One prism diopter will deviate light by 1 cm at a distance of 1 m, 2 prism diopters will deviate by 2 cm at a distance of 1 m, etc.

A lens that has the same curvature and power in all directions is called a *spherical lens*. This type of lens causes light to either converge (bend toward a focal point) or diverge (spread apart). The point within the lens that has no bending effect on light is called the optical center. This coincides to the thickest point of a plus lens or the thinnest point of a minus lens. It is not necessarily the geometric center of the lens.

Cylindrical lenses create a focal line instead of a focal point. This focal line is parallel to the axis of the cylinder, but the greatest power of the lens lies

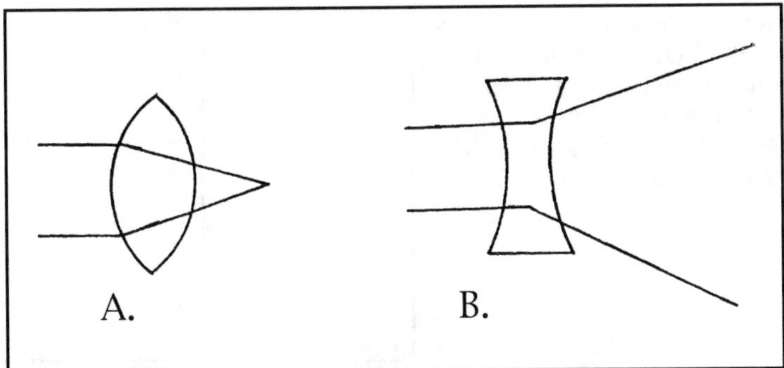

Figure 3-1. Light bent through a plus (A) and a minus (B) lens (drawing by Holly Hess. Reprinted from Ledford J. *Exercises in Refractometry*. Thorofare, NJ: SLACK Incorporated; 1990, with permission from Janice Ledford).

perpendicular to its axis in what is called the meridian of power (Figure 3-2). Thus cylinders must be referred to not only by power but by the direction of the axis. Cylindrical lenses also come in plus and minus form and are used to correct astigmatism.

Prescription Form

The power of any lens (spherical, cylindrical, or spherocylindrical—a combination of the two) must be put in written form if the lens is to be manufactured for a patient's eyeglasses. If the lens is spherical only, then the power may simply be written (example: +3.50 sph). If the lens is cylindrical or spherocylindrical, then the power and direction of the cylinder must be included as well in the following format: sphere power (listed as Plano [zero] if there is none) + cylinder power x cylinder axis. A cylindrical lens with a power of –1.75 at axis 90 would be written as: Plano – 1.75 x 90. A spherocylindrical lens of +2.25 sphere combined with a +1.00 cylinder at axis 172 would be written: +2.25 + 1.00 x 172.

Transposition is a way to change a prescription of one cylinder type into the other (ie, plus cylinder to minus or vice versa). Transposing is a three-step process. First, algebraically add the cylinder to the sphere to calculate the new sphere. Second, change the sign of the cylinder. Third, the axis is changed by 90 degrees (but cannot exceed 180 degrees—if the original axis exceeds 90 degrees, then subtract 90 degrees from the original axis).

For example, to transpose +3.50 – 1.50 x 95 to plus cylinder, the cylinder is algebraically added to the sphere [+3.50 + (-1.50)]. This gives us a new sphere value of +2.00. The sign of the cylinder is changed from minus to plus, becoming +1.50. The axis is changed by 90 degrees (the original axis exceeds 90, so use 95 minus 90). The new axis is 05. Thus, the plus cylinder form is +2.00 + 1.50 x 05.

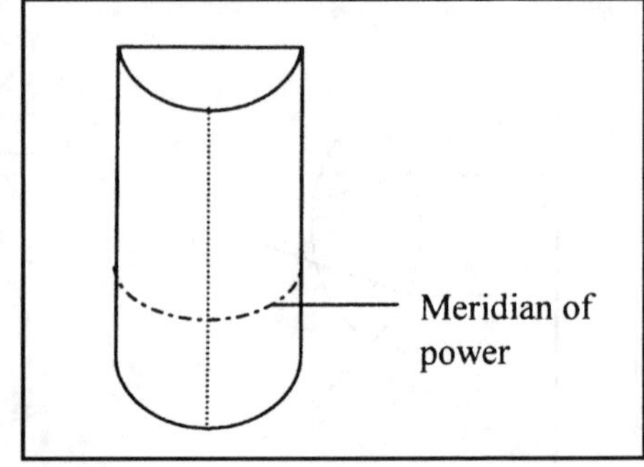

Figure 3-2. The power of a cylinder is 90 degrees away from its axis (reprinted with permission from Lens A. *Optics, Retinoscopy, and Refractometry*. Thorofare, NJ: SLACK Incorporated; 1999).

Spherical equivalent (SE) refers to the average of a spherocylindrical lens combination. Simply algebraically add half of the cylinder to the sphere, then disregard the cylindrical values. The SE will thus be the same whether plus or minus cylinder format is used. The SE is often used in contact lens fitting.

Induced Prism

When light does not pass through the optical center of a lens (the point where there is no change in vergence of light), prismatic effect is induced. The amount of prism induced can be determined using Prentice's rule (induced prism = decentration [in centimeters] x lens power [in diopters]). This is helpful for determining the amount of induced prism when the optical center of a lens is not aligned with the patient's visual axis. Just 1 D of vertical prism can cause diplopia or discomfort. (Base out prism is more easily tolerated due to a person's ability to converge.)

Physiologic Optics

Physiologic optics involves the mechanism, psychology, and physiology of vision and seeing. The eye is a compound lens system consisting of the cornea and crystalline lens surfaces. The power of this lens system and the axial length of the eye determine the refractive error of an eye. To help explain the optical system of the eye, the schematic eye (Gullstrand's is generally used) was developed to indicate the optical constants. It should be understood, however, that very few real eyes would duplicate the measurements noted in the schematic eye (Table 3-1; see also Figure 1-16).

Accommodation and refractive errors have been explained in Chapter 1. A mention of retinal image size is appropriate here. The size of the image on the retina is typically the same in each eye. Myopes, when wearing spectacles (and to a lesser degree, contact lenses), will see a smaller image than an emmetrope. Conversely, a hyperope tends to see a larger image. This variation in image size rarely poses a problem unless there is a difference in refractive error between the two eyes (anisometropia). Small amounts of anisometropia are

Table 3-1.
The Schematic Eye

Structure	Notes
Cornea	Index of refraction (IR) = 1.376 Radius of central anterior surface = 7.7 mm Radius of posterior surface = 6.8 mm Refractive power of anterior surface = +48.83 D Refractive power of posterior surface = -5.88 D Total refractive power = +42.95 D Central thickness = 0.5 mm
Pupil	"Ideal" size = 2 to 5 mm
Aqueous	IR = 1.336
Lens	IR of cortex = 1.386 IR of nucleus = 1.406 Overall IR = 1.42 Anterior radius of curvature (unaccommodated) = 10.00 mm Anterior radius of curvature (fully accommodated) = 5.33 mm Posterior radius of curvature (unaccommodated) = 6.0 mm Posterior radius of curvature (fully accommodated) = 5.33 mm Refractive power (unaccommodated) = +19.11 D Refractive power (fully accommodated) = +33.06 D Thickness of nucleus = 2.419 mm Overall thickness = 3.6 mm
Vitreous	IR = 1.336
Axial length	Overall eye length = 24.4 mm Distance from anterior K to anterior lens surface = 3.6 mm Distance from anterior K to posterior lens surface = 7.2 mm Distance from posterior lens surface to retina = 17.2 mm

Reprinted with permission from Ledford J. Certified Ophthalmic Medical Technologist Exam Review Manual. *Thorofare, NJ: SLACK Incorporated; 2000.*

usually well tolerated. However, when the difference exceeds 3 D, there is the potential for a noticeable difference in retinal image size (aniseikonia). Contact lenses are often used in such cases, since the lens is in contact with the eye and there is minimal effect on retinal image size. If contact lenses cannot be worn, the power of one (or both) of the spectacle lenses may have to be altered to lessen the aniseikonia.

Retinoscopy

- There are two basic varieties of streak retinoscopes available: those based on Copeland's design and all the others.
- A special filament in the bulb of the streak retinoscope creates the linear beam of light.
- For best results, the patient's fixating eye should be fogged with plus lenses to further prevent accommodation.
- The reflex (in the pupil) will move in either the same direction (with movement) as the intercept (on the face or phoropter) or in the opposite direction (against movement).
- Plus-powered lenses neutralize with movement. Minus-powered lenses neutralize against movement.
- The speed and brightness of the reflex increases as neutralization is approached.

Retinoscopy is used to objectively determine the refractive error of an eye. There are two principle types of retinoscope available: spot and streak. We will be describing the technique used in streak retinoscopy. One of the most important aspects of retinoscopy is holding the instrument properly. For convenience and efficiency, a one-handed method for holding the retinoscope must be used. It should be held so that the hand holding the retinoscope can also rotate the sleeve and slide it up and down.

The retinoscope should be held in the same hand as the eye that is being examined. Furthermore, the retinoscopist should use the same eye as the hand holding the scope. This will allow the patient to fixate on a distant target, which is important in order to control accommodation. For best results, the fixating eye should be fogged by placing a plus-powered sphere before the eye to further prevent accommodation.

Retinoscopy relies on a reflex from inside the eye. Movement of the reflex in the pupil is often seen when the streak of light from the retinoscope is moved. The intention of the retinoscopist is to completely fill the pupil and to stop the reflex from moving by using lenses placed in front of the eye. This process is called neutralizing the reflex.

The vergence of light from the retinoscope can be adjusted according to the position of the sleeve. Light rays from the retinoscope should be parallel when neutralizing the reflex. This is accomplished with a plane-mirror effect. Retinoscopes using Copeland's design have a plane-mirror effect when the sleeve is pushed all the way up (known as the up-position). The plane-mirror effect of retinoscopes using the alternate design is accomplished when the sleeve is in the down-position.

The distance from the retinoscope to the patient's eye is known as the working distance. Retinoscopy is generally performed at an arm's length from the refractor. The length of the average person's arm is 66 cm. The power of a lens that focuses parallel light rays at 66 cm is +1.50 D (D = 1/f). To allow the eye to focus at 20 feet (6 m), this power must be taken away from the gross retinoscopy result. This is done by dialing 1.50 D toward the minus, also known as "removing the working lens." Some retinoscopists do not have arms that are 66 cm long. If you are uncertain of your working distance, measure the distance and use a working lens, as noted in Table 3-2. Some retinoscopists prefer to use the "retinoscopy lens" (a +1.50 lens) built into most refractors.

The whole concept of retinoscopy is based on movement of the reflex. The objective is to find the lens(es) which will stop that movement. The two principal options for movement are "with" and "against." The light from the retinoscope is shone into the eye and is reflected by the retina. The image of this reflection in the pupil is known as the reflex. The light that falls on the iris, eye, phoroptor, etc is called the intercept. The reflex will move either in the same direction as the intercept (with movement) or in the opposite direction (against movement). If you see with movement, add plus-powered lenses. Conversely, against movement is neutralized with minus-powered lenses.

In certain cases, the angle of the reflex may appear to be skewed from that of the intercept (Figure 3-3). This signal indicates that astigmatism is present, and the axis of the primary meridian is not parallel to the axis of the intercept (discussed later).

In addition to the direction of movement, the retinoscopist should assess the speed and brightness of the reflex. A dull, slow moving reflex is seen when there is significant refractive error. In fact, a high refractive error may look neutral. When neutrality is approached, the reflex quickens and becomes brighter.

Neutrality is the point where the reflex appears to have no movement. When the intercept enters the pupil, the reflex fills the pupil. The reflex then disappears or blinks out when the intercept is moved off the eye.

The refractor is positioned so that the patient's pupils are centered in the apertures. A target is provided. The patient is instructed to look at the target and avoid looking at the examiner or the retinoscope (to prevent accommodation). The examiner positions him- or herself within a couple degrees of the patient's visual axis and an arm's length away. The patient should be told to blink periodically to keep the cornea from drying.

The first step in retinoscopy is to achieve with movement in all meridians, since with movement is more accurately neutralized than against movement. When against movement is seen at the start of retinoscopy, minus-powered spheres are added until with movement is seen. Plus-powered sphere is then added until the reflex is neutralized. The reflex will be neutralized at any axis when there is no astigmatism present.

There are not too many eyes that have absolutely no astigmatism. Try to think of the astigmatic eye as two separate eyes; you will neutralize one "eye" with spherical lenses and the other "eye" with cylindrical lenses.

Table 3-2.

Determining Working Lens Power

Distance to Retinoscope	Working Lens Power
80 cm (0.8 m)	+1.25 D
67 cm (0.67 m)	+1.50 D
57 cm (0.57 m)	+1.75 D
50 cm (0.5 m)	+2.00 D
44 cm (0.44 m)	+2.25 D
40 cm (0.4 m)	+2.50 D
33 cm (0.33 m)	+3.00 D
25 cm (0.25 m)	+4.00 D
20 cm (0.20 m)	+5.00 D
16 cm (0.16 m)	+6.00 D
10 cm (0.10 m)	+10.00 D

Reprinted with permission from Lens A. Optics, Retinoscopy, and Refractometry. *Thorofare, NJ: SLACK Incorporated; 1999.*

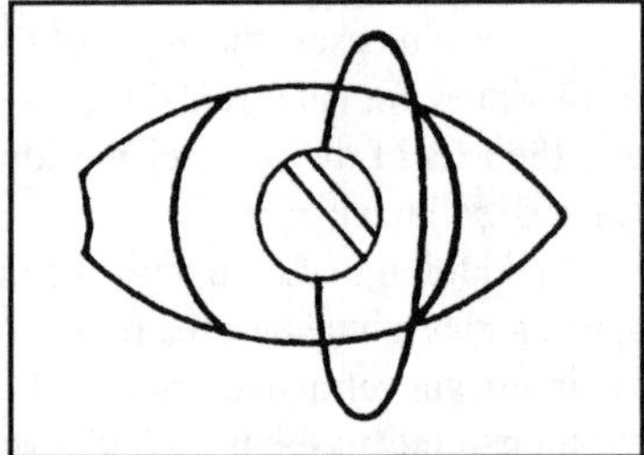

Figure 3-3. Misaligned streak (drawing by Holly Hess. Reprinted from Ledford J. *Exercises in Refractometry*. Thorofare, NJ: SLACK Incorporated; 1990, with permission from Janice Ledford).

The important thing to remember when neutralizing a reflex with cylindrical lenses is that the axis of the intercept, reflex, and cylinder must be parallel.

Locating the exact axis of a primary meridian can be difficult when there is nominal astigmatism present. Enhancing (narrowing) the intercept can be of some assistance. For Copeland-style retinoscopes, lower the sleeve slightly. For other retinoscope styles, raise the sleeve slightly. This narrowing of the intercept (and subsequently, the reflex) will make it easier to see the axis of the astigmatism.

How-To: Retinoscopy

Plus Cylinder:

- Evaluate reflexes for motion, axis, brightness, and width.
- Neutralize the least with (or most against) meridian first, using spheres only. This will be the meridian that has the widest, quickest with movement (or thinnest, slowest against movement).
- Turn the streak 90 degrees. You should still see with-movement. (If, when you turn your streak, you do not still have with-movement, you have selected the wrong meridian to neutralize first.)
- Position the axis on the phoropter to coincide with your streak. Add cylinder until this meridian is also neutral.
- Remove the working lens; refine via refractometry.

Minus Cylinder:

- Evaluate reflexes for motion, axis, brightness, and width.
- Neutralize the most with (or least against) meridian first. This will be the meridian that has the widest, quickest against movement (or thinnest, slowest with movement).
- Turn the streak 90 degrees. You should still see against-movement. (If, when you turn your streak, you do not still have against-movement, you have selected the wrong meridian to neutralize first.)
- Position the axis on the phoropter to coincide with your streak. Add cylinder until this meridian is also neutral.
- Remove the working lens; refine via refractometry.

Refractometry

- Refractometry refinement should be done in the following order: cylinder axis, cylinder power, and sphere power.
- For best results, the patient should understand what the examiner is trying to achieve during refractometry and how the he or she is expected to respond.
- The cross-cylinder usually causes the patient's vision to be slightly blurred; he or she should be made aware that this is normal and to choose which is the sharper of the *next* two choices.
- "Push plus" means to use the maximum amount of plus-powered sphere (or minimum minus-powered sphere) to achieve best acuity.

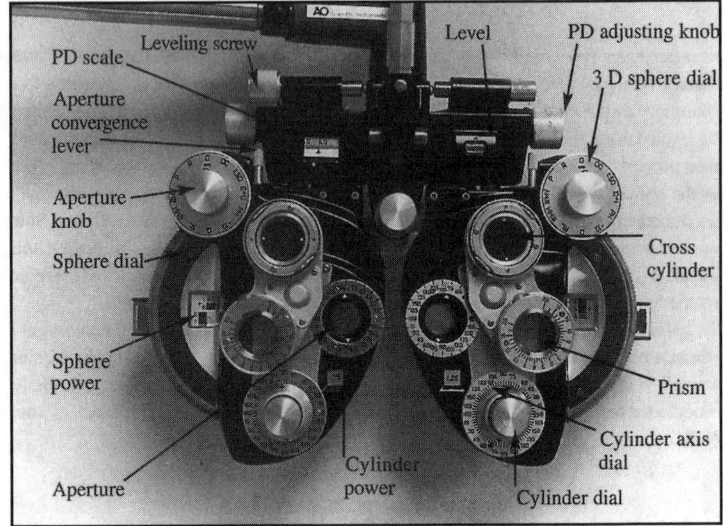

Figure 3-4. Refractor front (labeled) (photo by Jim Ledford. Reprinted from Ledford J. *Exercises in Refractometry.* Thorofare, NJ: SLACK Incorporated; 1990, with permission from Janice Ledford).

Refractometry is the measurement of the refractive error of an eye. The basic steps of refractometry can be described in a single sentence: estimate the spherical component, then refine the cylinder axis and power and, finally, refine the sphere power.

It is necessary to know the controls on the refractor before one performs refractometry (Figure 3-4). Not all refractors are the same, but they all have the same essential features. When the instrument is level, and the pupillary distance properly set, each eye should look through the center of the aperture.

How-To: Refractometry

Preliminaries:

- Explain the procedure to the patient.
- Occlude the eye that is not being tested.
- Determine the starting point: 1) retinoscopy, 2) autorefractor, 3) patient's habitual spectacles, or 4) refractometry results from a previous visit.

Gross Spheres:

- Show the patient a line of letters that is somewhat difficult to read.
- Add 0.50 D steps in the plus direction (ie, adding plus or reducing minus) **until** the patient states that the letters are more blurred. Once the letters blur, return to the previous setting.

(continued)

How-To: Refractometry (continued)

- If the letters have blurred after the initial addition of 0.50, return to the original setting and offer 0.50 in the minus direction (ie, adding minus or reducing plus).
- Each addition of minus-powered spheres should result in an improvement in the sharpness of the letters. This can be verified by asking the patient to read further down the eye chart as minus sphere is increased (or plus sphere is reduced). If he or she cannot read smaller letters, return to the previous setting.

Cylinder Refinement:

- Display letters that the patient can easily see.
- Position the cross-cylinder's knurled knob (used to flip the lens) parallel with the correcting cylinder axis.
- Ask the patient how the vision is affected with each flip of the cross-cylinder. If the patient prefers one choice over the other, position the lens with the patient's favored choice showing. Rotate the correcting cylinder axis several degrees toward the appropriate marker (white if using plus cylinder, red if using minus cylinder).
- This process is repeated until the patient either reports no change when the lens is flipped or repeatedly goes back and forth within a degree or two.
- Turn the cross cylinder so that the "P" (for Power) on the rim of the cross-cylinder is aligned with the axis.
- With each flip of the cross-cylinder, ask the patient how the vision is affected.
- If using plus cylinder and vision is better when the white marker (a dot or a line) is aligned with the correcting cylinder, cylinder power should be increased. Conversely, the red marker indicates the plus-cylinder power should be decreased. If using minus cylinder and vision is better when the red marker on the cross-cylinder is aligned with the correcting cylinder, cylinder power should be increased. Conversely, the white marker indicates the minus-cylinder power should be decreased.
- The process of adding or subtracting power is repeated until the patient indicates that both choices are equal or alternates between two choices repeatedly.

Fine Spheres:

- Remove the cross-cylinder, display the full acuity chart, and ask the patient to read the smallest line possible.

(continued)

How-To: Refractometry (continued)

- Offer 0.25 steps in a plus direction until the patient states that the line blurs. Once blurring occurs, return to the previous setting.
- If the first 0.25 step of plus causes the letters to blur, return to the first setting and then offer a 0.25 step of minus sphere. If the patient says this makes the letters more clear, he or she should "prove" it by reading more or smaller letters. If there is not an improvement in the number or size of letters read, go back to the original setting. Only continue to give 0.25 steps of minus as long as the patient really can see more or smaller letters.
- Repeat all steps for the other eye.

Add Power:

- Open both apertures.
- Have the patient hold the near target at the distance where he or she prefers to read.
- Add plus sphere to the distance correction to obtain sharpness. The lowest addition that provides clear vision should be used.

Unless otherwise noted, all text, tables, and figures are adapted or reprinted with permission from Lens A. Optics, Retinoscopy, and Refractometry. *Thorofare, NJ: SLACK Incorporated; 1999.*

CHAPTER 4

Frames and Lenses

Frames

Today's frames are a product of artists, craftsmen, and computer-aided design (CAD). Cellulose acetate (or zyl) is the most commonly used material for plastic frames. Monel is a corrosion-resistant alloy and is the most prevalent material used for metal frames. Frame materials are listed in Table 4-1.

Whether plastic or metal, ophthalmic frames are available in many different styles. Types of frames include full frame, combination frame, semi-rimless, full rimless or drill mount, and half-eyes (Figure 4-1).

Spectacle frames are made up of a frame front and two temples (Figure 4-2). The front contains two eyewires, a bridge, and end pieces (where the temples attach to the frame front). Plastic frames incorporate a saddle, modified saddle, keyhole, or adjustable bridge (nose pads) (Figure 4-3 and Table 4-2). Metal frames are constructed with adjustable nose pads, an unifit bridge, or a saddle bridge (Figure 4-4 and see Table 4-2). The five basic temple designs are shown in Figure 4-5 and discussed in Table 4-3.

The best frame for a patient complements his or her facial structure, requires minimal adjustments, and holds the lenses securely in place. The chosen frame will also positively affect the cosmetic appearance of the prescription lenses because of its shape and size.

The best way to control the finished look is to first imagine the thickness and curves of the lenses. For instance, a high minus lens will be thick on the edges and thin in the center; compounding this prescription with a high cylinder correction will add extra thickness to an area of the lens corresponding to the cylinder axis. A good choice for such a prescription is a small, rounded frame. Selecting a frame that meets this criteria will result in lenses that are as thin as possible; selecting a large, angular frame would result in much thicker and heavier lenses for the same correction.

Determining the patient's facial shape is the next step. The seven basic facial shapes are oval, round, triangle, long, square, inverted triangle, and

Table 4-1.

Frame Materials

I. Plastic

A. Cellulose acetate (zyl)

1. Features: Unique ability to slightly reduce in size to accommodate a lens that is edged a bit small or stretch to house a lens that is edged too large; lends itself well to coloration processes; most commonly used material for plastic frames.
2. Fitting notes: The plasticizers that keep the frame pliable are actually secreted from the plastic material as the frame ages. This can cause the material to become brittle, or may cause contact dermatitis in the patient.
3. Handling notes: Before adjusting, heat the material (preferably only the area that is to be adjusted) either in a bead pan or with an air blower. Overheating the frame can cause irreversible damage. Zyl is sensitive to some solvents, particularly acetone. When making lenses for an older zyl frame, it is always necessary to check the eyewires for cracks.

B. Cellulose propionate

1. Features: Lightweight and very strong; does not stretch or shrink much; difficult to scratch; color is applied *over* the material rather than part of the plastic, sealing in the plasticizers.
2. Fitting notes: Good choice for patients who have had allergic reactions to plastic frames in the past.
3. Handling notes: Very heat sensitive and damaged by temperatures over 105°F. Lenses should be "edged to size" for mounting. They can be permanently damaged by alcohol and/or acetone.

C. Carbon fiber graphite (Marchon, Melville, NY)

1. Features: Lightweight and stable with a very high tensile strength; transparent colors are not available; baked-on colored enamels are applied over the material in a wide variety of solid colors or with mottled color patterns.
2. Handling notes: Minimally affected by heat, so it is of little help to heat the frame before adjusting. Most frames have eyewires with screws, so the lenses are edged as they are for a metal frame. Not particularly sensitive to solvents such as alcohol or acetone.

D. Polycarbonate

1. Features: Impact-resistant; inherently soft and very easy to scratch.
2. Fitting notes: Safety frames.
3. Handling notes: Rinse well with water and use a mild cleaning solution to clean; easily scratched if wiped when dry; frame should fit well on the initial fitting. Adjustments are limited and heating the material will not add much flexibility. Lenses should be edged for a "cold mount." Acetone and alcohol should not be used.

E. Polyamide

1. Features: A type of nylon; very strong and lightweight in nature; easily tinted and available in a wide range of colors.

(continued)

Table 4-1. (continued)

Frame Materials

2. Fitting notes: Good choice for individuals who are sensitive to some types of plastic frames.
3. Handling notes: *Very* heat sensitive and frequently reduces in size when heated (beneficial if the lenses are edged slightly too small). Always edge lenses to size and cold snap into frame.

F. Optyl

1. Features: Hypoallergenic, lightweight, keeps its finish over time; available in a multitude of colors and with elaborate treatments; brittle.
2. Fitting notes: Good choice for patients sensitive to some types of plastic frames.
3. Handling notes: Returns to its original shape when thoroughly heated. Not easily damaged by excessive heat. For best results, heat only the portion of frame that is to be adjusted. Always heat the frame thoroughly to avoid breakage.

G. Nylon

1. Features: Does not shrink or stretch; virtually unbreakable; hypoallergenic; usually dark color.
2. Fitting notes: Sunglasses; men's frame styles.
3. Handling notes: Does not respond much to heat, thus nearly impossible to alter the adjustment. Edge the lenses for the exact size. Tendency to dry out, so occasionally soak in water overnight.

II. Metal

A. Monel

1. Features: Combination of nickel and copper; strong, stable; most common material used to produce metal frames; corrosion resistant; economical.

B. Nickel

1. Features: Strong; generally bends without breaking; also used with other metals to form alloys for fabrication of spectacle frames, such as stainless steel.
2. Fitting notes: Patients are frequently allergic to nickel products.

C. Nickel silver

1. Features: An alloy made of copper, zinc, silver, and nickel; also known as alpaca or German silver; strong, rigid; brittle, making it generally unsuitable for frame fronts or thin parts but improves durability when used as an inner core for plastic temples.

D. Phosphorous bronze

1. Features: Alloy comprised mostly of copper; also called phosphor bronze; flexible; susceptible to tarnishing; lustrous shine when polished.
2. Handling notes: Adjustments can be a problem because of its "springy" characteristic.

(continued)

Table 4-1. (continued)

Frame Materials

E. Stainless steel
   1. Features: An alloy comprised of manganese, nickel, iron, and chromium; strong even in thin, streamlined designs; corrosion resistant.
   2. Fitting notes: Good for people who work outdoors or who have had problems with frame corrosion due to perspiration; patients with known metal sensitivities are not likely to have problems with this material.
   3. Handling notes: Extreme temple adjustments can be a challenge because it is rigid and springy; frames should fit relatively well on the initial fitting.

F. Titanium
   1. Features: Highly corrosion resistant; incredibly lightweight; costly.
   2. Fitting notes: Difficult to know the percentage of titanium that is in a given style (an issue in metal allergies).
   3. Handling notes: A rigid material to work with.

G. Aluminum
   1. Features: Rarely used today; lighter than titanium; rigid.
   2. Handling notes: Difficult to adjust; nose pads are clamped onto the frame.

H. Beryllium
   1. Features: Strong; expensive; used in conjunction with other metals such as copper to form alloys; when mixed with copper, it forms a springy material that is well suited for temple production.

I. Cobalt
   1. Features: Expensive; used as part of an alloy to make a very strong and noncorrosive frame material; primarily used as a stabilizing interior metal on high quality frames; polishes nicely.

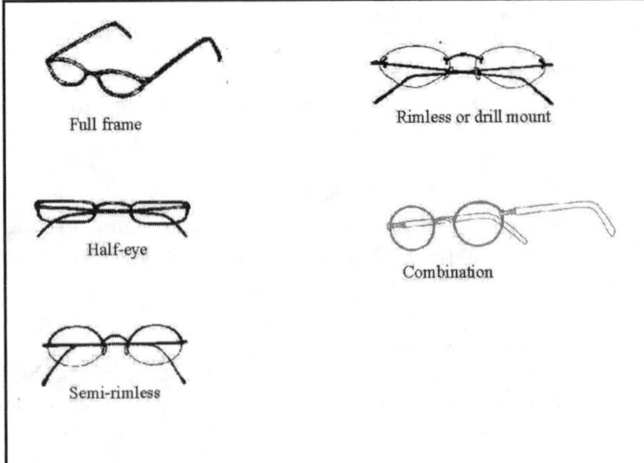

Figure 4-1. Frame styles (reprinted with permission from Carlton J. *Frames and Lenses*. Thorofare, NJ: SLACK Incorporated; 2000).

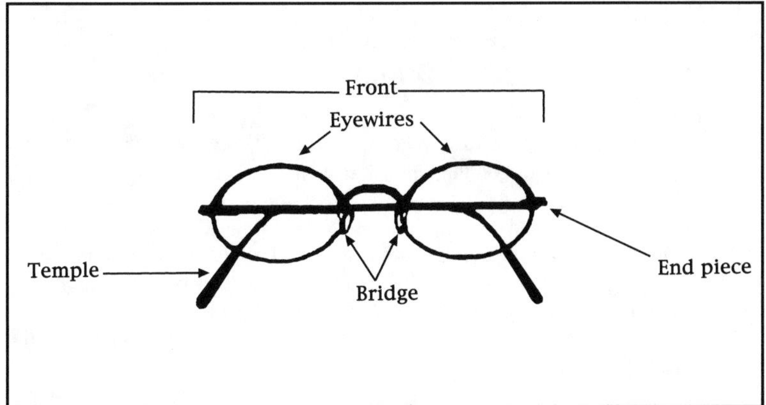

Figure 4-2. Parts of a frame (reprinted with permission from Carlton J. *Frames and Lenses*. Thorofare, NJ: SLACK Incorporated; 2000).

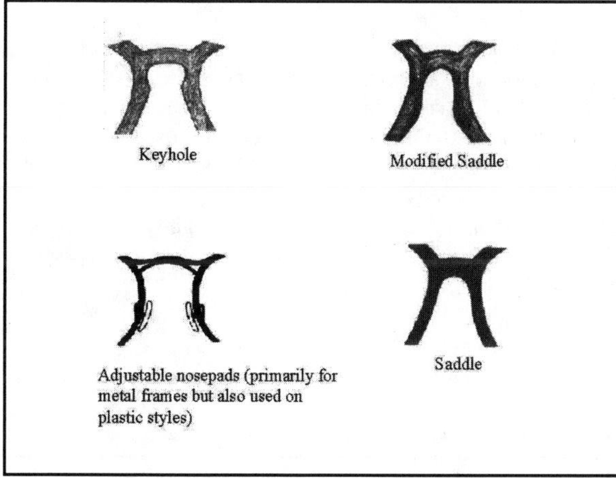

Figure 4-3. Bridge styles for plastic frames (reprinted with permission from Carlton J. *Frames and Lenses*. Thorofare, NJ: SLACK Incorporated; 2000).

Table 4-2.
Bridges

I. Plastic frames

A. Saddle

1. Features: Evenly distributes the weight of the spectacles on the top as well as sides of the nose.
2. Fitting notes: Best suited for patients sensitive to nose pads.

B. Modified saddle

1. Features: Offers built-up areas on either side of the bridge.
2. Fitting notes: Helpful when fitting patient with a very narrow nose.

Table 4-2. (continued)

Bridges

C. Keyhole
   1. Fitting notes: Good for a very thin nasal bridge; good choice if patient is sensitive to pressure on the top of the nose.

D. Adjustable (nose pads)
   1. Features: Weight of the glasses is balanced solely on the nose pads.
   2. Fitting notes: Good option for a very thin bridge or high cheekbones; may not be a good choice for heavy, high-powered lenses.
   3. Handling notes: Avoid heating the area where the nose pad guard arm is inserted into the plastic.

II. Metal frames
   A. Adjustable (nose pads)
      See D above.

   B. Unifit
      1. Features: Evenly distributes the weight of the glasses on the nasal bridge; mostly limited to men's styles, safety eyewear, and children's frames; most often made in silicon, some with a metal insert that allows for a long lasting, stable adjustment; acetate is sometimes used.
      2. Fitting notes: Good choice for safety frames and high-powered prescription dress lenses; excellent choice for children.
      3. Handling notes: An acetate unifit bridge can shrink slightly, resulting in a bridge that will not stay affixed to the frame. In this case, it is necessary to order a new bridge for the frame.

   C. Saddle
      1. Features: Supports the weight of the glasses mostly on the top of the bridge.
      2. Fitting notes: Not recommended for heavy, high-powered lenses.

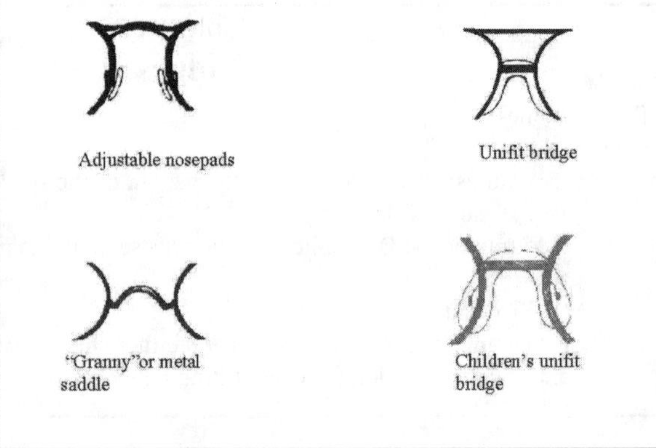

Figure 4-4. Bridge styles for metal frames (reprinted with permission from Carlton J. *Frames and Lenses.* Thorofare, NJ: SLACK Incorporated; 2000).

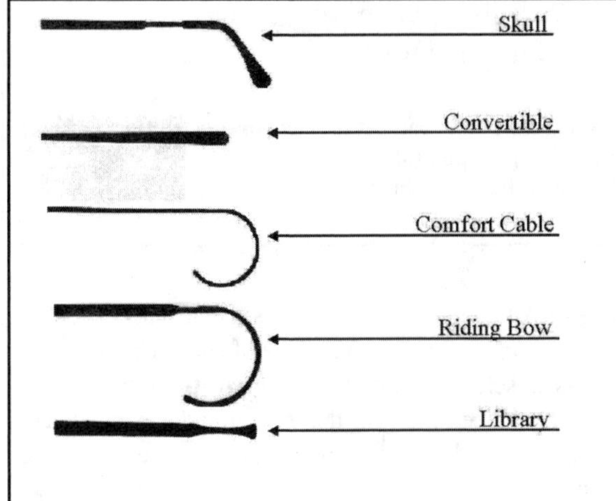

Figure 4-5. Temple styles (reprinted with permission from Carlton J. *Frames and Lenses*. Thorofare, NJ: SLACK Incorporated; 2000).

Table 4-3.

Temple Designs

A. Skull

1. Features: Closely follows the structure of the patient's ear.
2. Handling notes: Begin with a heated temple end; the bend should be a smooth curve and never "hooked"; follow the curve of the wearer's ear and do not put excessive pressure on the ear lobe or mastoid process.

B. Library

1. Features: Fits straight back and hugs patient's skull; quickly positioned on and off the face.
2. Fitting notes: Commonly seen on half-eye readers and military aviator frames.
3. Handling notes: Bow the temples in so that the tension will hold the frame in position against the head.

C. Convertible

1. Features: Can be adjusted straight back (like library temples) or behind the ear (like skull temples).

D. Comfort cable

1. Features: Metal coil temples that are very springy; quite effective at holding frame securely in place; can be shaped to fit either very tightly or loosely; encased in a flexible plastic temple cover for added comfort.
2. Fitting notes: Routinely used for children's frames and safety and sport styles.
3. Handling notes: To loosen the coil, simply bend the cable in its reverse direction; forming the coil into a smaller circle tightens the adjustment; jacket can be replaced. Simply cut off the old cable cover with chapel pliers and insert the cable into a new covering. Using an air blower, slightly heat the new sheath until it shrinks to the shape of the coil.

(continued)

Table 4-3. (continued)

Temple Designs

E. Riding bow

1. Features: Shaped to curl around the back of the ear; constructed from plastic.
2. Fitting notes: Children's, sport, and safety frames.
3. Handling notes: Can be difficult to adjust into a smooth curve; for best results, heat these temples thoroughly before shaping.

diamond (Figure 4-6). One trick to determine someone's facial shape is to have the patient trace his or her face on a mirror with a piece of soap. The basic rule of thumb for frame fitting is to select a frame that is opposite to the patient's facial shape. This results in a balanced look for the wearer and accentuates his or her positive features. Choosing a frame that is the same shape as the face emphasizes the facial shape.

Oval-shaped faces usually look good in any frame shape. This is the only facial shape that enjoys this advantage. Rounded faces look best in angular frames; frames that offer a high temple attachment are a plus. Square faces look best in round or oval-shaped frames; the goal here is to avoid angles. Faces that are long in shape take on a more balanced look by selecting styles with a small "B" measurement. (The "B" measurement is the deepest vertical measurement of the eyewire.) The smaller "B" measurement makes the length of the face appear shorter. Triangle, inverted triangle, and diamond-shaped faces are all very angular and appear softer in frames with shapes such as ovals or rounded designs. Rimless frames, as well as frames with delicate colors and features, are also a good choice for this group, as they soften the overall appearance of the face.

Most often there is not a frame that will meet each objective perfectly. The goal is to meet or exceed the patient's visual expectations while also enhancing the overall appearance of the patient and the lenses.

It is important to ask patients during the frame selection process if they have any known allergies to plastics or metals.

At this point it is necessary to select a lens material and multifocal style (if needed). Sometimes the lens material may dictate the frame style needed for a patient. An example would be glass lenses. Glass lenses are not suitable for mounting into drill mount frame styles. Likewise, progressive lenses are of little benefit if edged for a trendy frame with a very small "B" measurement. (Some lens manufacturers have recently addressed this problem by producing progressive lenses with a shorter corridor that are good choices for smaller "B" measurements. Ask your lens representatives for more information about these lenses.)

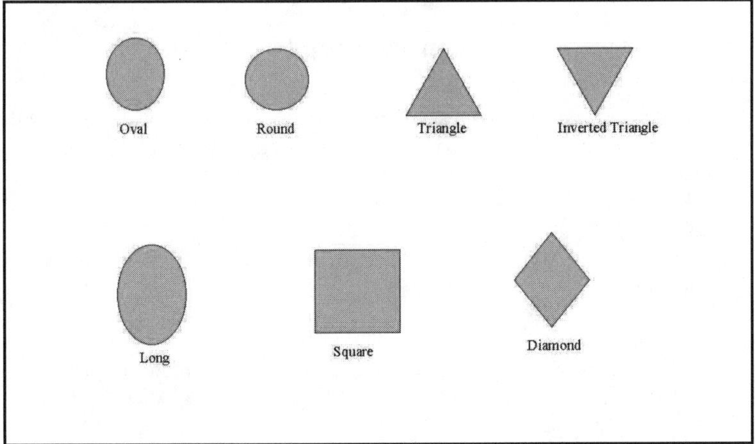

Figure 4-6. Common facial shapes (reprinted with permission from Carlton J. *Frames and Lenses*. Thorofare, NJ: SLACK Incorporated; 2000).

Lenses

- A spectacle lens consists of a transparent material that has two polished, opposing surfaces with the ability to focus light rays in an expected manner. (Optics are covered in Chapter 3.)
- The base curve of a spherical lens is ground on the front curve of the lens. Likewise, the base curve of spherocylindrical lenses (lenses that correct astigmatism) ground in minus cylinder (where the cylinder is ground on the backside of the lens) is also on the front surface of the lens.
- Safety lenses must have a minimum lens thickness of 3.0 mm (except lenses of +3.00 D or more, which must have a minimum thickness of 2.5 mm). They must also have the initials of the laboratory that manufactured them etched into the upper temporal edge.
- Lens styles and designs are available in many different materials (Table 4-4). Check lens availability guides to determine designs and materials.

Tinting lenses is easily accomplished by dyes. For the best results, frequently replace the dyes to produce accurate tint colors. Using filtered or distilled water further enhances the color and absorption of the tints. Plastic absorptive lenses can be tinted in a multitude of shades. Double-gradient tinted lenses have one color tint at the top of the lens and another color on the bottom half of the lens. Polycarbonate material generally takes only a tint of light to medium darkness. Overheating or attempting to tint a polycarbonate lens to a sunwear shade will most likely damage the lens.

Ultraviolet (UV) protection, which is important for all sunwear tinted lenses, is obtained by immersing absorptive lenses into a heated solution of UV filtering

Table 4-4.

Lens Materials

A. CR-39

1. Features: Plastic resin; most common lens material used today; lightweight and very stable; less likely to shatter than glass; readily accepts tints and coatings.
Index of refraction = 1.498
Abbe (Nu) value = 58
2. Fitting notes: Available in most lens styles, including single vision, bifocals, and multifocals.

B. Glass

1. Crown glass
    a. Features: Refracts light more purely than any other lens material.
    Index of refraction = 1.523
    Abbe (Nu) value = 59
    b. Fitting notes: Heavy; poses a safety risk, particularly for children and some occupations.
2. Photochromic glass
    a. Features: Lenses change from light inside to dark outside.
    b. Fitting notes: Darkens in color depending on the degree of UV rays striking the lens surface, thus it will turn dark even on a cloudy day.

C. Transitions (Pittsburgh Plate Glass Industries, Pittsburgh, PA)

1. Features: A resin lens; darkens and lightens depending on the amount of UV light that is striking the front lens surface; available in several different colors.

D. High index

1. Features: Made of denser materials than more conventional materials, thus the lens is thinner and lighter; available in plastic resins and glass.
Indices of refraction:
    High index 1.56 (resin) = 1.556
    High index 1.60 (resin) = 1.60
    High index 1.66 (resin) = 1.66
Abbe (Nu) values:
    High index 1.56 (resin) = 39
    High index 1.60 (resin) = 37
    High index 1.66 (resin) = 32
    High index glass = 25
2. Fitting notes: It is important to know if the lenses are decentered or laid out "on center"; if "on center" it is necessary to keep the frame size to a minimum to guarantee that the job will cut out after decentering the lenses. It is *always* beneficial to select smaller frames when it comes to lenses with higher powers. Maximize the overall appearance by controlling either the center thickness of minus lenses or the edge thickness of plus lenses; grind as thin as possible based on the recommendations of the manufacturer.

E. Polycarbonate

1. Features: Extremely lightweight; high refractive index; produces thinner lens than conventional materials; very soft; impact-absorbing; difficult to polish.

(continued)

Table 4-4. (continued)
Lens Materials

Index of refraction = 1.586
Abbe (Nu) value = 31
2. Fitting notes: Some patients (especially in the higher minus powers) may complain of peripheral chromatic aberration.
3. Handling notes: Acetone will crack the surface; tint and neutralize with dye pots at a lower temperature than standard to avoid crazing or splitting. Chromatic problems with polycarbonate (or any other ultra-high refractive index material such as 1.66) can be minimized if a) the optical centers of the lenses are specified and ground into the correct position, b) the monocular pupillary distance (PD) is correct (for single vision and progressive styles only), and c) the frame size is kept to a minimum.

chemicals. (Polycarbonate and some high-index lenses inherently provide UV protection due to the material.) Once the lenses are immersed for the required period of time (dependent on the chemical manufacturer), they are capable of absorbing UV up to 400 nm.

Antireflective coating reflects a substantial amount of visible light, allowing more light to transmit through the lens, which enhances the wearer's vision. Antireflective coating also diminishes the amount of light that is reflected from the lens surface. Because antireflective coating is superb at transmitting additional light through the lens material, it is best to specify that the lens be clear, ie, with no additional tinting. Patients should be advised that antireflective coated lenses should be cleaned with solutions that are approved for this type of coating.

Lens materials, especially those with a high refractive index, often cause *chromatic aberration* (color dispersion) through the periphery of the lens. The Abbe value (or Nu value) indicates the ability of a lens material to purely refract white light without chromatic aberration. A high Abbe number indicates that the material is not likely to cause chromatic problems.

The *index of refraction* is a ratio obtained by dividing the speed that light travels through a specific material into the speed that light travels through air. Light travels slower through some materials than others, depending on the density of the material. The denser the material, the slower light travels through that material. The slower that light travels through a specific material, the higher the material's refractive index and the greater its refracting ability.

The best (and least distorted) vision with an ophthalmic lens is obtained by matching the patient's visual axis with the *optical center* of the lens. (The visual axis is an imaginary line from a viewed object to the fovea.) When alignment is accurate, the patient looks directly through the optical center of the lens without the presence of any unwanted vertical or horizontal prism. (See Chapter 3, Induced Prism.)

Single vision lenses correct vision for one focal length. *Bifocal* lenses correct vision at two distances, usually with a prescription for distance vision at the top of the lens and a segment at the bottom of the lenses for close work (Figure 4-7). A conventional *trifocal* lens has a distance portion, an intermediate segment (usually calculated for 30 inches away, generally half the bifocal power), and a bottom segment to correct vision at 16 inches away (Figure 4-8). An *occupational* lens usually has a bifocal at the top and bottom, or a bifocal at the top and a trifocal at the bottom (Figure 4-9).

Progressive lenses are aspheric lenses with no segment line. They consist of distance, intermediate, and near zones (Figure 4-10). The power differences between the zones are achieved through slight, gradual changes in power.

Manufacturers offer many different progressive designs, each of which performs uniquely. Designs that offer a wide reading area but a more narrow intermediate area are called "hard designs." A hard design has a vast amount of change over a small area but can also have peripheral problems and increased peripheral cylinder aberrations. A soft design has a wide intermediate zone with a more narrow reading area. This would be beneficial for a computer user who can benefit from a wider intermediate field. A soft design has a slight amount of change over a small area, resulting in less noticeable peripheral cylinder aberrations.

Patients with high cylinder corrections (over 2.00 D) sometimes have difficulty adjusting to progressive lenses. Patients should be informed that their best vision with progressives is achieved through the central portion of the lenses. Objects viewed through the periphery of the lenses are generally not quite as clear as objects seen through the central portion.

Progressive lenses have etchings engraved into the front lens surface to indicate the particular lens design, as well as the power of the near addition. These etchings are more easily viewed if held up to a bright light. When the markings are placed on a template (provided by the manufacturer), verification markings can be drawn onto the lens (Figure 4-11). Just above the fitting cross is an arch. It is within this arch that the distance lens power should be verified with the lensometer.

Corrective curve lenses, unlike flat lenses that produce significant peripheral problems, couple specific base curves with a given prescription to produce a lens that will have minimal spherical aberration, chromatic aberration, distortion, and cylindrical aberration.

Aspheric lenses are mathematically enhanced to produce improved peripheral optics. The curvatures of an aspheric design change in the outer portions of the lens. This produces better peripheral vision, a flatter and thinner lens, and an increased field of vision. This is especially true with mid- to high-powered lenses. In addition, the size of the patient's eyes appear more normal than with conventional base curves. They are available in plastic resins (conventional or high index) in a multitude of single vision and multifocal lens styles.

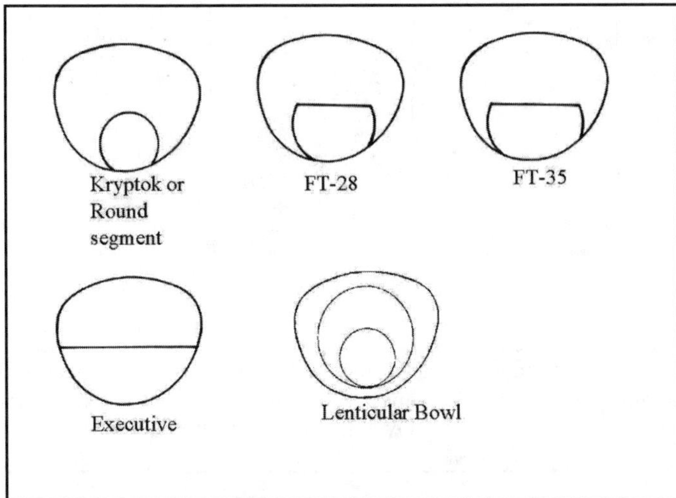

Figure 4-7. Bifocal styles (reprinted with permission from Carlton J. *Frames and Lenses*. Thorofare, NJ: SLACK Incorporated; 2000).

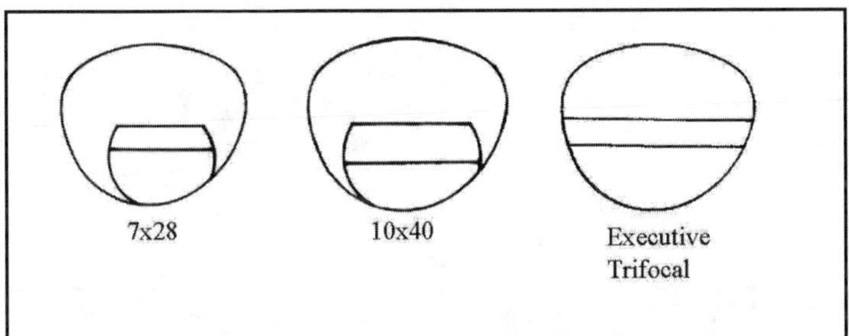

Figure 4-8. Trifocal styles (reprinted with permission from Carlton J. *Frames and Lenses*. Thorofare, NJ: SLACK Incorporated; 2000).

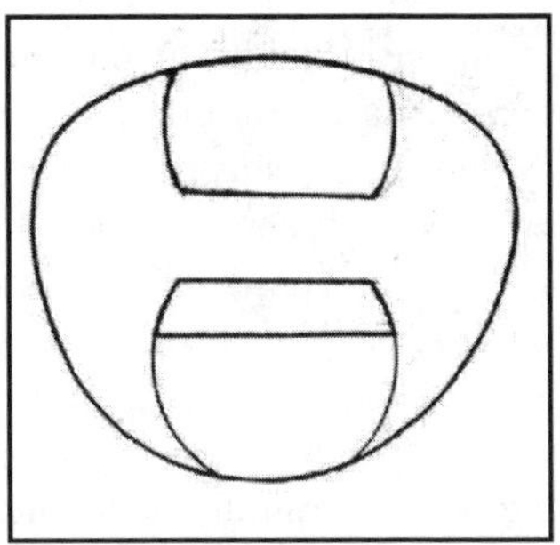

Figure 4-9. Occupational lens (reprinted with permission from Carlton J. *Frames and Lenses*. Thorofare, NJ: SLACK Incorporated; 2000).

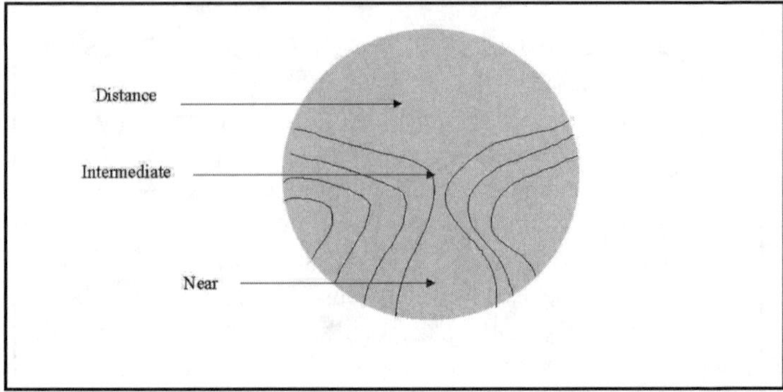

Figure 4-10. A progressive lens consists of three primary zones: distance, intermediate, and near (reprinted with permission from Carlton J. *Frames and Lenses*. Thorofare, NJ: SLACK Incorporated; 2000).

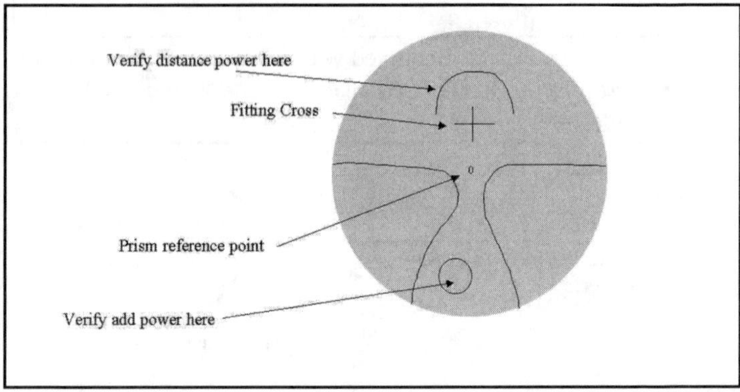

Figure 4-11. Progressive lens with verification markings (reprinted with permission from Carlton J. *Frames and Lenses*. Thorofare, NJ: SLACK Incorporated; 2000).

A *myodisc* or *blended myodisc* lens is generally considered for high minus powers beginning at –12.00 D. It is a lenticular lens with a carrier and produces a clear central area for vision with a significantly thinner lens edge. The major drawback to this lens style is that it offers very little peripheral vision, and patients may complain of "tunnel vision." When selecting a frame style for this lens, it is important to choose a sturdy frame with a heavy eyewire and deep lens groove.

Another lens for high myopia is the *biconcave* lens, which is concave and ground on both the front and back surface, resulting in an overall thinner and lighter-weight lens. Unfortunately, biconcave designs offer less peripheral clarity. The best frame selection for such a lens is a sturdy plastic frame or metal style that is specially designed for high minus lenses.

The American National Standards Institute, Inc (ANSI) safety standard states that approved *safety* lenses must have a minimum thickness of 3.0 mm. The exception is lenses of +3.00 D or more, which must have a minimum thickness of 2.5 mm. The lenses must also have the initials of the laboratory that manufactured them etched into the upper temporal edge. ANSI-approved safety lenses are to be mounted only in approved Z-87 frames. ANSI-approved frames must have Z-87 stamped on the frame front as well as on the temples. No other combination of frame and lenses denotes ANSI-approved safety eyewear. Any material can be used for safety lenses; however, polycarbonate is the safest lens material on the market and is virtually shatterproof when the thickness rules for safety eyewear are followed.

Single vision or multifocal patients who are anisometropic (have unequal refractive powers in the two eyes, particularly when one eye requires a plus correction and the other eye requires a minus correction) often need a lens with a specially ground lens, called a *slab-off*. The unbalanced refractive powers of the two lenses, especially if the difference between the two corrections is greater than 1.50 D, cause prismatic problems at near. Because of this, the patient is not able to achieve binocular vision (or one fused image) when reading with the glasses. A slab-off lens remedies this problem by correcting vertical prism imbalances. A lens with slab-off treatment has a fine, raised horizontal line across the lens. If the lens is a bifocal, the line appears equal with the segment line

Optical Instrumentation and Measurements

The *lensometer* is used to determine the spherical power, cylinder power, axis, pupillary measurement, and optical center of a lens. It is also used to determine the degree and direction of prism.

How-To: Lensometry

- *Focus the eyepiece.* To focus the eyepiece, first turn the power wheel to 0. Then turn the eyepiece to its most plus position. Inspect the reticule (the image of circles and numbers inside the instrument). Adjust the eyepiece by turning it slowly toward minus until the numbers and circles appear sharp and focused. Stop as soon as the reticule is clear and goes no further.
- *Place the frame on the carriage,* making sure that both eyewires are even.
- *Locate the optical center* of the lens by finding the central point at which the cross hairs meet. Lock the lens into place with the lens holder.
- *Determine if the lens is spherical or spherocylindrical.* While looking through the eyepiece, turn the power drum until you obtain a clear image of the mires. Next, rotate the axis wheel while continuing to inspect the

(continued)

How-To: Lensometry (continued)

mires through the eyepiece. Do the lines break, come into sharp focus, then break again as you turn the axis wheel? If the mires do not change, the lens is spherical (see A). If they do change, the lens is spherocylindrical (see B).

- *Read the power of the lens.*

A. *Neutralizing a spherical lens:* Adjust the frame on the carriage until the optical center of the lens is well-centered when viewed through the eyepiece. Turn the power drum until the mires are clear and sharp. Read the diopter power from the power drum.

B. Neutralizing a spherocylindrical lens:

1. Place the frame on the carriage and position the glasses with the optical center of the strongest lens in the center of the reticule.
2. In the optical shop, lenses are always neutralized in minus cylinder. This means that it is necessary to turn the power drum *away* from you when obtaining the cylinder correction of a lens. (Conversely, when neutralizing the lens in plus cylinder, you must turn the power wheel *toward* you.) Turn the axis wheel until the sphere lines, which are the thinnest lines on most lensometers, are unbroken. Then turn the power wheel until the lines focus clearly. Note the power indicated on the power drum; this is the spherical power of the lens.
3. Rotate the power wheel *away* from you until the cylinder lines, which are usually the thickest lines, come in clearly. If the cylinder lines only come in clearly when you rotate the power wheel toward you, you must then turn the *axis* wheel until the mires come in clearly when you rotate the power drum *away* from you. This will be a 90-degree change in axis. You have obtained the minus cylinder correction when the thickest lines are sharp and unbroken. Note the power on the power wheel. If the cylinder lines are not perfectly straight, turn the axis wheel until they become very crisp and intact.
4. Determine the cylinder power of the lenses. The cylinder power is the difference between the spherical reading and the cylinder reading on the power wheel.
5. To complete the neutralization of the lens, note the reading on the axis wheel.

(continued)

How-To: Lensometry (continued)

C. Determining the power of the add (if present):

1. Move the lens up slightly so that the bifocal portion of the lens is resting on the lens stop. Clamp the lens down using the lens holder, and rotate the power wheel until the sphere lines come in clearly. Note the spherical reading.
2. Now calculate the difference between the bifocal power and the distance spherical power. This is the add power. The midrange portion of a trifocal can be similarly read and is usually half of the bifocal power.

Note: When reading the bifocal power of a high plus lens (over +3.00), turn the glasses so that they are facing you and read the front vertex power of the lens (distance portion). Then move the lens up slightly and read the bifocal power. Subtract the distance reading from the near reading (as above) to determine the true add power.

D. *Prism*:

1. Make sure that both eyewires are in an even position on the carriage. *Ground-in prism* generally cannot be made to center in the reticle. Instead, the optical center will intersect one of the rings on the reticule, which are numbered to indicate the degree of prism diopter.
2. The direction of a prism is determined by its base. The reticule is divided into four quadrants (Figure 4-12). To calculate the direction of the prism, determine in which quadrant the optical center appears, as well as its relationship to the bridge of the frame.
3. Use the prism compensating device (located close to the eyepiece) to inspect lenses with a high degree of prism correction (over 5.00 D). First move the device into the appropriate position: 180-degree position for horizontal prism or 90-degree position for vertical prism. Rotate the silver knob on the prism compensating device until the optical center (OC) of the lens is centered in the reticle. The prism scale on the device indicates the degree of prism present in the lens.
4. *Induced prism* can often be moved to different positions on the reticule (unlike ground-in prism). First align the optical center in the middle of the reticule and read the power. Then use Prentice's rule (Chapter 3) to determine the amount of induced prism. When determining the direction of induced prism, it may be helpful to remember that lenses are really prisms connected either base to base (plus lenses) or apex to apex (minus lenses). It is sometimes useful to actually draw the situation on paper to assess the placement of the optical center and the resultant direction of the induced prism.

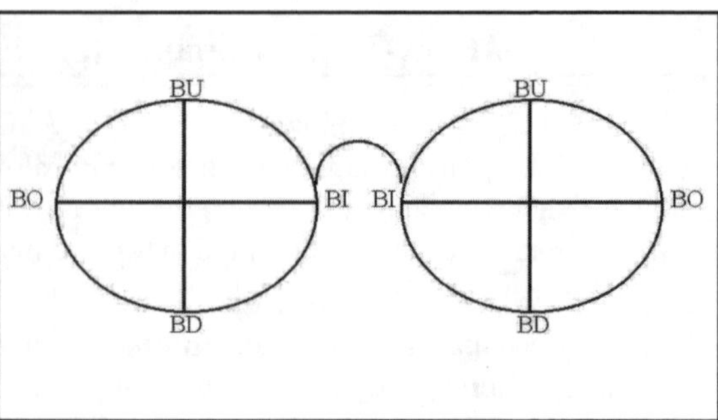

Figure 4-12. Determining prism direction (reprinted with permission from Carlton J. *Frames and Lenses.* Thorofare, NJ: SLACK Incorporated; 2000).

The pupillary distance (PD), also known as the interpupillary distance (IPD), is the distance between the visual axis of each eye. To ensure that the optical center of the lens is ground to coincide with the patient's visual axis, it is necessary to measure the PD in millimeters. In addition, a monocular PD is needed when ordering progressive lenses or when ordering lenses with a high refractive index. Both of these measurements can be obtained by using a millimeter ruler or a corneal reflection pupillometer (CRP).

How-To: Pupillary Distance

Binocular Pupillary Measurement:

- Position yourself directly in front of the patient. Place the millimeter ruler on the patient's bridge and close your right eye.
- Ask the patient to look directly at your open eye. Align the 0 on the ruler with the *outside edge* of the patient's right pupil.
- Without moving the ruler, close your left eye and open your right eye. Note the number on the ruler at the *inside* edge of the patient's left pupil.

Note: This method is inappropriate if the patient's pupils have been dilated.

Monocular Pupillary Measurement:

- Position yourself directly in front of the patient, no farther than 16 inches away.
- Place the spectacle frame on the patient's face and inspect the frame's adjustment. Correct any adjustment problems before continuing with the measurement.
- Close your left eye and ask the patient to look directly at your open eye. Using a grease pencil or a marker, dot the center of the patient's left pupil on the demo lens.

(continued)

How-To: Pupillary Distance (continued)

- Close your right eye and open the left. Ask your patient to look directly at your open eye and place a mark on the demo lens in the center of the patient's right pupil.
- Remove the frame and draw a vertical line at the center of the bridge with your grease pencil. Consider this point to be 0. Measure from the 0 point horizontally to each dot to determine the monocular PD for each eye.

Corneal Reflection Pupillometer:

- Clean all areas of the pupillometer that come into contact with the patient's face with an alcohol wipe.
- Ask the patient to assist you in holding the pupillometer up to his or her face. (It is sometimes helpful to instruct the patient to hold the pupillometer as if using a pair of binoculars.)
- Adjust the knob on the top of the pupillometer to the infinity position (∞).
- Looking through the eyepiece, move the sliding pieces beneath your thumbs so that the vertical lines inside the pupillometer are aligned with the light reflexes on both corneas.
- Turn the instrument over and take note of the measurements. The pupillometer will give you the binocular dimension (usually in the center) plus the monocular calculations for each eye.

The *vertex distance* (VD) is the distance (in millimeters) between the back surface of an ophthalmic lens (as measured during the examination) and the patient's cornea. This measurement is especially important for lenses of + 5.00 D or greater. A distometer is a calibration tool that is used to determine this measurement (Figure 4-13).

The *Boxing System* (Figure 4-14) is the preferred means of obtaining necessary frame and lens measurements.

How-To: Vertex Distance

The Distometer:

- Ask the patient to close his or her eyes.
- Gently place the stationary foot of the distometer against the closed lid (see Figure 4-13). Do not press on the globe.
- Slowly press the plunger until the arm of the device touches the backside of the lens. Note the vertex measurement in millimeters on the scale.
- Make sure that you are measuring through only one thickness of the lid, not folded over tissue. Some distometers automatically compensate for

(continued)

How-To: Vertex Distance (continued)

the thickness of the eyelid. If your distometer does not compensate for the lid thickness, add 1 mm to the measurement.

Note: The initial distometer reading is taken during the examination, using the phoropter or trial frames used during refractometry. A second reading may be taken when the patient selects new frames.

The Rotary Chart:

- On the rotary chart, use the red scale for minus lenses or the black scale for plus lenses. Turn the chart until the prescribed spherical power of the lens aligns with the vertex distance used during refractometry.
- Without moving the dial, find the vertex distance of the new spectacles. The recalculated lens power is adjacent to the spectacle vertex distance.

Note: The rotary chart is used to compensate for any variance between the vertex distance used when the patient is refracted vs. the new frames he or she has selected.

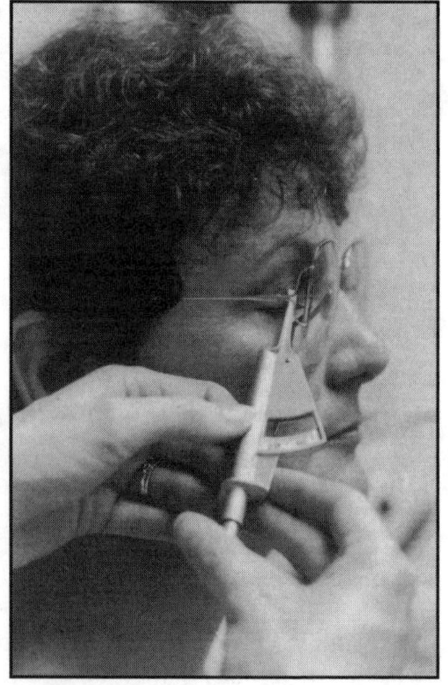

Figure 4-13. Measuring vertex distance (photo by Jim Ledford. Reprinted from Ledford J. *Exercises in Refractometry*. Thorofare, NJ: SLACK Incorporated; 1990, with permission from Janice Ledford).

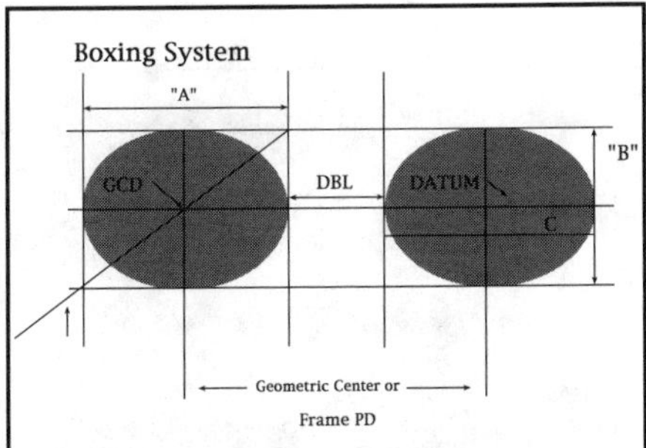

Figure 4-14. The Boxing System (reprinted with permission from Carlton J. *Frames and Lenses*. Thorofare, NJ: SLACK Incorporated; 2000).

How-To: The Boxing System

- The A measurement refers to the eye size of the frame. Determine the A measurement by using a millimeter ruler to measure horizontally inside one of the eyewires from side to side. Add 1 mm to this measurement to account for the groove inside the eyewire.
- The B measurement is the vertical measurement. Calculate the B measurement by using a millimeter ruler to measure vertically inside the deepest portion of the eyewire from top to bottom. Add 1 mm to this number to account for the groove inside the frame.
- The C measurement refers to the datum line measurement.
- The ED measurement is the effective diameter of a lens, taken by measuring from one corner of the lens opening to the opposite edge. Add 1 mm to this figure to account for the groove inside the frame.
- The DBL (distance between lenses) is the width of the bridge. Calculate this figure by measuring the distance between the eyewires at the narrowest point of the bridge with a millimeter ruler.
- The GCD (geometric center distance) or the frame PD is the DBL added to the A measurement. Measure from the inside of the bridge, across the lens opening, to the inside of the eyewire close to the temple.
- The minimum blank size is determined by adding the ED measurement with the total amount of decentration plus 2 mm for edging purposes. (The total amount of decentration is figured by adding the A measurement to the DBL measurement, then subtracting the patient's PD.)
- The frame difference is the difference between the A and B measurements.

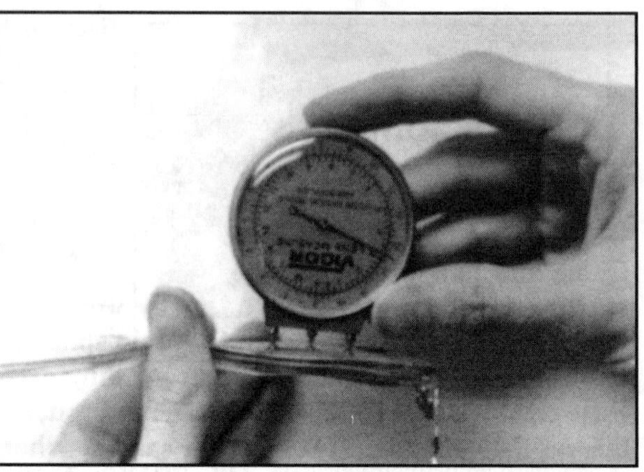

Figure 4-15. Using Geneva lens clock (photo by Jim Ledford. Reprinted from Ledford J. *Exercises in Refractometry.* Thorofare, NJ: SLACK Incorporated; 1990, with permission from Janice Ledford).

The *lens clock*, also known as the *Geneva lens measure*, is an instrument used to determine the base curvature of an ophthalmic lens. The face of the clock has diopter powers in red and black. When reading the front curve of a lens, the black numbers are used. The red numbers are used if reading the back curve of a lens.

How-To: Geneva Lens Measure

- Prior to testing lenses with the clock, "clock" the curvature of a flat surface. If the lens clock reads zero, then the instrument is working accurately.
- While holding the lens or glasses firmly in one hand, use the other hand to press the lens clock gently against the surface of the lens, making sure that the center pin is depressed against the lens (Figure 4-15). To obtain an accurate reading, the placement of the lens clock should be along the 90-degree meridian of the lens (horizontally across the lens) and should not contact a multifocal segment of any kind (flat top or progressive).
- The measurement is read directly off of the clock face.

Prior to *dispensing*, the following items are to be inspected for accuracy:

- power
- PD
- segment style
- segment height
- tinting
- coatings
- lens size
- lens mounting
- safety engravings (when necessary)
- cosmetic appearance
- standard adjustment

Unless otherwise noted, all text, tables, and figures are adapted or reprinted with permission from Carlton J. Frames and Lenses. *Thorofare, NJ: SLACK Incorporated; 1999.*

CHAPTER 5

Ocular Disorders

Disorders are divided into systems, then presented in alphabetical order.

Skin and Eyelids (Table 5-1)

It is important to have any suspicious growths of the skin and eyelids checked by a physician. Often a biopsy is performed to determine whether or not the lesion is cancerous.

Table 5-1.
Skin and Eyelid Disorders

Clinical Entity	Features	Notes
Actinic keratosis	Patchy, scaly, and irregular Tan, ivory, or yellow	Also called climatic keratopathy Precancerous
Basal cell carcinoma	Malignant a. Raised, ulcerated, pearly surface b. Flat and leathery	Type b more likely to invade deeper tissues Metastitic spread is rare Treatment: surgical excision, cryotherapy, radiation
Blepharitis	Swollen, congested, and red lid margins; lid crusting; itching	Treatment: lid hygiene, antibiotic ointment
Chalazion	Swollen, painful, and inflamed lid with cyst formation	Chronic inflammation of a meibomian gland Treatment: warm compresses, antibiotics, incise, and curettage

(continued)

Table 5-1. (continued)

Skin and Eyelid Disorders

Clinical Entity	Features	Notes
Dermatochalasis	Redundant skin of upper lid	May interfere with peripheral vision
Ectropion	Lid falls away from the globe	Usually the lower lid May cause conjunctival and/or corneal exposure
Entropion	Inward-turning of the lid	Usually the lower lid Lashes may brush globe May cause corneal damage
Hemangioma	Bright red growth	Composed of small, dilated blood vessels Usually regresses with age
Herpes zoster ophthalmicus	Blisters on skin Sometimes involves the cornea, sclera, ciliary body, or optic nerve	Also called shingles Treatment: antiviral drugs
Hordeolum	Lid swelling with abscess	Also called a stye Treatment: warm compresses, antibiotic ointment
Melanoma	Pigmented or nonpigmented lesion	Biopsy to confirm diagnosis Prognosis depends on degree of tissue invasion Treatment: total excision
Milia	Small, round, white, slightly elevated cysts	Treatment: removal (may be considered cosmetic)
Nevi	Benign, flat, pigmented	Watch for changes
Ptosis	Upper lid margin is abnormally low	If severe, may cover pupil and interfere with vision

(continued)

Table 5-1. (continued)
Skin and Eyelid Disorders

Clinical Entity	Features	Notes
Squamous cell carcinoma	Usually develops from actinic keratosis	Greater malignant potential Treatment: wide surgical excision
Trichiasis	Lashes grow inward toward the eye	Often results from lid scarring Causes corneal irritation May cause corneal ulceration
Xanthoma	Yellowish fatty deposits on the upper and lower lids	Also called xanthelasma May be associated with high blood fat levels Treatment: trichloracetic acid, carbon dioxide snow, surgery

Lacrimal Apparatus and Orbital Disorders (Table 5-2)

Table 5-2.
Lacrimal Apparatus and Orbital Disorders

Clinical Entity	Features	Notes
Canaliculitis	Persistent discharge, red eye, itching, epiphora, swelling, and inflammation in nasal canthus	Inflammation of canaliculus
Dacryocystitis	Pain, edema, epiphora, and redness at inner canthus	Treatment: hot compresses, antibiotic drops, systemic antibiotics, incise, and draine
Endophthalmitis	Unilateral edema, poor vision, redness of the lids and conjunctiva, vitreous haze	Response to infection, trauma, immune reaction, and physical or chemical change Treatment: antibiotic and/or antifungal agent

(continued)

Table 5-2. (continued)
Lacrimal Apparatus and Orbital Disorders

Clinical Entity	Features	Notes
Exophthalmus	Abnormal protrusion of eyeball	May be due to thyroid lid retraction, scleral show, corneal exposure Measured and monitored with exophthalmometer
Nasolacrimal duct obstruction	Tearing and mattering	Occurs in 30% of newborns Treatment: massage, topical antibiotics, probe, and irrigation
Prolapsed tear gland	Yellow glob under upper lid	Lacrimal gland has dropped down between the sclera and bulbar conjunctiva Reassure; there is no dysfunction
Sympathetic ophthalmia	Early symptoms may include slight pain, photophobia, lacrimation, disturbances in accommodation, and decreased vision	Late complication of penetrating injury in injured **and** non-injured eye Uveitis can lead to blindness May occur 6 to 12 months after original injury Treatment: enucleation of injured, blind eye; steroids

Conjunctival and Scleral Disorders (Table 5-3)

Table 5-3.
Conjunctival and Scleral Disorders

Clinical Entity	Features	Notes
Allergic conjunctivitis	Itching, mild to moderate infection, swelling of the conjunctiva, lacrimation, and mucus discharge	Hypersensitivity to foreign substance Treatment: topical sodium cromoglycate and corticosteroid

(continued)

Table 5-3. (continued)

Conjunctival and Scleral Disorders

Clinical entity	Features	Notes
Bacterial conjunctivitis	Gritty sensation, conjunctival injection, and purulent discharge	Treatment: topical antibiotics, hygiene
Conjunctival nevi	Flat pigmented lesions	Usually present at birth and darkens during adolescence Those appearing in late adolescence may become malignant
Conjunctivitis	See type (allergic, viral, etc)	
Episcleritis	Simple: acute onset of redness Nodular: red raised area near limbus	Inflammatory process Treatment: topical steroids
Giant papillary conjunctivitis	Papillae under upper lid (1 mm or larger) Conjunctiva swollen and irritated	Associated with contact lens wear Treatment: evaluate care regime, change lens materials
Pinguecula	Yellowish conjunctival mass nasally	Frequently caused by wind and dust Never invades the cornea
Pterygium	Triangular wedge of conjunctiva progressing onto the cornea	May progress onto visual axis, threatening vision Common in tropical climates Treatment: excision (recurrence is common)
Scleral degeneration	Small, round, gray areas (usually 2 to 3 mm in diameter)	No symptoms or complications

(continued)

Table 5-3. (continued)

Conjunctival and Scleral Disorders

Clinical entity	Features	Notes
Scleritis	Severe pain, tenderness, tearing, redness	Tissue destruction causes or associated with conditions include keratitis, uveitis, glaucoma, cataract, retinal detachment Treatment: topical and/or systemic steroids; systemic NSAIDs
Subconjunctival hemorrhage	Bright red area under the conjunctiva	Bleeding due to a ruptured conjunctival blood vessel
Vernal conjunctivitis	Itching, redness, lacrimation, and mucus discharge	Limbal: papillary enlargement on limbal conjunctiva with concretions near limbus Palpebral: cobblestone papillae on tarsal conjunctiva Treatment: topical sodium cromoglycate and corticosteroid
Viral conjunctivitis	Follicles, watery discharge, and superficial punctate keratitis	Adenoviruses are most common Treatment: topical antivirals

Corneal Disorders (Table 5-4)

Table 5-4.

Corneal Disorders

Clinical Entity	Features	Notes
Acanthamoeba	Persistent keratitis (may look dendritic in early stages), redness, pain; in late stages: ringshaped infiltrate, anterior chamber reaction	Organism found in nonsterile solutions (as for contact lenses) and swimming environments Highly resistant to treatment *(continued)*

Table 5-4. (continued)

Corneal Disorders

Clinical Entity	Features	Notes
Arcus senilis	Cloudy ring around limbus	Also called gerontoxan Benign fat deposit May be associated with high blood fat levels
Dystrophy	Corneal clouding Decreased vision	Corneal tissue undergoes atrophy or regression Affects various corneal layers Inherited, usually shows up in later life Treatment varies: topical sodium, K transplant, bandage contact lens
Edema	Photophobia, halos, redness, discomfort Hazy corneal tissues	Swelling of the cornea caused by disturbance in endothelium's pump action Causes include degeneration, dystrophy, trauma, glaucoma, uveitis, keratitis
Exposure keratitis	Irritation, inflammation	Corneal drying due to incomplete lid closure Treatment: topical lubricants, tape lid shut, lid surgery
Guttata	"Wart-like" deposits on backside of cornea	Patients usually over 40 years of age Can destroy or compromise endothelial cells, producing edema
Infiltrates	Grayish-white, punctate, oval, or stellate If infectious: pain, photophobia, discharge, redness, anterior chamber (A/C) reaction If sterile: no staining or discharge, minimal discomfort or A/C reaction	Subepithelial inflammatory cells; usually do not stain May be infectious or noninfectious (sterile)

(continued)

Table 5-4. (continued)

Corneal Disorders

Clinical Entity	Features	Notes
Keratitis	Lack-luster cornea, infiltrates, surface lesions, pain Often accompanied by conjunctivitis	Causes include fungi, viruses, bacteria Treatment depends on cause
Keratoconjunctivitis sicca	Irritation, redness, photophobia, mucus strands, contact lens intolerance	Also called dry eye Decreased tear producttion Superficial punctate staining Most seen in menopausal women Associated with Sjögren's syndrome, rheumatoid arthritis, lupus, thyroid imbalance, diuretics, antihistmines, blood pressure meds, birth control pills Treatment varies: topical lubricants, punctal occlusion, humidifiers, vitamins
Keratoconus	Decreased vision Increased astigmatism Reduced corneal sensitivity	Also called ectactic dystrophy Central cornea thins and bulges forward Progresses at varying rates Treatment: rigid contact lens, K transplant
Krukenberg's spindle	Vertical pigment deposits on central endothelium	May be benign or associated with glaucoma
Neovascularization	Vessel encroachment onto cornea	Caused by hypoxia Often associated with contact lens wear

(continued)

Table 5-4. (continued)

Corneal Disorders

Clinical Entity	Features	Notes
Pannus	Vessels and fibrous tissue infiltrating the cornea	Degenerative type associated with late bullous keratopathy Inflammatory type associated with trachoma
Ulcers	Pain, redness, surface corneal lesion, infiltrates	May be caused by bacteria, fungi, viruses, chemical, or physical insult Treatment varies with cause

Uveal Tract, Pupil, and Anterior Chamber Disorders (Table 5-5)

Table 5-5.

Uveal Tract, Pupil, and Anterior Chamber Disorders

Clinical entity	Features	Notes
Adie's tonic pupil	Pupil reacts poorly to light and slowly to near	Caused by damage to short ciliary nerves True tonic pupil will constrict to topical methacholine
Anisocoria	Unequal pupil sizes	May be genetic or caused by trauma, chemicals, or medications
Argyll Robertson syndrome	Pupil fails to respond to direct and consensual light; reaction to accomodation is normal	Usually caused by syphilis
Horner's syndrome	Ptosis, miosis, and anhydrosis on affected side	Caused by damage to CN III Dilates poorly to topical cocaine

(continued)

Table 5-5. (continued)

Uveal Tract, Pupil, and Anterior Chamber Disorders

Clinical entity	Features	Notes
Hyphema	Red pool in inferior anterior chamber	Accumulation of blood Usually associated with trauma May be associated with iritis, neovascular glaucoma, iridocyclitis, or tumors
Hypopyon	White pool in inferior anterior chamber	Accumulation of white blood cells Associated with trauma, iritis, ulcers, or keratitis May be infective or sterile
Iris coloboma	Fissure in iris, ranging from a notch to half or more of iris	Fetal fissure defect
Iris melanoma	Arise from pre-existing nevus vascular; increase in size	Rare Usually metastatic, can be life-threatening Early treatment: excision Late treatment: enucleation
Iris synechiae	Anterior: iris adheres to cornea or angle structures; irregular pupil shape Posterior: iris adheres to lens; irregular pupil shape	Caused by inflammation Secondary glaucoma may develop Treatment: dilation, anti-inflammatories
Iritis	Pain, photophobia, ciliary flush, cells in anterior chamber, miosis, blurred vision, tearing, precipitates on posterior cornea	Also called anterior uveitis Treatment: topical anti-inflammatories and dilation Inflammation of iris

(continued)

Table 5-5. (continued)

Uveal Tract, Pupil, and Anterior Chamber Disorders

Clinical entity	Features	Notes
Marcus Gunn pupil	Diminished pupil reaction to direct light Normal consensual response	Also called afferent pupillary defect Caused by impaired retinal or optic nerve function Vision usually decreased
Narrow angles	Lack of adequate space between cornea and iris	May be genetic More common in hyperopes More common in women May lead to angle-closure glaucoma in later life
Pars planitis	Blurred vision, floaters	Also called intermediate uveitis Inflammation of pars plana Usually associated with multiple sclerosis Usually bilateral Treatment may include steroids or NSAIDs
Uveitis	Minimal pain, redness, photophobia, blurred vision	Also called posterior uveitis Inflammation of the uvea May be associated with systemic inflammatory diseases, Herpes zoster or simplex, trauma Treatment may include steroids or NSAIDs

Vitreous and Retinal Disorders (Table 5-6)

Table 5-6.
Vitreous and Retinal Disorders

Clinical Entity	Features	Notes
Asteroid hyalosis	No symptoms	Also known as Benson's disease Clumps of calcium deposits suspended in the vitreous Usually occurs in the elderly
Background diabetic retinopathy	Visual impairment varies	Distinguished by microaneurysms, hemorrhages, cotton-wool spots, exudates, intraretinal shunt vessels, and venous bleeding
Choriodal nevus	No symptoms	Flat, benign lesion in choroid May be pigmented
Flashes	"Flashing lights," especially in dim lighting	Result from traction on the retina
Floaters	"Specks, bugs, webs, hairs" in patient's line of vision	Caused by clumps of protein that cast shadows on retina Common in myopes and elderly Usually benign Can be associated with retinal detachment
Hypertensive retinopathy	Visual impairment varies	Group I: narrow and straightened vessels, copper-wire appearance Group II: vessels begin to leak, hemorrhages Group III: retinal edema, hemorrhages, cotton-wool spots, branch retinal vein occlusion (BRVO)

(continued)

Table 5-6. (continued)
Vitreous and Retinal Disorders

Clinical Entity	Features	Notes
Hypertensive retinopathy		Group IV: disc edema
Macular degeneration	Varying visual impairment at near; peripheral vision remains largely intact	Also called age-related macular degeneration or senile macular degeneration Caused by breakdown of macular tissue as retinal blood vessels sclerose Most common in elderly Can be hereditary
Proliferative diabetic retinopathy	Visual impairment varies	Abnormalities in vessels, retinal surface, or vitreous cavity; neovascularization Vitreous hemorrhages and traction retinal detachments may occur
Retinal detachment	"Missing" areas of vision; floaters, flashes; decreased vision	Retina separates from underlying retinal pigment epithelium (RPE) May be associated with myopia, trauma, aphakia, inflammation Treatment: laser or conventional surgery
Retinitis	Haze, loss of central vision, floaters	Inflammation of retina Cause is usually infective May include retinal detachment, hemorrhage, scarring Treatment: varies; antibiotic, pars plana vitrectomy

(continued)

Table 5-6. (continued)
Vitreous and Retinal Disorders

Clinical Entity	Features	Notes
Retinoblastoma	White pupillary reflex Strabismus	Malignant retinal tumor Usually ocurrs in children Treatment: radiation or enucleation
Retinopathy of prematurity	Visual impairment varies	Thought to be caused by O_2 administered at premature or underweight birth Retinal neovascularization, twisted and dilated retinal blood vessels, peripheral retinal detachment Treatment: cryotherapy, laser, vitreoretinal surgery
Vitreous detachment	Floaters and flashes	Detachment of the vitreous from underlying retina Common in myopes and elderly people Can be a precursor of retinal detachment

Optic Nerve Disorders (Table 5-7)

Table 5-7.
Optic Nerve Disorders

Clinical Entity	Features	Notes
Atrophy	Blind spots in vision, loss of color perception	Degeneration of optic nerve fibers May be hereditary or related to glaucoma or other disease processes Treatment depends on underlying cause

(continued)

Table 5-7. (continued)

Optic Nerve Disorders

Clinical Entity	Features	Notes
Coloboma	Visual impairment varies	Fissure in lower segment of optic nerve head Fetal fissure defect Often associated with detachment at macula in later life
Cupping	Visual impairment varies	Excavation of optic disc due to elevated intra-ocular pressure, thus associated with glaucoma Measured as cup-to-disc ratio (see Figure 1-13)
Ischemic optic neuropathy	Sudden vision loss or transient vision loss, blind spots in the periphery, temporal headache	Nerve tissue degeneration due to blocked arteries in the optic nerve Often associated with temporal arteritis, diabetes, hypertension Treatment: oral steroids in decreasing dose
Optic neuritis	Symptoms vary, may include: pain, decreased vision, transient vision loss, blind spots	Inflammation or degeneration of optic nerve Often associated with multiple sclerosis Other causes may include medications or unknown Treatment varies with cause
Papilledema	Transient blurring episodes, diplopia, loss of peripheral vision, headache	Also called choked disc Caused by increased intracranial pressure May be associated with head injury or infection Cannot occur if optic atrophy is present Treatment: lower intercranial pressure

Neurological Conditions (Table 5-8)

Table 5-8.
Neurological Conditions

Clinical Entity	Features	Notes
Fourth nerve palsy	Diagonal double vision (may resolve with head tilted toward one shoulder)	Also called trochlear nerve palsy May be associated with head injury, multiple sclerosis, myasthenia gravis, tumor, aneurysm, diabetes Treatment: patching, prism, surgery after 6 months
Nystagmus	Blurred vision, oscillopsia, head tilt or turn, amblyopia	Involuntary, rhythmic movements of one or both eyes There are nearly 40 types May be congenital or acquired Movement may decrease or stop in one position of gaze
Seventh nerve palsy	Partial or full facial paralysis on the affected side, inability to close eye on affected side	Also called Bell's palsy, facial palsy, facial nerve palsy Affects orbicularis muscle Cause unknown No treatment except for corneal exposure and dryness Recovery varies
Sixth nerve palsy	Horizontal diplopia (may resolve with head turned to right or left)	Also called abducens nerve palsy May be associated with head injury, hypertension, migraine, arteriosclerosis, viral infection, diabetes, others

(continued)

Table 5-8. (continued)

Neurological Conditions

Clinical Entity	Features	Notes
Sixth nerve palsy		Treatment: patching, prism, surgery after 6 months
Strabismus	Abnormal eye position	Misalignment of eyes caused by problem with extraocular muscles or nerves See Chapter 12
Third nerve palsy	Double vision (may resolve in right or left gaze), ptosis, enlarged pupil, cycloplegia	Also called oculomotor nerve palsy Can affect the superior rectus (SR), inferior rectus (IR), medial rectus (MR), inferior oblique (IO), and levator muscles May be associated with diabetes, multiple sclerosis, hypertension, head injury, viral infection, aneurysm Treatment: prisms, patching, surgery after 6 months

Unless otherwise noted, all text, tables, and figures are adapted or reprinted with permission from Gwin N. Overview of Ocular Disorders. *Thorofare, NJ: SLACK Incorporated; 1999.*

CHAPTER 6

Cataract and Glaucoma

Cataract

- The human lens is a clear, avascular structure responsible for focusing light precisely on the retina.
- Lens cell division and growth is a lifelong process.
- The lens fibers formed earliest make up the hard central lens nucleus. Fibers formed later in life make up the softer outer lens cortex.
- Lens opacities form as the result of any process that disrupts either the lens architecture or the physiology necessary to maintain transparency.
- Classification systems of cataracts are based on cause, location, onset, stage of development, or descriptive appearance (Table 6-1).
- Clinically significant cataracts are those where the lens opacity affects some aspect of visual function, having an impact on patient lifestyle.
- There is no single exam sequence for all cataract patients. Though many standard tests and questions are necessary, each exam is tailored specifically to the patient based on the history and exam findings that arise (see Table 20-1).
- When surgery is considered, all risks, benefits, consequences, and alternatives must be discussed in detail with the patient (see Chapter 18).
- Extracapsular surgery is a means of removing the opacified lens while leaving the lens capsule in place. Phacoemulsification uses ultrasonic waves to fragment the opacified lens and liquify its contents (see Table 18-6).
- The two parts of an intraocular lens are the optic (the actual prescription lens) and the haptics (which provide physical support).
- Cataract surgery can be performed under three types of anesthesia: general, local, or topical.
- The incision used during cataract surgery varies in placement, size, shape, and construction depending on surgeon preference, surgical technique, and size of intraocular lens.

Table 6-1.
Classification of Cataracts

I. Classification by location

Type	Location	Notes
Anterior sub-capsular (ASC)	Just beneath the anterior capsule	
Cortical	Lens cortex	Usually appear as vacuoles or clefts in the beginning, then expand to spoke-like
Lamellar (Zonular)	Within one layer of the nucleus	
Nuclear	Central nucleus	Most often associated with aging
Polar	Anterior or posterior pole	Usually congenital
Posterior sub-capsular (PSC)	Just beneath the posterior capsule	More common than ASC Typically related to toxicity, disease, or aging changes Tend to advance rapidly
Pyramidal	Anterior polar opacity that actually protrudes forward into the anterior chamber	Usually congenital
Sutoral	Within the nucleus at the point where the ends of the individual lens fibers come together	Visual effect usually minimal

II. Classification by age of onset

Type	Onset	Notes
Congenital	Birth	Generally not progressive Usually visually insignificant If significant, surgery is indicated at an early age One-third are hereditary
Senile	Adult	Most common type of cataract Result of aging Usually bilateral Usually progresses slowly but is unpredictable *(continued)*

Table 6-1. (continued)

Classification of Cataracts

Type	Onset	Notes
Senile		"Second sight" results from a myopic shift

III. Classification of a senile cataract

Type	Characteristics	Notes
Incipient	Earliest visible lens changes Early brunescence or peripheral cortical opacities appear	Vision rarely affected
Immature	Progression of incipient changes Diffuse opacities Lens begins to swell	Lens may remain at this stage for a long period of time Early visual interference
Mature	Subcapsular, nuclear, and cortical opacities now involve the whole lens Lens continues to swell Intumescent: water content at maximum Brunescent: brown Nigrescent: black	Vision significantly affected
Hypermature	Dehydration and lens degradation is extreme Lens shrinks, capsule wrinkles	
Morganian	Lens nucleus is very dense and shrunken, and sinks down into liquified cortex	

IV. Classification by cause

Type	Cause	Notes
Complicated (secondary)	Associated with, or resulting from, other intraocular disease	Not to be confused with so-called "secondary cataract," which refers to capsular opacity in pseudophakia Usually present as PSCs Most commonly associated with uveitis

(continued)

Table 6-1. (continued)
Classification of Cataracts

Type	Cause	Notes
Metabolic	Systemic dysfunction or disease	Diabetes is the most common cause; also found in mytonic dystrophy, Marfan syndrome, Down syndrome
Toxic	Chemicals, poison, and therapeutic drugs	Corticosteroids (well-documented cause of PSC), miotics, amiodarone, gold Intraocular antibiotics
Traumatic	Result from disruption in lens physiology or architecture by external force	Usually due to penetration or concussion directly to the globe Also caused by radiation, ultraviolet or infrared light, extreme temperature, and electrical shock Cataract can advance very quickly, occurring immediately or within several days

- Cataract surgery may be combined with refractive, corneal transplant, or glaucoma surgical procedures.
- Pharmaceuticals commonly employed in cataract surgery include those that fight infection, reduce inflammation, and control intraocular pressure (IOP) (see Chapter 17).

Glaucoma

- The circulation of the aqueous generates the IOP.
- IOP is measured with a device called a tonometer (Table 6-2) (see also How To's: Calibrate Goldmann Tonometer through Schiotz Tonometry [Chapter 8]).
- Elevations of IOP may damage the optic nerve (Figure 6-1), causing visual field loss and producing the clinical condition of glaucoma.
- The specific patterns of field loss are so classically related to glaucoma that the disorder can practically be identified by the appearance of the visual field alone. Subtle field changes may sometimes be detected before any change in the cupping of the optic disc is seen.
- Early field defects in glaucoma appear as a nasal step. As further damage occurs, the step will extend and eventually connect to the blind spot in an arcuate pattern (Bjerrum's scotoma). Another common glaucomatous field

Table 6-2.
Measurement of IOP

I. Applanation

Method	Notes
Goldmann	The industry standard; accurate for high and low measurements Topical anesthetic and fluorescein dye are required Not portable Tip must be cleaned between patients
Noncontact	No anesthetic or dye is necessary A superb screening device Accuracy diminishes as the IOP increases
Perkins	Topical anesthetic and fluorescein dye are required Portable Takes considerable practice Tip must be cleaned between patients

II. Indentation

Method	Notes
Schiotz	Topical anesthetic is required Portable Must use weights that came with instrument Must be cleaned between patients Can be sterilized in the autoclave Repeat measurements can be less reliable Errors induced by scleral rigidity factors
Tactile	An estimate at best

III. Other

Method	Notes
Mackey-Marg	Combination of applanation and indentation methods Bulky but portable Uses disposable membrane-like tip covers Provides a printout of the reading Provides the most accurate readings on damaged corneas
Manometry	The only direct method of measuring IOP (a needle is inserted into the anterior chamber)
Tonography	Research device for measuring aqueous outflow Topical anesthetic is required

(continued)

Table 6-2. (continued)
Measurement of IOP

Method	Notes
Tonography	Electronic tonometer is placed on the eye for 4 minutes; the IOP is continuously recorded on a graph during the test time Used only in research settings
Tono-Pen XL (Intermedics Intraocular, Pasadena, Calif)	Combination of applanation and indentation methods Portable, completely hand-held, and easy to use Uses disposable membrane-like tip covers Most accurate in the normal ranges

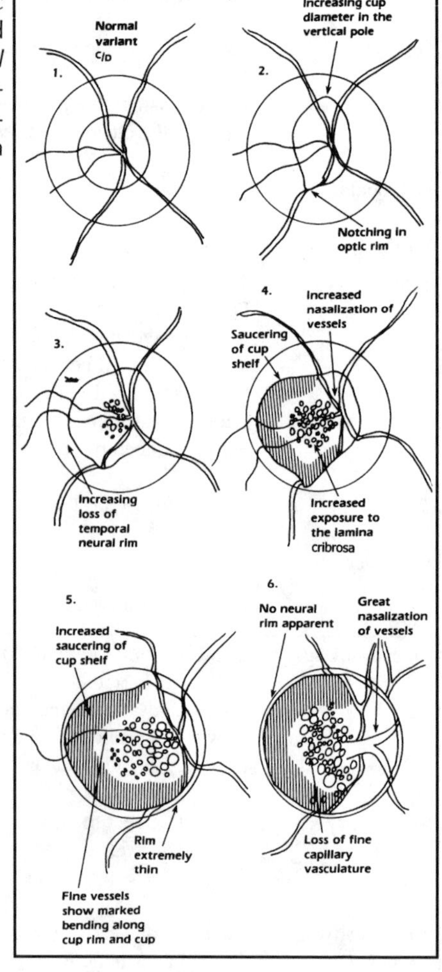

Figure 6-1. Progression of optic cupping in glaucoma (reprinted from Nemeth SC, Shea CA. *Medical Sciences for the Ophthalmic Assistant*. Thorofare, NJ: SLACK Incorporated; 1988, with permission from Sheila Nemeth).

Table 6-3.
Provocative Tests

Type	Scenario	Results
Dark room provocative test	Patient stays in a dark room for 1 hour with eyes open	If IOP rises from baseline measurement, angle closure may be occurring
Prone provocative test	Patient lies face-down for 45 minutes	If IOP rises from baseline measurement, angle closure may be occurring
Water provocative test	Patient drinks 2 to 4 quarts of water in 15 to 20 minutes	If IOP rises into high 20s or more, open-angle glaucoma probably exists

defect is a comma-shaped extension of the physiologic blind spot (Seidel's scotoma). These defects coincide with the pattern of damage that occurs along the optic nerve fibers.

- In certain cases, the physician may need to find out if the patient's eye(s) can be forced or *provoked* into having elevated IOP. There are several such provocative tests (Table 6-3).
- There are various types of glaucoma (Tables 6-4 and 6-5) with varying methods of treatment.

Table 6-4.

Types of Glaucoma

I. Primary open angle

Etiology	**Risk Factors**	**Symptoms**	**Treatment(s)**
Aqueous fails to drain out of a normal-looking angle	African ancestry > age 40 High myopia Positive family history	Onset: none Later: tunnel vision, blindness	Topical (see Tables 17-21 and 17-22) Oral Surgical: (see Table 18-5) laser trabeculoplasty trabeculectomy drainage implant cyclodestruction

II. Secondary open angle

Etiology	**Types**	**Treatment**
Caused by other ocular or systemic pathology (see Table 6-5 for causes)	Pigmentary Hemolytic Exfoliation Pseudoexfoliation Phacolytic Lens-induced Pupillary block Neovascular Inflammatory	Treatment is typically directed at the underlying cause Traditional glaucoma treatments are also used to lower the IOP

III. Angle closure

Etiology	**Risk Factors**	**Symptoms**	**Treatment**
Peripheral iris blocks access of aqueous humor to the trabecular meshwork	Hyperopia Nanophthalmos Swollen lens Plateau iris Mydriasis Trauma	Ciliary flush Pain Blurred vision Mid-dilated pupil with minimal or no reaction to light Steamy cornea Halos Elevated IOP	Emergency: drugs (hyperosmotics, aqueous suppressants, and miotics) Definitive: laser iridectomy

IV. Congenital

Cause	**Signs/Symptoms**	**Notes**
Isolated: Abnormal development of the trabecular meshwork not associated with other ocular anomalies or diseases	Tearing Photophobia Blepharospasm Buphthalmos	Surgical treatment is primary: goniotomy, trabeculotomy Treatment via medication, see Tables 17-21 and 17-22 *(continued)*

Table 6-4. (continued)
Types of Glaucoma

Cause	Signs/Symptoms	Notes
Other:		
Associated with other ocular anomalies or diseases	Same as above	Associated disorders include: aniridia, Marfan syndrome, congenital cataract, Sturge-Weber syndrome, neurofibramatosis, Down syndrome Treatment as above

Table 6-5.
Situations Associated With Secondary Glaucoma

Ocular	Systemic	Medicinal
Angle recession	Ankylosing spondylitis	Amphetamines
Aphakia	Asthma	Anticholingerics (atropine, belladonna)
Central retinal vein occlusion	Congenital rubella	Reserpine
Dislocated lens	Diabetes	Systemic steroids
Exfoliation syndrome	Emphysema	Topical corticosteroids
Flat anterior chamber	Leukemia	Tricyclic antidepressants (amitriptyline)
Hypermature cataract	Marfan syndrome	

Reprinted with permission from Duvall BS, Lens A, Werner EB. Cataract and Glaucoma for Eyecare Paraprofessionals. *Thorofare, NJ: SLACK Incorporated; 1999.*

Unless otherwise noted, all text, tables, and figures are adapted or reprinted with permission from Duvall BS, Lens A, Werner EB. Cataract and Glaucoma for Eyecare Paraprofessionals. *Thorofare, NJ: SLACK Incorporated; 1999.*

CHAPTER 7

Emergencies in Eyecare

Triage (Table 7-1)

- Triage is the screening of patients to determine the urgency of their situation.
- The purpose of triage is to ensure that patients with the most serious complaints are seen or referred promptly.
- Conditions may be rated as emergent (to be seen immediately), urgent (to be seen same or next day), or elective (or routine exam within 1 to 2 weeks).
- Each practice or clinic should set up specific protocols and procedures regarding triage.
- The anxiety of the patient also plays a key role in how soon he or she should be seen.

Table 7-1.
Triage

I. Emergent
   A. Emergent 1: treatment within minutes
      1. Chemical burns
      2. Sudden, painless loss of vision
      3. Penetrating injuries
   B. Emergent 2: treatment within hours
      1. Acute ocular trauma, including blunt trauma, especially if accompanied by visual loss or visual abnormality
      2. Foreign body (FB) or corneal abrasion caused by a foreign body
      3. Recent onset of eye pain with or without redness
      4. Recent onset of flashing lights or floaters
      5. Pain or redness with contact lens usage
      6. Monocular patients with ocular complaints
      7. Postoperative patients with ocular complaints

(continued)

Table 7-1. (continued)

Triage

II. Urgent: Seen the same or next day
- A. Recent onset of double vision
- B. Sudden onset of ptosis (droopy lid)
- C. Photophobia (light sensitivity)
- D. Distorted vision for less than 2 weeks
- E. Eye pain for more than 48 hours but less than 1 week
- F. Colored halos around lights

III. Elective/nonemergent: Seen within 1 to 2 weeks
- A. Gradual visual loss for more than 3 weeks
- B. Headaches not accompanied by other symptoms
- C. Eye itching, tearing, or discharge for more than 3 weeks
- D. Mild redness for more than 3 weeks not accompanied by other symptoms
- E. Masses on lids
- F. Broken glasses

Injuries and Emergencies of the Lids and Lacrimal System (Table 7-2)

Table 7-2.

Injuries and Emergencies of the Lids and Lacrimal System

Situation	Category	Notes
Chemical burns	Emergent 1	Irrigate for 20 minutes at the scene, another 20 minutes upon arrival at office; globe may be protected by blink reflex
Lid lacerations	Emergent 2	High risk of infection; lacrimal system may be involved; globe may be involved
Thermal burns	Emergent 2	Later swelling may prevent good exam; strong blink reflex generally protects the globe
Blunt trauma	Emergent 2	Risk of orbital fracture, anterior segment involvement, and retinal damage

(continued)

Table 7-2. (continued)
Injuries and Emergencies of the Lids and Lacrimal System

Situation	Category	Notes
Preseptal cellulitis	Urgent	Symptoms: swelling and infection of lid tissue; urgent to rule out orbital cellulitis
Entropion, ectropion, and trichiasis	Nonemergent	Patient discomfort may indicate need for same-day appointment
Eyelid tumors	Nonemergent	These are usually not painful; biopsy can be scheduled in 1 to 2 weeks
Hordeolum/chalazion	Nonemergent	Patient discomfort may indicate need for earlier appointment
Nasolacrimal duct obstruction	Nonemergent	Patient discomfort may indicate need for earlier appointment

Emergencies and Injuries of the Orbit (Table 7-3)

Table 7-3.
Emergencies and Injuries of the Orbit

Situation	Category	Notes
Blow-out fracture	Emergent 2	Caused by blunt trauma; IO and IR muscles may herniate into the sinus cavity, producing limited range of motion and diplopia
Intraorbital foreign body	Emergent 2	Often not immediately evident; combined with other trauma; type of FB determines eye's reaction: organic material carries high rate of intolerance and infection, copper is not tolerated, glass and plastic are generally inert
Orbital cellulitis	Emergent 2	Infection of orbital tissues; emergent because it can be life-threatening if infection spreads to brain

(continued)

Table 7-3. (continued)

Emergencies and Injuries of the Orbit

Situation	Category	Notes
Orbital cellulitis		Symptoms: swelling, redness, proptosis, pain, fever, headache, diplopia, restricted eye movement

Emergencies and Injuries of the Conjunctiva, Sclera, and Cornea (Table 7-4)

Table 7-4.

Emergencies and Injuries of the Conjunctiva, Sclera, and Cornea

Situation	Category	Notes
Chemical burn	Emergent 1	Irrigate for 20 minutes at the scene, another 20 minutes upon arrival at office Bases (alkalis) tend to penetrate the ocular tissues, and are more damaging than acids
Conjunctival laceration	Emergent 2	May be accompanied by subconjunctival hemorrhage (SCH), uveal prolapse Rule out intraocular foreign body
Corneal abrasion	Emergent 2	Symptoms: FB sensation to severe pain, redness, photophobia, tearing
Corneal graft rejection	Emergent 2	Can occur weeks to years after surgery Symptoms: redness, photophobia, decreased vision, pain
Corneal laceration	Emergent 2	May be partial or full thickness Rule out intraocular foreign body
Foreign body	Emergent 2	May become lodged on corneal or conjunctival surface Important to ascertain patient's activity at the time of injury

(continued)

Table 7-4. (continued)

Emergencies and Injuries of the Conjunctiva, Sclera, and Cornea

Situation	Category	Notes
Foreign body		Symptoms: FB sensation/pain, redness, tearing, photophobia, blurred vision Rule out intraocular foreign body
Thermal burn	Emergent 2	Cornea usually protected by the blink reflex
Episcleritis	Urgent	Inflammation of episclera Urgent because of association with scleritis Symptoms: sudden onset redness, photophobia, mild pain, purple nodules (when chronic)
Gonococcal conjunctivitis	Urgent	Severe infection, can lead to corneal ulceration, perforation, and blindness Symptoms: copious purulent discharge, chemosis, papillae
Keratitis	Urgent	Corneal inflammation, may result in corneal ulceration Causes include: viral, bacterial, or fungal organisms; chemical or physical injury; ultraviolet light exposure; contact lens-related Symptoms vary, but include: pain, redness, photophobia, tearing
Radiation burn	Urgent	Ultraviolet radiation damage usually associated with exposure to sunlight, sunlamps, or welding arcs Symptoms usually start 6 to 10 hours after exposure Symptoms: FB sensation to severe pain, redness, photophobia, decreased vision

(continued)

Table 7-4. (continued)

Emergencies and Injuries of the Conjunctiva, Sclera, and Cornea

Situation	Category	Notes
Recurrent corneal erosion	Urgent	Healing epithelium is continually stripped off May be associated with previous corneal insult Symptoms: FB sensation or pain on awakening, redness, photophobia, tearing
Scleritis	Urgent	Inflammation of sclera Can lead to scleral thinning, perforations, loss of vision, loss of eye Symptoms: gradual onset, severe deep pain, redness, photophobia, tearing, decreased vision, inflamed blood vessels
Viral conjunctivitis	Urgent	Urgent because it is highly contagious Symptoms: watery discharge, swollen lids, eye and lid redness, irritation, itching
Conjunctivitis	Nonemergent	While there may be some discomfort, usually the symptoms will come and go without medical treatment; gonococcal and viral forms require more immediate attention

Emergencies and Injuries of the Lens (Table 7-5)

Note: Once we move beyond the external eye, triage becomes more difficult because the injury may not be immediately apparent to the patient or caregiver. Thus, the categorization of emergent, urgent, and nonemergent are difficult to call. In many cases, these situations are accompanied by external trauma and can be triaged in that way.

Table 7-5.
Emergencies and Injuries of the Lens

Situation	Category	Notes
Subluxation	Dependent on cause; emergent 1 or 2 if associated with trauma	If caused by trauma, patient should be evaluated for other signs of ocular injury Treatment may include correction of new refractive error, lasering of the zonules, or lens extraction
Total dislocation	Dependent on cause; emergent 1 or 2 if associated with trauma	Dislocation into the anterior chamber may cause pupillary block and angle closure glaucoma, necessitating removal of the lens Dislocation into the vitreous often causes no secondary complication and may require no treatment
Traumatic cataract	Emergent 1 or 2 depending on type of trauma	Trauma is the most common cause of unilateral cataract May be caused by contusion, concussion, laceration, intraocular FB, or radiation

Emergencies and Injuries of the Uveal Tract (Table 7-6)

Table 7-6.
Emergencies and Injuries of the Uveal Tract

Situation	Category	Notes
Choroidal prolapse	Emergent 1	Prolapse of uveal material through a laceration in the sclera Symptoms: black-brown "ooze" on scleral surface, peaked pupil If uveal tissue is exposed to the atmosphere for more than 1 hour, the chances of developing sympathetic ophthalmia are greatly increased
Sympathetic ophthalmia	Emergent 2	Bilateral panuveitis where an uninjured eye "sympathizes" with its injured fellow Often occurs between 2 to 8 weeks of original injury, or within 1 year

(continued)

Table 7-6. (continued)

Emergencies and Injuries of the Uveal Tract

Situation	Category	Notes
Sympathetic ophthalmia		Trauma seems to be healing, but injured eye develops pain, photophobia, and decreased vision Uninjured eye then also develops pain, photophobia, and decreased vision Severe vision loss or blindness may result
Hyphema	Emergent 2 or urgent, depending on cause	Bleeding into the anterior chamber Usually a result of trauma May be accompanied by elevated IOP
Iritis	Urgent (unless there is trauma)	Inflammation of the iris Can be precipitated by trauma or systemic inflammatory processes Symptoms: pain, redness (limbal), tearing, photophobia Signs: constricted pupil, cells, and flare in anterior chamber See also Table 7-8
Uveitis	Urgent (unless there is trauma)	Inflammation of the posterior uvea Can be precipitated by trauma or systemic inflammatory processes Symptoms: pain, redness, blurred vision, photophobia If severe, may result in: synechiae, cataracts, macular edema, corneal edema, secondary glaucoma, retinal detachment

Emergencies and Injuries of the Vitreous and Retina (Table 7-7)

Table 7-7.
Emergencies and Injuries of the Vitreous and Retina

Situation	Category	Notes
Central retinal artery occlusion	Emergent 1	Cuts off blood supply to most of the retina; if restored within 30 minutes there is a chance of saving some vision Symptoms: sudden, painless, acute loss of vision
Central retinal vein occlusion	Emergent 2	Vision in area through which the vein passes is affected Symptoms may go unnoticed at first; vision may be lost in peripheral spots; central vision may be affected
Endophthalmitis	Emergent 2	Infection of vitreous and surrounding tissues Usually caused by bacteria, especially after penetration via trauma or surgery Can destroy the eye within days Symptoms: pain, redness, sudden onset of reduced vision
Intraocular foreign body	Emergent 2	Often not immediately evident; combined with other trauma Type of FB determines eye's reaction Organic material carries high rate of intolerance and infection, copper is not tolerated, glass and plastic are generally inert
Posterior vitreous detachment (PVD)	Emergent 2	Emergent 2 status is because the symptoms of PVD are the same as those for RD Symptoms: floaters and flashes
Retinal hemorrhage	Emergent 2	Symptoms: blurred or blocked vision Occurs in trauma, diabetes, wet macular degeneration, other

(continued)

Table 7-7. (continued)

Emergencies and Injuries of the Vitreous and Retina

Situation	Category	Notes
Retinal tears and detachments	Emergent 2	Symptoms: floaters, flashes, curtain over vision, loss of vision
Vitreous hemorrhage	Emergent 2	Symptoms: floaters, flashes, dark spots in vision, decreased vision Especially common in trauma and diabetics
Macular hole	Urgent	Urgent status if there is a sudden onset of central vision change Initially, patient may notice slight visual disturbances or decreased vision
Papilledema	Urgent	Swelling of the optic disc due to increased intracranial pressure Symptoms: transient vision loss and/or diplopia, headaches, nausea

The Red Eye (Table 7-8)

- The red eye is a pathological condition in which the blood vessels of the conjunctiva or ciliary body become dilated. This can signify a serious vision-threatening condition or a superficial transient irritation.
- Tissues of the lids, lacrimal systems, and orbit may also become red and inflamed due to pathological conditions.
- The most common causes of the red eye are irritation and infection. Other causes include allergic reaction, disease, and trauma.
- Eye redness with itching usually indicates allergy.
- Eye redness with an acute onset of a poking or sticking pain suggests the presence of a foreign body.
- Eye redness with deep, internal pain can signify glaucoma, uveitis, or scleritis.
- Eye redness with burning, irritation, and/or a gritty feeling suggests a superficial condition of the lids, conjunctiva, or cornea.

Table 7-8.

Red Eye Differential Diagnosis

	Conjunctivitis	**Iritis**	**Acute Angle-Closure Glaucoma**	**Keratitis, Corneal FB**
Vision	Normal to blurring that clears with blinking	Mild blurring	Considerable blurring or haziness; halos around lights	Mild blurring
Pain	None to minor discomfort, burning or grittiness	Moderate to aching	Severe aching	Sharp pain or FB sensation
Discharge	Dependent on type: Mucopurulent—bacterial Watery—viral Watery/stringy—allergic	None	None	None to mild
Pattern of redness	Palpebral conjunctiva and/or diffuse conjunctiva	Conjunctival circumcorneal pattern	Diffuse conjunctiva with prominent circumcorneal pattern	Conjunctival circumcorneal pattern
Pupils	Normal, reactive	Constricted—may be slightly reactive	Dilated, fixed	Normal to constricted, reactive
Cornea	Clear	Clear to slightly hazy	Hazy	Possible visible FB opacification, abnormal light reflex, fluorescein staining
IOP	Normal	Normal to low	High	Normal
Other		Photophobia	Possible nausea and vomiting	Possible photophobia

Reprinted with permission from Hargis-Greenshields L, Sims L. Emergencies in Eyecare. *Thorofare, NJ: SLACK Incorporated; 1999.*

First Aid and Office Emergencies

- Every employee should regularly update his or her basic first aid skills and cardiopulmonary resuscitation (CPR) certification.
- Every person working in the office, regardless of his or her position, needs to know where the crash cart is kept.
- Someone should be assigned the duty of checking the cart every month to make sure that all supplies are present, in good condition, and unexpired (Table 7-9).
- Everyone in the office needs to know the emergency response phone numbers, whether it be 911 for an external response team or an internal number for larger facilities who have their own emergency response teams.
- While all ocular emergencies must be treated by an MD, we need to be aware of what we should and should not do in the event of an ocular emergency.

How-To: Handle Ocular Emergencies

- Have the proper emergency supplies on hand and readily accessible.
- Have sterile (unopened) eye drops and ointments on hand for use when dealing with a traumatized eye (however, do not use until instructed to do so by the physician).
- Lightly patch the eye and get assistance if uncertain what to do. The exception to patching is a chemical splash or protruding foreign body.
- Continue the irrigation process for any chemical splash immediately upon the patient's arrival for a period of at least 20 minutes. (The patient should have started this process before coming to your office.)
- Tell the patient that the doctor will do everything possible to help him or her.
- Do not tell the patient that everything will be "all right."
- Do not put pressure on a traumatized eye.
- Do not instill eye medications unless instructed to do so by the physician.
- Do not use any ophthalmic instruments on a traumatized eye.

Cardiopulmonary Resuscitation

- CPR alone is not usually enough to save a life.
- Early activation of the EMS system is essential.
- The primary goal of CPR is to provide oxygen to the heart, brain, and other vital organs until advanced medical treatment can be applied.

Table 7-9.

The Office Crash Cart

I. Items for establishing an intravenous line
- IV needles
- IV tubing
- Tourniquets
- Alcohol wipes
- Tape
- Gauze
- Scissors
- IV solution bags, such as dextrose and saline

II. Items used for suction
- Suction tips
- Tubing
- Catheters
- Lubricating jelly
- Suction machine

III. Items used to restore respiration
- Oxygen masks
- Barrier masks
- Nasal cannulas
- Bite blocks
- Oxygen tank

IV. Miscellaneous items
- Blood pressure cuff
- Stethoscope
- Gloves
- Sharps container
- Various drugs such as epinephrine and Benadryl (Warner-Lambert, Morris Plains, NJ)
- Bottled eye wash
- Topical anesthetic
- Lid speculum
- Sterile cotton-tipped applicators

How-To: One-Rescuer CPR: Adult

- Establish unresponsiveness. Shake gently and shout, “Are you OK?”
- Activate EMS system—phone first.
- Position victim.
- Establish an airway.

(continued)

How-To: One-Rescuer CPR: Adult (continued)

- Assess breathing. Look, listen, and feel (3 to 5 seconds). If breathing, place victim in the recovery position and monitor breathing and pulse.

If not breathing:

- Give two slow, full breaths (1.5 to 2 seconds per breath).
- Assess pulse at the carotid artery (5 to 10 seconds).

If there is a pulse, continue rescue breathing at a rate of one breath every 5 seconds (approximately 12 breaths per minute).

If there is no pulse:

- Locate landmarks and position hands over lower half of the sternum.
- Begin chest compressions counting one-and-two-and-three-and... to establish a rhythm. The chest should be depressed 1.5 to 2 inches at a rate of 80 to 100 compressions per minute.
- Give 15 compressions.
- Give two ventilations.
- At the end of four cycles of 15 compressions and two ventilations, check for the return of a pulse.

If there is a pulse but no breathing, rescue breathe at a rate of one breath every 5 seconds.

If there is no pulse, resume CPR starting with two ventilations followed by chest compressions.

- Repeat the sequence of 15 compressions and two ventilations.
- Assess for pulse and return of breath every few minutes.

Entrance of Second Layperson Rescuer:

- The layperson is taught only the one-man CPR technique. If a second rescuer appears and is not identified as a health professional, he or she should:
  - Identify him- or herself.
  - Ask if EMS has been activated and call 911 if necessary.
  - Check for carotid pulse.

How-To: Two-Rescuer CPR (Healthcare Professionals Only): Adult

- Follow procedure for one-person CPR.
- Second person identifies him- or herself by stating "I know CPR, I can help."
- Ask if EMS system has been activated. If not, call 911.
- Take a position on the opposite side of the victim from the first rescuer.
- First rescuer discontinues compressions. Second rescuer palpates the carotid artery (5 seconds).

If there is no pulse, state "No pulse, resume CPR," and give a breath.

- First rescuer resumes compressions at a rate of 80 to 100 per minute, at a ratio of five compressions to one ventilation.
- Second rescuer ventilates every five compressions and palpates the carotid pulse during chest compressions to evaluate the effectiveness of the compressor.
- When the compressor tires, he or she should call for a switch during counting (switch-and-two-and-three-and…).
- Second rescuer finishes with a ventilation and moves to the chest to find hand positions.
- First rescuer moves to the head and checks for carotid pulse.

If there is no pulse, first rescuer states "No pulse, resume CPR," and gives a breath.

- Repeat compression/ventilation sequence until help arrives.

How-To: One-Rescuer CPR: Child (1 to 8 Years)

- Establish unresponsiveness. Shake gently and shout, "Are you OK?"
- Call out for help.
- Position the victim.
- Establish an airway using head tilt-chin lift method.
- Assess breathing. Look, listen, and feel.

If breathing, place the victim in the recovery position and monitor breathing and pulse.

If not breathing:

- Give two slow breaths, 1 to 1.5 seconds per breath.
- Assess pulse at the carotid artery.

(continued)

How-To: One-Rescuer CPR: Child (1 to 8 Years) (continued)

If there is a pulse, continue rescue breathing at a rate of one breath every 3 seconds and monitor the pulse.

If no pulse:

- Locate landmarks and position the heel of one hand over the lower sternum.
- Begin chest compressions at the rate of 80 to 100 compressions per minute and a ratio of five compressions to one ventilation.
- After 1 minute of CPR, phone fast for the EMS system (call 911).
- On returning to the victim, check the carotid pulse.

If there is a pulse, continue rescue breathing at a rate of one breath every 3 seconds and monitor the pulse.

If no pulse:

- Continue chest compressions and ventilation sequence.
- Check for the return of spontaneous breathing and pulse every few minutes until the EMS arrives.

How-To: One-Rescuer CPR: Infant (Less than 1 Year)

- Establish unresponsiveness. Shake gently and shout, "Are you OK?"
- Call out for help.
- Position the victim on his or her back on a firm surface (supporting the head and neck).
- Establish an airway using head tilt-chin lift method (take care not to hyperextend the neck).
- Assess breathing. Look, listen, and feel.

If breathing: place the victim in the recovery position, maintain an open airway, and monitor breathing and pulse.

If not breathing:

- Give two gentle breaths, covering the nose and mouth (1 to 1.5 seconds per breath).
- Assess pulse at the brachial artery inside the upper arm.

If there is a pulse, continue rescue breathing at a rate of one breath every 3 seconds and monitor the pulse.

(continued)

How-To: One-Rescuer CPR: Infant (Less than 1 Year) (continued)

If there is no pulse:

- Locate landmarks by placing two fingers one finger-width below the imaginary nipple line.
- Begin chest compressions at a depth of 0.5 to 1 inch per compression, at the rate of 80 to 100 compressions per minute and a ratio of five compressions to one ventilation.
- Do 20 cycles of compressions and ventilations (roughly 1 minute of CPR).
- After 1 minute of CPR, phone fast for the EMS system (call 911).
- Return to the victim and check the brachial pulse.

If there is a pulse, continue rescue breathing at a rate of one breath every 3 seconds and monitor the pulse.

If there is no pulse:

- Continue chest compressions and ventilations sequence.
- Check for the return of spontaneous breathing and pulse every few minutes until the EMS arrives.

Unless otherwise noted, all text, tables, and figures are adapted or reprinted with permission from Hargis-Greenshields L, Sims L. Emergencies in Eyecare. *Thorofare, NJ: SLACK Incorporated; 1999.*

CHAPTER 8

Basic Procedures

Evaluating the Patient

- Treat every patient with respect.
- Always protect the patient's privacy and preserve confidentiality.
- A complete and accurate history is the foundation of the examination (Tables 8-1 and 8-2).
- An examination strategy will streamline data collection and lessen test contamination (Table 8-3).

Table 8-1.
Patient History

Chief complaint
- Symptoms
- Onset
- Duration
- Cause (if known)
- Prior treatment
- Special tests and results
- Course of any prior episodes

Past ocular history
- Infections
- Injuries
- Surgery
- Treatment
- Contact lenses
  - Type
  - Wearing time
  - Cleaning regimen
  - Comfort, vision
  - Replacement schedule

(continued)

Table 8-1. (continued)

Patient History

- Family medical history (parents, siblings, children)
  - Ocular
    - Cataract
    - Glaucoma
    - High myopia
    - Strabismus
    - Retinal problems
    - Other
  - Major disorders
    - Hypertension
    - Diabetes
    - Heart disease
    - Cancer
    - Other
- Medications (see also Table 8-2)
  - Prescription drugs
    - Systemic
      - Oral
      - Injectable
      - Patches
      - Inhalants
    - Ocular (note name and dosage; with glaucoma medications, note time last used)
  - Over-the-counter
- Allergies/drug reactions
  - Medications
  - Contactants
  - Food
  - Environmental
- Interim history (on return visits)
  - Improvement
  - Treatment verification
  - New problems
  - Changes in medications
  - Changes in general health

Table 8-2.
Common Prescription Abbreviations

q	every
qd	once daily
bid	twice daily (every 12 hours)
tid	three times daily (every 8 hours)
qid	four times daily (every 6 hours)
h	hour
q 2h	every 2 hours
hs	bedtime (hour of sleep)
soln	solution (drops)
ung	ointment
gtt	drop
mg	milligram
mL	milliliter

Reprinted with permission from DuBois L. Basic Procedures. *Thorofare, NJ: SLACK Incorporated; 1998.*

Table 8-3.
Exam Strategy

A. Update medical record

B. History (see Table 8-1)

C. Routine eye exam:
- Visual acuity (with and without correction, each eye individually plus both eyes together as per office protocol; pinhole as indicated)
  - Distance
  - Near
- Lensometry
- Assessment of refractive error
  - Keratometry
  - Retinoscopy
  - Refractometry
- Pupil function
- Ocular motility
- Miscellaneous tests as needed (color vision, etc)
- Slit lamp exam
- Measurement of IOP
- Dilation
- Retinal exam

D. Suspected binocular function problems:
- Fusion
  - Stereo tests
  - Worth four-dot test (W4D)
  - Haploscopic devices (synoptophore/troposcope)

(continued)

Table 8-3. (continued)

Exam Strategy

Alignment

Control: cover/uncover (or single cover test)

Direction: cross cover test

Size: prism measurements (prism and cover; see also How-To: Prism and Cover Measurements, Chapter 12).

Visual acuity; remainder of exam proceeds as in C above

Notes—Avoiding examination contamination:

- All binocular tests must be performed before the patient undergoes tests requiring covering one eye or removing glasses.
- All tests of visual function, refractometry, and pupil function must be performed before the patient's pupils are dilated.
- Corneal sensation and reflex tearing must be tested before an anesthetic drop is placed in the eye.
- All tests of visual function and refractometry must be performed before contact tonometry or other corneal contact tests.
- Evaluating the surface of the cornea (keratometry, topography, etc) should be done before contact tonometry or other corneal contact tests.

Visual Acuity

Visual acuity is tested at every visit. Some tests give better data than others (Table 8-4 A). If the eyechart cannot be read, move to other tests (Table 8-4 B). Choose tests and targets appropriate for the patient's ability (Table 8-4 C).

How-To: Visual Acuity

Distance Vision:

- Distance testing is performed in dim illumination so that the pupil is not stimulated to constrict (which increases the depth of focus and artificially improves the acuity).
- Occlude one eye. (By convention, the right eye is usually tested first.) Be sure that occlusion is complete and that the patient is not peeking.
- Show the patient whole lines of letters, not isolated letters. (This is especially significant when testing children, because those with amblyopia are better able to identify single letters and end letters of a line than letters bound on two sides by other letters. This is called the crowding phenomenon.)
- Record the last full line read correctly, plus the number of figures read correctly on the next line (Example: 20/40 +3). Also note if the test was done with or without correction.

(continued)

How-To: Visual Acuity (continued)

- The test is sometimes performed binocularly as well.

Near Vision:

- Near vision is measured at a standard distance of 14 inches. This test is done in bright illumination.
- If the test is to be done with correction and it is appropriate, have the patient use his or her reading glasses or bifocals.
- Fully occlude one eye.
- Record the last full line read correctly plus the number of figures read correctly on the next line. Also note if the test was done with or without correction.
- With very young children, the examiner can present uniform small objects and record the size of the object that the child can see well enough to pick up ("picks up 3 mm object").
- The test is sometimes performed binocularly as well.

Table 8-4.

Vision Testing

A. Vision tests from most to least sophisticated

1. Snellen letters
2. Snellen numbers
3. Lea symbols matching test
4. HOTV matching test
5. Tumbling E
6. Allen pictures (held together)
7. Teller acuity cards
8. Fix and follow
9. Central steady maintained

B. Vision test progression (if patient is unable to perform first test, move to second, etc)

1. Optotype chart (see A, above)
2. Move patient closer to chart; be sure to record new test distance
3. Count fingers (give farthest distance at which patient can accurately identify)
4. Hand motions (give farthest distance at which patient can accurately identify)
5. Light projection (patient must be able to discern direction from which light is projecting; ie, right, left, upper, lower)
6. Light perception (simple discernment that light is on or off)
7. No light perception (even to noxious light; ie, indirect ophthalmoscope at full blast)

(continued)

Table 8-4. (continued)
Vision Testing

C. Vision tests for illiterates
1. Numbers (many illiterates know numbers)
2. Landolt rings
3. Pictures and geometric shapes
4. Tumbling E

- If vision improves with the use of a pinhole, there may be some amount of uncorrected refractive error present. If the pinhole does not improve the patient's acuity, then some nonrefractive problem such as macular degeneration may be responsible for the decreased vision.
- There are two categories of factitious visual loss: malingering and hysterical. The malingering patient deliberately feigns visual loss for some kind of personal or financial gain such as monetary compensation or to get attention. Hysterical visual loss usually results from emotional distress.
- Suspicious situations that suggest factitious vision loss:

  Findings do not add up:

  "Poor vision" with perfect stereopsis

  "Inability" to see color plates

  No improvement with pinhole (in absence of pathology)

  Mobility and activity do not match claim of poor vision

  Potential gain:

  Pending litigation

  Worker's compensation

How-To: Factitious Visual Loss

Evaluating the Suspected Malingerer:

- Start with small letters on the eye chart and work your way **UP**; patient may tire and begin seeing letters on a level that was previously denied.
- Check stereo acuity. Perfect stereopsis cannot exist unless both eyes can see.
- Perform Polaroid vectograph or other instrument that presents different optotypes to each eye. If patient identifies all letters, vision is present in both eyes. (Note: patient must keep both eyes open to avoid detecting the "trick.")
- W4D is useful when patient is claiming **no** vision in one eye. While it does not give a level of acuity, if patient identifies all the lights, then vision is present in both eyes. (Note: patient must keep both eyes open to avoid detecting the "trick.")

(continued)

How-To: Factitious Visual Loss (continued)

- Use the phoropter. Open both apertures and put +3.00 in front of the "good" eye, nothing in front of the "low vision" eye. Ask patient to read letters on the distant chart. Since the "good" eye is fogged, vision is possible only through the "bad" eye. (Note: patient must keep both eyes open to avoid detecting the "trick.")
- Have the patient slowly read a small line of numbers on a near card with both eyes open and introduce a 4 diopter prism base-out in front of one eye, then the other. Watch the patient's eyes; a seeing eye behind the prism will shift in to fuse with the other eye. If both eyes do this, it indicates both eyes see the small numbers equally well.
- Use the optokinetic nystagmus (OKN) drum. Turn the drum slowly in front of the patient's eyes; a seeing eye automatically follows the stripes on the drum. While the patient is watching the turning drum, alternately cover the patient's eyes. If one eye truly cannot see, it will stop moving. The size of the stripes or figures on the drum will indicate the level of vision.
- Use the optokinetic tape. Have the patient cover the "good" eye. Without warning, suddenly present the tape and move it left to right, right to left. A seeing eye will automatically follow the stripes on the tape. (Obviously this does not quantify vision, it merely shows that it exists.)
- In a child with little or no refractive error and unexplained poor vision, see if a –0.12 trial lens will "magically" improve the patient's vision.

Evaluating Hysteria:

- Confrontation or tangent screen fields show a tubular or spiral result in hysteria. Test is first performed at standard distance. Test distance is then doubled. In a true visual field loss, the defect will enlarge with the decreased distance. In hysteria, it often remains the same size as the original test.

Keratometry

- Keratometry measures only the central 3 mm of the cornea.
- Corneal epithelial irregularities may render the mires unfocusable.
- When the surface of the cornea has been altered (as in refractive surgery), the keratometry readings are no longer accurate.

How-To: Keratometry

- Focus the eyepiece before beginning the measurement. Use the occluder or a blank piece of paper as a "screen" in front of the barrel. Turn the eyepiece to the most plus position. Looking through the eyepiece, slowly turn it toward the minus just until the targets are clear. Stop.
- Wipe patient contact areas with alcohol. Make sure the patient is comfortable while positioned at the instrument.
- The patient should be instructed to look at the target in the instrument, at the center of the circle, or at the reflection of his or her own eye at all times. If the patient's vision is extremely poor, or if he or she does not seem to understand where to look, a penlight can be shown through the eyepiece. (This cannot be done during the reading, but it will give the patient an idea of where to fixate.) The patient should also be reminded to blink normally throughout the test, as this helps keep the corneal surface smooth. A drop of artificial tears may be needed if the cornea is dry, but the eyes should be gently blotted before taking the reading.
- Align the barrel so the target is visible on the right eye. You should be able to see the three mires. If they are blurred or doubled, use the focusing knob or joystick to move the barrel until they are single and in sharp focus. Finer adjustments of the barrel position should place the cross hairs in the center of the lower right circle. Keep the mires centered and focused at all times.
- If the three circles are not completely separated from each other, turn the horizontal dial on the left and the vertical dial on the right to move the circles apart. Loosely lock the instrument to avoid accidentally misaligning it during the measurement.
- To begin the measurement, rotate the keratometer barrel either clockwise or counterclockwise to align the crosses of the two lower circles so that they are exactly opposite each other. The left horizontal dial is then turned so that the crosses are moved toward each other until they are superimposed and appear to be a single cross connecting the two circles.
- Next, turn the right vertical dial to superimpose the dashes between the upper and lower circles on the right so that it appears to be a single dash. During both of these maneuvers, the mires must be kept centered on the patient's cornea and sharply focused.
- Once the crosses and dashes have been superimposed, the measurements can be read directly from the instrument. The numbers indicated on the horizontal and vertical dials are recorded in diopters, and the two axes corresponding to the two dioptric powers may be read from the axis dial.

(continued)

How-To: Keratometry (continued)

- By convention, the lower number, corresponding to the flattest corneal meridian, and its axis are written first.

  Example: OD 42.25 x 175 / 43.50 x 85
- There is a shorthand version of this reading that leaves out the axis of the flatter meridian, making the assumption that the two readings will always be 90 degrees apart.

  Example : OD 42.25 / 43.50 x 85
- Make a note regarding the quality of the mires and patient cooperation.

Informal Visual Fields

- Informal visual fields (confrontation and Amsler grid) are screening tests for visual system problems.
- Defects that respect the vertical or horizontal meridian should be further investigated with formal visual fields (see Chapter 11).
- The Amsler grid is a near test designed to evaluate the central 20 degrees of the visual field.

How-To: Confrontation Fields

Static Testing:

- Sit directly in front of the patient, 2 or 3 feet apart (about an arm's length), with your eyes on the same level.
- Ask the patient to cover his or her left eye with the palm of the hand, being sure not to apply pressure to the eye.
- Close your right eye and instruct the patient to look only at your open eye at all times. (In this way, the assistant's normal field of vision corresponds to the patient's and serves as the comparison for the test.)
- Present one to four fingers in each of the four quadrants of the visual field and ask the patient to report the number of fingers being shown without looking directly at them. The fingers are presented midway between the patient and the assistant so each can see the targets equally well.
- The test is performed separately on each eye.
- This gross static test (ie, the fingers do not move once presented) can detect differences in the visual field from side to side (hemianopias) and above and below (altitudinal or arcuate).
- Record the visual field from the patient's point of view.

(continued)

How-To: Confrontation Fields (continued)

Kinetic Testing:

- Sit directly in front of the patient, 2 or 3 feet apart (about an arm's length), with your eyes on the same level.
- Ask the patient to cover his or her left eye with the palm of the hand, being sure not to apply pressure to the eye.
- Close your right eye and instruct the patient to look only at your open eye at all times. (In this way, the assistant's normal field of vision corresponds to the patient's and serves as the comparison for the test.)
- Move your fingers from the far periphery toward the center in each quadrant. Except for the inferotemporal quadrant, the fingers should not be immediately visible. The patient is instructed to report when the fingers first come into view.
- If the patient's visual field is normal, this point will be about the same time as the examiner sees the fingers.
- Kinetic visual field testing (a moving target) can establish gross peripheral boundaries, the size of large blind spots, or respect for the vertical or horizontal meridians.

Variations:

- Present fingers in two quadrants at once and ask the patient to count the total number seen. If the targets are presented on either side of the vertical midline and the patient sees only the fingers on one side, this suggests hemianopic loss on the other side. Similarly, fingers seen only below the horizontal midline when they are presented both above and below suggests a superior altitudinal defect. This method may be more sensitive for discovering hemianopias or altitudinal defects.
- Use a brightly colored object, such as a red-topped eyedrop bottle, as the target. Ask the patient if the color differs when the red top is shown on one side versus the other. Differences in actual color or brightness in one area of the visual field demonstrates loss of at least some of the normal perception of that color. This method may be better for detecting differences in sensitivity.

How-To: Amsler Grid

- The patient should wear his or her near correction and hold the grid at 14 inches. Cover one eye.
- Tell the patient to look at the central dot and to continue to do so even when asked about other parts of the grid.
- Ask the patient:
  a. Do you see the central dot?
  b. As you look at the central dot, are you aware of all four corners?
  c. Are all the lines straight and square?
  d. Are there any gaps or blank areas on the grid?
- Repeat with the other eye.
- If the patient gives answers indicating abnormalities, have him or her sketch or circle the distorted area(s) directly on the grid. Be sure to label the grid with patient name, date, and eye.

The Pupil Evaluation (Tables 8-5 and 8-6)

- Check pupils on every new patient and patients with recent visual loss.
- Test response prior to instillation of any eye drops.
- Unusual pupil function can also be observed with the slit lamp.

How-To: Pupil Evaluation

General Notes:

- Use a bright light.
- Dim the room lights.
- Patient fixates on distant target.

Procedure for Direct Light Response:

- Shine light into eye, slightly off center. That pupil should constrict.
- Record as an estimate of briskness on a scale of 1 to 4.

Procedure for Consensual Response:

- Shine light into eye, slightly off center. The fellow pupil should constrict.
- When light source is removed, both pupils should dilate.

Swinging Flashlight Test to Evaluate for Relative Afferent Pupillary Defect (RAPD) or Marcus Gunn Pupil:

- The light is presented to one eye, and its direct response is noted.

(continued)

How-To: Pupil Evaluation (continued)

- The light is quickly moved across the bridge of the nose to the other eye. There should be little or no constriction of the second pupil because it is already consensually constricted. However, the second pupil may dilate or constrict relative to the first pupil under the following conditions:

    a. If the first pupil constricts little or not at all and the second pupil-constricts to direct stimulation, then there is an afferent problem in the first eye. With the second eye constricted to the light stimulus, the first eye's pupil should now be consensually constricted.

    b. If the first pupil constricts fully and the second pupil dilates to direct stimulation, then the second eye has a RAPD and has been constricted consensually. The first pupil will now be relatively dilated in consensual response with the defective pupil.

- Note: This RAPD is demonstrated by moving the light source rapidly back and forth between the two eyes and noting each pupil's response relative to the other. The pupil that dilates with direct stimulation has an afferent defect relative to the other pupil. Both pupils may have an afferent problem, but they are usually asymmetric, and a RAPD can be elicited in the inferior eye.

Evaluating Near Response:

- Because there is only one instance where the light response and near response differ (Argyll Robertson pupil, see Table 8-6), it is not necessary to test the near reaction if the light reaction is intact.
- Patient begins by looking at distant target. Hold a near target about 12 inches from the bridge of the patient's nose, a bit below the line of vision.
- Watching the pupils, ask the patient to shift focus from the distant target to the close one. The pupils should constrict briskly.
- If using the penlight as a near target, normal pupils should remain at least as small as they were under direct light stimulation.

Table 8-5.
Pupil Evaluation

Indications
New patients
Patients with recent vision loss
Elements
Size
In dim illumination, the average pupil diameter is 3 or 4 mm *(continued)*

Table 8-5. (continued)

Pupil Evaluation

Pupils smaller than 2 mm are miotic
Pupils larger than 6 mm are mydriatic
Pupils should be equal in size
Anisocoria (unequal pupil size)

- Difference should be further evaluated in both dark and bright room illumination
- If difference is greater in dark illumination, then it is likely that the dilator muscle of the eye with the smaller pupil is not working properly
- If difference is greater in light illumination, the sphincter muscle of the larger pupil is probably at fault
- If one pupil remains the same size in light and dark conditions, the iris muscles themselves may have been affected by trauma or drugs
- When one or both pupils are fully dilated and nonreactive (blown pupils), consider this an emergency after ascertaining that drugs or previous injury are not the cause

Shape
Both pupils should be round
The pupils are normally centered or a little nasal in the iris

Direct light response
When exposed to a light source, the pupil should constrict briskly

Consensual light response
The consensual response is the simultaneous and equal response of one pupil when the other pupil is being stimulated by direct illumination or a near target

Near response (if the light reaction is abnormal)
When shifting focus from a distant target to the near one, the pupils should constrict briskly

Table 8-6.

Characteristics of Pupillary Disorders

	Size	Shape	Light Rx	Consensual	Near Rx
Afferent					
Marcus Gunn	Normal	Normal	Dilation	Normal	Normal
Efferent					
A. Parasympathetic					
III nerve palsy	Widely dilated	Normal	None	None	None
Adie's pupil	Dilated	Irregular	Slow	Slow	Gradual/slow
Argyll Robertson pupil	Miotic	Irregular	None	None	Normal
B. Sympathetic					
Horner's syndrome	Miotic	Normal	Normal	Normal	Normal

(continued)

Table 8-6. (continued)
Characteristics of Pupillary Disorders

	Size	Shape	Light Rx	Consensual	Near Rx
Other					
Physiologic anisocoria	Unequal	Normal	Normal	Normal	Normal
Fixed pupil (amaurotic)	Dilated	Round/oval	None	None	None

Reprinted with permission from DuBois L. Basic Procedures. *Thorofare, NJ: SLACK Incorporated; 1998.*

Near Point of Accommodation (NPA)

NPA is a monocular test of the eye's ability to maintain clear focus on a near object. It is defined as the closest point that a target is seen clearly and represents the maximum accommodation that the eye can naturally exert. Because accommodation is a function of the performance of the ciliary muscle coupled with the elasticity of the lens itself, the NPA and accommodative reserve diminish with age (Table 8-7).

How-To: Near Point of Accommodation

- The patient must be wearing his or her full distance correction; the bifocal should not be used.
- Instruct the patient to cover one eye and look at an accommodative target (no larger than 20/40 size on a near card). Move the target slowly toward the patient's open eye until the patient reports that the target is no longer clear. This point is the NPA and is measured from the cornea to the target at the blur point.
- The NPA may be recorded in centimeters or diopters. The Prince rule, a bar ruler often attached to the front of the phoropter, has both metric and dioptric markings.
- Occasionally, accommodation may be so low that the NPA is too remote for the patient to be able to distinguish the target. In this instance, place a plus lens over the distance correction that is just strong enough to make the target clear at arm's length. The NPA is measured in the same manner as previously described, but the amount of the added plus lens must then be subtracted from the final dioptric NPA.

Notes:

- The NPA should be about the same for each eye, assuming that the natural lens is present in both eyes.

(continued)

How-To: Near Point of Accommodation (continued)

- If the NPA is significantly unequal, recheck the distance correction for an undiscovered refractive error in one eye.
- An eye that has undergone cataract extraction (whether pseudophakic or aphakic) has no accommodative ability.
- The NPA is no longer obtainable once the pupils have been dilated.

Table 8-7.
Normal Accommodative Decline with Age

Age	5	10	15	20	25	30	35	40	45	50	60
NPA (D)	16	14	12	10	8.5	7	5.5	4.5	4	2.5	1

Reprinted with permission from DuBois L. Basic Procedures. *Thorofare, NJ: SLACK Incorporated; 1998.*

Near Point of Convergence (NPC)

The eyes are essentially parallel when viewing a distant object. In order to maintain the image of a near object on both foveas, the eyes must converge (ie, move toward the midline). The nearer the object, the more convergence must be exerted to maintain single vision. The closest point at which the eyes can maintain single vision by exerting maximum convergence is called the NPC. In young people, the NPC may be as close as the nose, but as with accommodation, the point becomes more remote with age (although not to the same extent).

How-To: Near Point of Convergence

- The patient should keep both eyes open and use distance correction (not bifocal or reading glasses). Instruct the patient to maintain fixation on the target.
- Slowly move the target toward the bridge of the patient's nose. The patient is to report first when the target becomes blurred (the endpoint of accommodative convergence), and then when the target becomes double.
- The nearest point where the target is still single, the NPC, is measured in centimeters.
- Sometimes patients will not be able to appreciate double vision or cannot distinguish between a blurred image and a double image. In this case, observe the patient's eyes throughout the test. The eyes will move toward each other. As the eyes reach and then exceed maximum convergence, one eye will drift outward. This point is a reasonable objective estimation of the NPC.

(continued)

How-To: Near Point of Convergence (continued)

Notes:

- The normal value for children is 5 to 10 cm, but adults may have an NPC more remote than 10 cm.
- In some patients with convergence insufficiency, the NPC may exceed 25 cm.
- Insufficient convergence is frequently seen in young adults whose reading or other near vision demands suddenly increase.
- A remote NPC and/or insufficient convergence reserves may lead to asthenopic symptoms. Convergence exercises, prescribed and monitored by an eyecare professional, are generally highly effective in improving convergence function and relieving symptoms.

Tonometry

- Tonometry measures intraocular pressure (IOP) in millimeters of mercury.
- Measurement of IOP is vital in diagnosing and monitoring glaucoma (see Chapter 6).
- Repeat any readings that seem unusual.
- Wash hands before and after touching the patient.

How-To: Calibrate Goldmann Tonometer

- Insert the attachment piece into the calibration port above the dial on the right side, and position the bar so that the middle etched line is aligned with the attachment calibration line. At each calibration point, the tonometer head should rock back and forth within ±1 mm Hg of that point.
- Rotate the dial to the zero mark. As the dial nears the zero mark, the tonometer head will tilt slightly. Rotating the dial slightly away from zero will cause the head to move back.
- Set the calibration bar to the next line, and rotate the dial to the 2 gm (20 mm Hg) mark, again causing movement of the tonometer head.
- Set the bar at the end line, and rotate the dial to 6 gm (60 mm Hg).
- If the tonometer head does not respond properly, the whole unit must be sent to the manufacturer for recalibration.

How-To: Goldmann Tonometry

- Make sure the tonometer is calibrated (How-To: Calibrate Goldmann Tonometer) and disinfected. (The head can be soaked in 3% hydrogen peroxide or a 1:10 dilution of household bleach for 10 minutes, then rinsed thoroughly with water and blotted dry.)
- Wipe areas of patient contact on the slit lamp with alcohol.
- Instill fluorescein/topical anesthetic. Position the patient at the slit lamp. He or she should be comfortable and not straining. Loosen tight collars.
- Rotate the cobalt filter into place. Open the slit beam to its widest point. Use the lowest magnification. The light source should be at about 60 degrees. Move the tonometer into place.
- Ask the patient to open wide and look straight ahead, or at a fixation target.
- Move the tonometer forward until contact is made.
- Observe the mires through the ocular. Manipulate until mires are positioned centrally, pulling slightly off the cornea during these adjustments.
- Rotate the measuring drum until the mires are positioned properly, with the inside edge of each circle just touching (Figure 8-1).
- Record the measurement by multiplying the visible number by 10 (ie, 2 = 20). Each line represents 2.

How-To: Clean and Calibrate Schiotz Tonometer

Cleaning:

- Disassemble the instrument by removing the weight at the top of the plunger—it snaps or screws off—and allow the plunger to fall into the hand or onto a tissue.
- Clean the cylinder with a pipe cleaner soaked in alcohol. Wipe the footplate with alcohol.
- Set the instrument aside to dry thoroughly, because any alcohol remaining on the instrument will damage the corneal epithelium.
- Clean the plunger with alcohol and set aside on a sterile pad to dry thoroughly. Do not touch the footplate or plunger with bare hands once they have been cleaned.
- Once dry, reassemble the instrument in reverse order, placing the notched end of the plunger into the cylinder and reattaching the weight to hold it in place.

(continued)

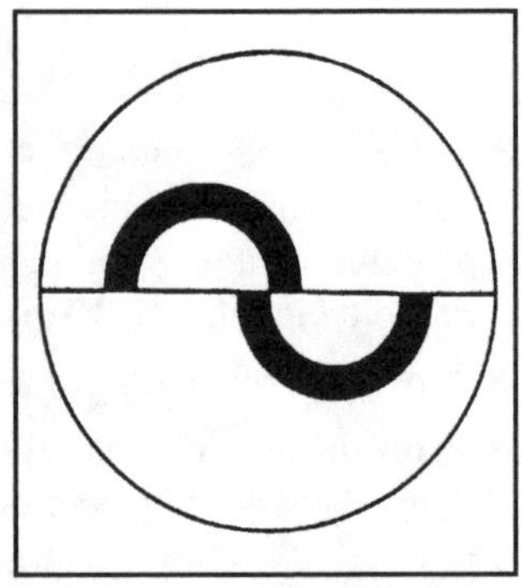

Figure 8-1. The proper position of the mires for taking an IOP reading with the Goldmann tonometer (reprinted with permission from Duvall BS, Lens A, Werner EB. *Cataract and Glaucoma for Eyecare Paraprofessionals*. Thorofare, NJ: SLACK Incorporated; 1999).

How-To: Clean and Calibrate Schiotz Tonometer (continued)

- Sterile caps that are discarded after each patient may be used to cover the footplate. If these caps are used, the instrument does not have to be cleaned between each patient but should be cleaned at the beginning of each day.
- The instrument is made entirely of metal, so it can also withstand steam sterilization and noncorrosive chemical disinfection.

Calibrating:

- Wipe the test plate clean before each use.
- Rest the tonometer perpendicularly on the test block. The needle should indicate zero on the left end of the scale.
- If it does not register zero, a small screw at the base of the needle can be loosened to rezero the needle. The needle itself should be perfectly straight because bending it will give a false reading.

How-To: Schiotz Tonometry

- Make sure the instrument is disinfected and calibrated. At this point the standard 5.5 weight should be on the instrument. (Use only the weights provided with that particular instrument.)
- Recline the patient. Instill topical anesthetic.
- Instruct the patient to look straight up or at a fixation target.
- Hold the tonometer in the right hand by the two curved arms attached to the side of the cylinder. Turn the scale mount so that the scale is facing you.
- Use the left hand to gently hold the lids of the patient's right eye apart, anchoring them against the orbital rim so that no pressure is applied to the globe. The hand holding the tonometer can rest on the patient's cheek or forehead for stabiiity.

(continued)

How-To: Schiotz Tonometry (continued)

- Gently lower the tonometer onto the eye so that the footplate rests on the central cornea and the instrument is perpendicular.
- Lower the cylinder slightly, so that the tonometer is resting on the eye and you are providing only lateral support. The cylinder should neither lift up nor press down on the footplate at this point.
- Looking straight at the scale, note the needle position. Remove the instrument from the eye.
- The scale readings do not indicate IOP in mm Hg, but must be converted according to a table provided with the instrument. The scale readings are inversely proportional to the IOP; lower numbers indicate higher pressures.

Ocular Motility

- Range of motion (ROM) testing evaluates all six muscles of each eye.
- The eyes should also be evaluated for the presence of a manifest (obvious) or latent (hidden) deviation.
- A manifest deviation is called a tropia and is observable at all times. Tropias are categorized according to the position of the deviated (nonfixing) eye: an in-turned eye is esotropic, an eye deviated out is exotropic, and when one eye is higher than the other, it is termed hypertropic. The classifications and their notations are listed in Table 8-8.
- A latent deviation is called a phoria and is observable only during testing. They are also classified as per Table 8-8.
- The cover-uncover test will detect the presence of a phoria or a tropia, depending on which eye is being observed.
- The alternate cover (cross-cover) test does not distinguish between a phoria and a tropia, but does bring out the maximum deviation.
- Sometimes a deviation is consistently observable only temporarily, such as when fusion has been broken and recovery is difficult. In this instance, the tropia is designated as intermittent.
- The site of a deviation is best measured with prisms (see How-To in Chapter 12), but it can also be estimated with the Hirschberg or Krimsky tests.

How-To: Range of Motion

- Use a near target. A muscle light is good, because you can evaluate the pupillary reflexes at the same time.
- While the patient holds his or her head stationary facing you, direct the patient to follow the target with the eyes only. *(continued)*

How-To: Range of Motion (continued)

- As the patient's eyes reach each of the positions shown in Figure 8-2, evaluate whether the two eyes' rotation to that position has been symmetrical and whether each eye moves to the full extent of each position.
- If the two eyes' ROM is equally full, the test is complete. Document that the ROM is normal.
- If one eye has failed to complete a full rotation in any direction, the opposite eye should be covered, and the weak eye should be moved to the fullest possible extent in the direction of the weakness.
- The weakness is recorded on a scale of 0 (no weakness/full range of motion) to -4 (maximum weakness/no movement) for each of the six cardinal positions of gaze as compared to the rotations of the normal eye.

Table 8-8.
Classification of Common Ocular Deviations

Deviation of Eye	Classification	Notation
In	Esotropia/esophoria	ET/E
Out	Exotropia/exophoria	EX/X
Up	Hypertropia/hyperphoria	HT/H
Down	Hypotropia	hT

Reprinted with permission from DuBois L. Basic Procedures. *Thorofare, NJ: SLACK Incorporated;1998.*

How-To: Hirschberg and Krimsky Measurements

Hirschberg:

- Direct the patient to look at the muscle light.
- Note where the reflexes fall. Normal corneal reflexes may not be centered in the pupil but may appear decentered nasally.
- If the corneal light reflex in one eye is shifted, a manifest deviation is present. The amount of deviation can be estimated by the Hirschberg method: 1 mm of deviation from the symmetric position is equal to about 15 prism diopters of tropia (Figure 8-3).

Krimskey:

- Direct the patient to look at the muscle light.
- Select a prism based on the Hirschberg estimates.

(continued)

How-To: Hirschberg and Krimsky Measurements (continued)

- Hold the prism over the patient's preferred eye with the *apex* pointing in the direction of the eye's deviation (**not** in the direction of the light's displacement). If neither eye seems to be preferred, then the prism may be held over either eye.
- Observe the position of the reflexes now. Add or subtract prism power until the reflexes fall on the normal position.

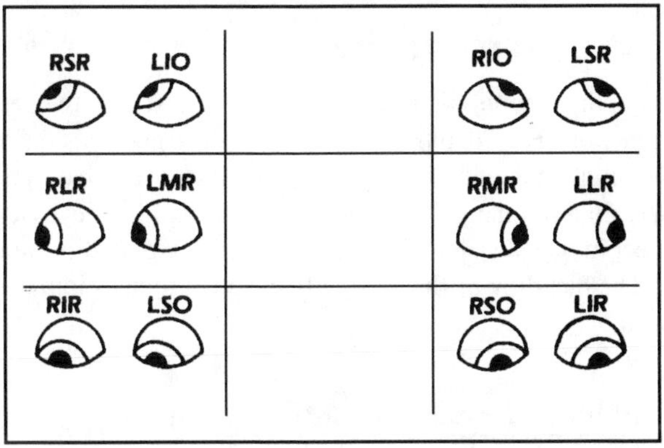

RSR LIO RIO LSR
RLR LMR RMR LLR
RIR LSO RSO LIR

Figure 8-2. Pairs of yoke muscles responsible for moving eyes into various positions of gaze (reprinted with permission from Hansen VC. *A Systematic Approach to Strabismus*. Thorofare, NJ: SLACK Incorporated; 1998).

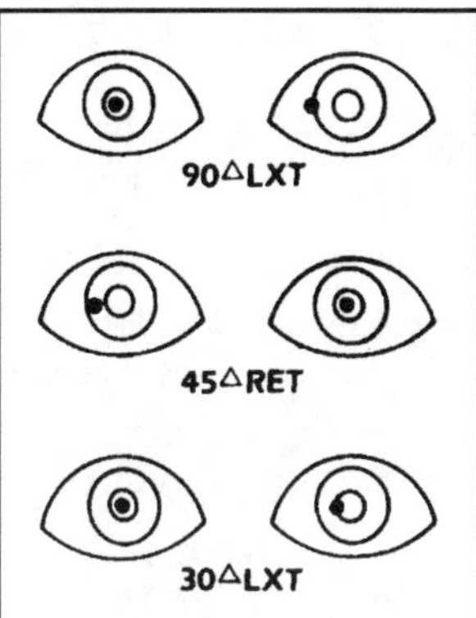

Figure 8-3. Hirschberg measurements: 90 PD LXT—light reflex of the left eye deviates to the nasal limbus (top). 45 PD RET—light reflex of the right eye temporal iris (middle). 30 PD LXT—light reflex of the left eye deviates to the nasal pupillary border (bottom) (reprinted with permission from *A Systematic Approach to Strabismus*. Thorofare, NJ: SLACK Incorporated; 1998).

How-To: Cover Test (Cover/Uncover Test)

- Have the patient fixate on either a distant or near target while you cover one eye.
- If the uncovered eye moves to pick up fixation (assuming at least some macular vision) when the other eye is covered, there is a tropia present.
- If the uncovered eye does not move when the first eye is covered, cover the second eye and observe the movement of the first eye. Evaluate according to the flow chart (Table 8-9).
- If a deviation is found, it can be measured using prisms and the cover test.

Stereoacuity

The evaluation of depth perception (stereoacuity) is the most sensitive test of binocular visual function. Fine depth perception requires good vision in both eyes, good ocular alignment, and visual fields (from both eyes) that overlap each other centrally. In a normal person, when the foveas of both eyes are fixed on the same object in visual space, the brain melds the slightly different views from each eye. The blending of these slightly different images into one produces the perception of depth.

How-To: Depth Perception and Stereopsis

Gross Depth Perception:

- Patient is given two pencils, one in each hand, and asked to touch the pencil points together.
- A person without stereopsis will not be able to move the pencils so that the points are touching.

Measuring Stereoacuity Using Polarized Glasses:

- Patient wears habitual correction and uses bifocal or reading glasses if appropriate. (Polarized glasses are placed over habitual correction, if used.)
- Patient is requested to identify figures of graded arc. (Instruct the patient to point at the figures; oils from fingers may soil the targets, and repeated pressing may alter the test booklet.)
- The last figure (circle or animal) correctly identified is the measure of a patient's level of stereoacuity and can be documented according to the test pamphlet.

Notes:

- It is important that nothing has been done prior to the test that might possibly interfere with fusion. Glasses should not be removed, neither eye should be occluded.
- The patient should be allowed to use an abnormal head position if this permits the best possible binocular function.

Table 8-9.
Decision Tree for Evaluating Ocular Balance

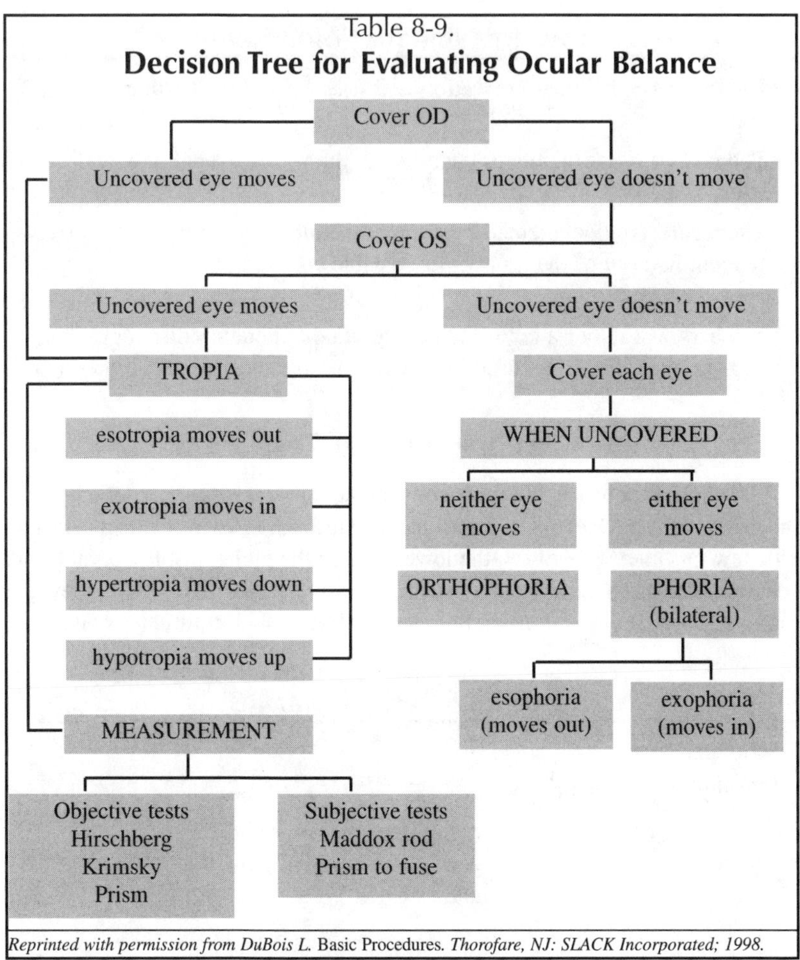

Reprinted with permission from DuBois L. Basic Procedures. *Thorofare, NJ: SLACK Incorporated; 1998.*

Color Vision Plates

The color vision test most often used in the office is the Ishihara pseudoisochromatic plates. These plates have colored dots that form numbers against a dotted background of another color. The first plate in the booklet is a test plate that is easy to distinguish and intended to show the patient how the test works. A person with normal color vision will be able to identify most of the remaining numbers; one or two of the plates are difficult for most people and do not distinguish between normal and abnormal color vision. A color deficient person will either misidentify certain numbers or not see them at all. This test will show complete color blindness or red-green confusion but does not quantify color deficiencies.

How-To: Ishihara Color Plates

- Patient wears habitual correction and uses bifocal or reading glasses if appropriate.
- The patient views the plates under good illumination separately with each eye.
- The results are documented by noting the number of color plates correctly identified out of the number of possible correct answers.
- For young or illiterate patients, there are some plates that do not have test numbers, but rather a colored line that winds through a different colored background. These are used by having the patient trace the colored line.

Schirmer Tear Test

The Schirmer test is the most convenient way to assess tear deficiency in the office setting. One end of a sterile, standardized, filter paper strip is inserted a few millimeters between the lower lid and the globe, just temporal to the cornea. The strips remain in place for 5 minutes. At that point, they are removed and the amount of wetting is measured with a millimeter rule.

How-To: Schirmer Tear Test

Schirmer Test I:

- **No** topical anesthetic is used.
- The strips are inserted a few millimeters between the lower lid and the globe, just temporal to the cornea. The patient is instructed to keep the eyes gently closed for 5 minutes.
- The strips are then carefully removed, and the length of the strip that has become moistened with tears is measured.

Notes:

- The irritation caused by the paper strip causes reflex tearing.
- A normal eye should produce enough tears to wet at least 10 mm of the strip in 5 minutes.

Schirmer Test II:

- Topical anesthetic is instilled.
- The strips are inserted a few millimeters between the lower lid and the globe, just temporal to the cornea. The patient is instructed to keep the eyes gently closed for 5 minutes.
- The strips are then carefully removed, and the length of the strip that has become moistened with tears is measured.

(continued)

How-To: Schirmer Tear Test (continued)

Notes:

- This test measures baseline tear function.
- There is usually less paper strip wetting than in Test I.

Vital Signs

Occasionally, it is necessary for the eyecare professional to monitor a patient's vital signs. This includes measuring blood pressure, taking the pulse, and counting respirations.

How-To: Blood Pressure

- The pressure cuff is firmly secured (but not tight) around the patient's upper arm.
- The patient should have his or her arm extended, palm up, so that the flat surface of the stethoscope membrane can be held firmly against the inner elbow.
- With the stethoscope earpieces in place, the stethoscope membrane against the patient's inner elbow, the cuff gauge visible, and the bulb valve in the closed position (ie, air can be pumped into but cannot escape the cuff), begin to pump air into the cuff by repeatedly squeezing the bulb.
- At a point usually between 80 and 110 mmHg on the gauge, the heartbeat will become audible. Enough air must be pumped into the cuff so that this sound is no longer heard.
- Barely open the bulb valve to allow the air in the cuff to escape slowly.
- Listen carefully, note the number on the gauge at which the heartbeat first becomes audible again; this is the systolic pressure and is usually 110 to 140 mmHg.
- Continue to slowly let air out of the cuff and note the gauge reading at which the heartbeat sound again disappears; this is the diastolic pressure (normally 70 to 90 mmHg).
- The blood pressure is recorded with the higher number (systolic pressure) over the lower number (diastolic pressure), as in 134/86. Documentation should include which arm was used and the patient's position (sitting, reclining, etc) during the test.

How-To: Heart Rate and Respirations

Heart Rate:

- Place your first two fingers—never the thumb—over the lateral aspect of the patient's inner wrist (the palm is turned up). The heartbeat can be felt in the groove between the outer wrist bone and the central cords.
- Once the pulse is identified, the number of beats in a minute is counted using a watch with a second hand. The normal adult heart rate is about 72 beats/minute (HR = 72).

Respirations:

- While still pretending to measure pulse, shift your attention to the rise and fall of the patient's chest as each breath is taken and exhaled. Either the inhalation or the exhalation should be counted, not both.
- The number of breaths in a minute is counted using a watch with a second hand. Normal adult respiration is about 18 breaths/minute (R = 18).

How-To: Temperature

- Between patients, clean thermometer with a disinfectant solution.
- When ready for use, grasp the clear end of the thermometer firmly and shake the mercury down into the reservoir.
- The liquid reservoir end of the thermometer is placed under the patient's tongue and allowed to remain there with the mouth closed until the column has reached its maximum height (usually in 3 or 4 minutes).
- The top of the column is read against a scale printed on the glass. The normal temperature is about 98.6°F.
- If the reading is not at least 98°F, the thermometer should be repositioned under the patient's tongue for another minute or two to make sure the temperature is accurate.

Unless otherwise noted, all text, tables, and figures are adapted or reprinted with permission from DuBois L. Basic Procedures. *Thorofare, NJ: SLACK Incorporated; 1998.*

CHAPTER 9

Instrumentation

General Preventative Maintenance

- Maintain equipment records and manuals.
- Keep equipment covered or properly stored at night.
- Small instruments should be stored, preferably in the original box or case, in drawers.
- Turn illuminated equipment off when not in use.
- Unplug instruments prior to any maintenance.
- Allow bulbs to cool before handling.
- Do not get fingerprints on bulbs.
- Follow accepted cleaning and maintenance procedures.
- Never spray or pour cleaning solutions directly on equipment or pieces; moisten a lint-free cloth or lens wipe instead.
- Use a rechargeable instrument all day long—do not recharge in between use.

Instruments Used in Determining Visual Acuity (Table 9-1)

- Keep instruments free from dust and fingerprints.
- Change the projector bulb with great care.
- Front surface mirrors must be gently cleaned to protect silver coating.
- Oil and dirt from fingers can damage color vision plates and caps.

Table 9-1.

Instruments Used in Determining Visual Acuity

Equipment: Projector
Purpose: Used to project symbols onto a screen to obtain a subjective visual acuity.
Maintenance: Dust housing with a soft cloth; lens can be dusted with canned air, a camel hair brush, or lens solution.
Other notes: The manual that accompanies the projector has projection brackets that can be used to obtain proper image size when the distance from the patient to the chart is not 20 feet. Another method of determining symbol size is to calculate the appropriate symbol height using the following formula:

$$\frac{\text{the size of 20/200 symbol needed (x)}}{\text{9 cm}} = \frac{\text{patient distance}}{\text{20 ft}}$$

Equipment: Projector slides
Purpose: Used in projectors; adult, pediatric, and vectograph slides are available.
Maintenance: Carefully wipe the glass surfaces with a clean, dry lens wipe; never place the slide under running water or spray solutions on it.

Equipment: Screens
Purpose: Used to reflect the light and symbols from a projector.
Maintenance: Clean with a mild soap solution if it is a washable type; frequent wiping and washing will erode the surface.

Equipment: Front surface mirrors
Purpose: Used to artificially extend exam rooms less than 20 ft long in order to obtain standardized visual acuities.
Maintenance: Remove dust particles with canned air, an ear bulb, or a camel hair brush; stubborn stains or fingerprint oils can be removed by this method: 1) moisten cotton and dab over the mirror, 2) take another piece of cotton and dip it into cream of tartar, 3) blot the entire surface, reapplying the cream of tartar to the cotton as necessary, 4) take a dry piece of cotton and blot excess moisture off of the mirror, use as many pieces of cotton as necessary, 5) after blotting excess moisture, take another piece of cotton and begin to gently wipe in small circles until the cream of tartar comes off; each cleaning removes a small amount of silver—clean the mirrors only when absolutely necessary.

Equipment: Distance and near vision charts
Purpose: Used for measuring visual acuity.
Maintenance: Laminated cardboard or plastic can easily be washed with a mild soap solution.

Equipment: Brightness acuity tester
Purpose: Provides objective measurements of functional visual acuity in different light conditions.
Maintenance: The reflector can be removed and washed with a mild nonabrasive soap or detergent that does not contain lanolin or hand lotion; pat or air-dry.

(continued)

Table 9-1. (continued)

Instruments Used in Determining Visual Acuity

Equipment: Vision screener
Purpose: A portable screening system for measuring visual acuity.
Maintenance: Use a lens wipe to clean viewing lenses; each slide can be removed and cleaned with a lens tissue or a lens cleaning towelette.

Equipment: Color plates and test books
Purpose: Used to determine color blindness.
Maintenance: Oils and dirt from fingers can soil the plates over time—instruct the patient to identify the shapes on the plates verbally without actually touching the plates.

Equipment: Farnsworth dichotomous 15 and 100 hue
Purpose: Used to determine color vision anomalies.
Maintenance: Oils and dirt from fingers can soil the caps over time—instruct the patient to handle the sides of the caps.

Equipment: Optokinetic drum
Purpose: Used to determine the presence of visual acuity; used to evaluate neurological disorders.
Maintenance: Wipe clean with a mild soap solution if needed.

Equipment: Optokinetic tape
Purpose: Used to determine the presence of visual acuity; used to evaluate neurological disorders.
Maintenance: Replace if fabric becomes soiled.

Instruments Used to Determine the Refractive State of the Eye (Table 9-2)

Table 9-2.

Instruments Used to Determine the Refractive State of the Eye

Equipment: Phoropter
Purpose: Used to determine refractive error via a system of rotating lenses.
Maintenance: Lenses are protected when the dials are set to zero; professional maintenance required, or lenses can be cleaned as they are rotated through the opening (canned air, camel hair brush, lint-free cloth moistened with lens cleaner); face shields can be washed with soap and water, soaked in alcohol, or sterilized in an autoclave.

(continued)

Table 9-2. (continued)

Instruments Used to Determine the Refractive State of the Eye

Equipment: Autorefractor
Purpose: Used to automatically determine the refractive measurement of the eye.
Maintenance: Forehead rest, chin rest, and face shields should be cleaned with an alcohol wipe between patients; otherwise, professional maintenance is called for.

Equipment: Streak or spot retinoscope
Purpose: Used to objectively determine the refractive power of the eye.
Maintenance: Leave the retinoscope out of the charger during daily use to discharge the battery; always place the instrument upright, never on its side (this can warp the filament).

Equipment: Lensmeter/lensometer
Purpose: Used to measure the spherical and cylindrical power and the axis of the cylinder in a spectacle or contact lens, as well as optical center and prism.
Maintenance: Eyepiece must be focused for each individual user; clean eyepiece lens with canned air, lens wipe, or camel hair brush; marking pens should be cleaned periodically with an alcohol wipe.

Equipment: Automatic lensmeter
Purpose: Computerized device used to obtain objective spectacle measurements.
Maintenance: Wipe with a damp cloth; ink pen tips should be wiped periodically with alcohol; nosepiece cover occasionally needs to be replaced.

Equipment: Trial frame
Purpose: An adjustable frame that is used with trial lenses when measuring the patient for spectacle lenses.
Maintenance: Wipe with a soft cloth; avoid dropping; nose rest should be cleaned with an alcohol wipe between patients.

Equipment: Trial lenses
Purpose: A set of lenses used to measure the refractive state of the eye.
Maintenance: Can be cleaned with a glass cleaner and a soft cotton cloth.

Equipment: Cross cylinder
Purpose: A compound lens used to refine the axis and power of the cylinder when performing refractometry.
Maintenance: Wipe with a damp cloth; do not use harsh detergents or rub vigorously.

Equipment: Distometer
Purpose: Used to measure vertex distance.
Maintenance: Do not drop; wipe footplate with alcohol between patients.

Instruments Used to Evaluate Motility and Binocularity (Table 9-3)

Table 9-3.

Instruments Used to Evaluate Motility and Binocularity

Equipment: Loose prisms and prism bar
Purpose: Used to quantify extraocular muscle deviations.
Maintenance: Clean with a soft, lint-free cloth; do not use alcohol on plastic prisms; glass cleaner may be used on glass prisms.

Equipment: Rotary or Risley prism
Purpose: Used to quantify extraocular muscle deviations.
Maintenance: Clean with a soft, lint-free cloth; do not immerse in cleaner (this will loosen the mounting).

Equipment: Stereopsis tests
Purpose: Used to measure stereopsis and depth perception.
Maintenance: Constant pushing and touching of circles can disrupt the symbols; patients should be asked to point instead.

Equipment: Maddox rod
Purpose: Used to dissociate the eyes to evaluate extraocular muscle deviations.
Maintenance: Plastic carrier can be washed with a mild soap solution or wiped with an alcohol wipe.

Equipment: Worth 4 dot
Purpose: Used to determine visual functions, fusion, suppression, and/or diplopia.
Maintenance: Occasionally dust off the dots using a cotton swab; remove batteries if not in constant use.

Equipment: Bagolini lenses
Purpose: Used to determine normal and abnormal retinal correspondence.
Maintenance: Clean with lens wipe and lens cleaner.

Instruments Used in Glaucoma Evaluation (Table 9-4)

- Proper tonometer calibration is crucial when determining the intraocular pressure (IOP).
- Disinfection is important to prevent transfer of infection between patients.
- Always thoroughly dry any probe tip before touching the cornea.

Table 9-4.

Instruments Used in Glaucoma Evaluation

Equipment: Schiotz tonometer
Purpose: Portable device used to measure IOP via indention.
Maintenance: The plunger is removed from the barrel and cleaned with alcohol, or both parts can be soaked in 3% hydrogen peroxide (a pipe cleaner works well to clean the inside of the barrel); can also be heat sterilized; the test plate should be wiped with alcohol and allowed to dry completely.

Equipment: Goldmann applanation tonometer
Purpose: Used to measure IOP via applanation.
Maintenance: The head can be soaked for 10 minutes in 3% hydrogen peroxide, one part household bleach to 10 parts water, or a similar disinfectant that will not damage the plastic prism (the etching marks on the prism will eventually bleach out if the entire head is left in a solution over a long period of time); the prism should be rinsed and dried with a cotton ball after disinfecting; calibration should be performed on a regular basis (professional maintenance required if calibration is off).

Equipment: Noncontact tonometer (NCT)
Purpose: Used to measure IOP via applanation but does not contact the eye.
Maintenance: At the start of each day, check the air nozzle by firing an air pulse without a patient in place; the chin cup and forehead rest can be cleaned with an alcohol swab between patients; otherwise, professional maintenance is required.

Equipment: Tono-Pen XL
Purpose: Portable device used to measure IOP via a combination of applanation and indentation.
Maintenance: Before using each day, before storage at night, and when a good calibration cannot be obtained, insert the probe tip into the optical quality gas can nozzle, spray for 2 seconds, and wait for 3 to 4 minutes before checking the instrument's calibration; calibrate once a day before the first use; otherwise, professional maintenance is required.

Equipment: Perkins hand-held applanation tonometer
Purpose: Portable device used to measure IOP via applanation.
Maintenance: Same as Goldmann tonometer.

Equipment: Pneumotonometer
Purpose: Used to measure IOP via applanation.
Maintenance: Clean the tip with an isopropyl alcohol pad after each patient use and allow to dry thoroughly; both the tip and membrane can be soaked in alcohol for 10 minutes for a weekly routine cleaning; dust periodically with a lint-free cloth; check the vents on the filter access door for dust; change both filters twice a year.

(continued)

Table 9-4. (continued)

Instruments Used in Glaucoma Evaluation

Equipment: Goldmann 3 mirror lens
Purpose: Used in conjunction with the slit lamp to view the trabecular meshwork and the anterior chamber angle.
Maintenance: Clean immediately after use; wash with soap and water, then soak in 3% hydrogen peroxide, one part household bleach to 10 parts water, or a similar disinfectant (soaking should only be allowed for 10 to 20 minutes), rinse with distilled water, and dry with a soft cloth.

Instruments Used in Visual Field Testing (Table 9-5)

Table 9-5.

Instruments Used in Visual Field Testing

Equipment: Tangent screen
Purpose: Used to determine the visual field status in the central 30 degrees of the visual field.
Maintenance: Whisking the screen occasionally with a soft brush; targets can be washed with a mild soapy water (oils from fingers can soil the targets).

Equipment: Bowl-type perimeters
Purpose: Used to test both the peripheral and central visual fields.
Maintenance: Chin and forehead rests should be wiped with alcohol between each patient; the outside of the instrument can be dusted with a soft, lint-free cotton cloth; to clean the inside surface, first blow dust out of bowl with canned air (stubborn dust or debris can be removed with a camel hair brush); projection arm should be lubricated twice a year with a small drop of thin oil; the lamp housing should be cleaned with a blast of canned air; the lower surface of the condenser lens can be removed and wiped with a soft cloth; bowl illumination should be calibrated before each patient, with the patient seated in front of the perimeter; target illumination should be performed at the beginning of each day.

Equipment: Automated perimeter
Purpose: Used to test both the peripheral and central visual fields via automation.
Maintenance: The outside of the machine can be dusted with a soft cloth; use only static wipes to clean the screen of the CRT; the light pen tip can be cleaned using a cotton swab and alcohol; the patient response button should be cleaned with soap and water, alcohol, or a spray cleaner; disk drives should be cleaned at least three times a year depending on use; evaluate the stimulus of the perimeter once a week (stimulus should have crisp edges with no blurring or inconsistencies); otherwise, professional maintenance is required.

Instruments Used in the Retinal Exam (Table 9-6)

- A blast of canned air should be used regularly to keep all lenses dust-free.
- Never use regular tissues to clean delicate ophthalmic lenses.
- Never boil or autoclave ophthalmic lenses.

Table 9-6.
Instruments Used in the Retinal Exam

Equipment: Direct ophthalmoscope
Purpose: A hand-held instrument used to view the internal structures of the eye.
Maintenance: Keep the ophthalmoscope set to the zero viewing lens to keep lenses clean; the lenses should be cleaned by a professional; if the instrument contains a front surface mirror, clean it as described in Table 9-1.

Equipment: Indirect ophthalmoscope
Purpose: Used to view the internal structures of the eye stereoscopically.
Maintenance: Eyepieces are cleaned with a blast of canned air or wiped with alcohol (for stubborn marks); the front surface mirror should be cleaned as described in Table 9-1; the headband can be wiped with alcohol; headband cushions can be removed and cleaned with soap and water.

Equipment: Laser and diagnostic lenses
Purpose: Used for fundus viewing for examination and treatment.
Maintenance: To clean lenses that do not contact the eye, use canned air, a bulb syringe, a lens brush or lens paper; to maintain lenses that touch the eye, rinse the lens after each use in tepid water and a mild dishwashing liquid or contact lens cleaner, rinse the lens well, and dry with a soft nonlinting cloth (never use alcohol, hydrogen peroxide, or acetone); to disinfect a diagnostic contact lens, soak in a 2% aqueous solution of glutaraldehyde for 20 to 25 minutes or use a fresh solution of hypochlorite in a 1:10 dilution for 5 to 10 minutes—either of these two methods must be followed by a thorough, brisk rinse with running water, dry with a lint-free cloth; to sterilize, use standard ethylene oxide gas procedures with aeration up to but not exceeding 130°F; a lens that dislodges from its holder can be reattached by the manufacturer.

Instruments Used in the Contact Lens Exam (Table 9-7)

Table 9-7.
Instruments Used in the Contact Lens Exam

Equipment: Slit lamp
Purpose: Used to provide a magnified stereoscopic view of the eye's exterior, surface, and anterior segment.
Maintenance: The painted external parts of the instrument can be dusted with a soft lint-free cloth; canned air is useful to get dust out of the tiny crevices; front surface mirrors are cleaned as described in Table 9-1; lenses are cleaned with canned air or a camel hair brush; plastic (not rubber) chin and forehead rests should be wiped with alcohol between patients; to clean the gliding plate, wipe the plate with an alcohol wipe (every five cleanings, spray a small amount of silicone on the plate).

Equipment: Placido disc
Purpose: Used to evaluate the regularity of the anterior surface of the cornea.
Maintenance: Oils from fingers will mar disc; depending on the material of the disc, wipe with a soft cloth; if fingerprints appear, wipe gently with a slightly damp cloth.

Equipment: Keratometer (ophthalmometer)
Purpose: Used to measure the curvature of the cornea's anterior central zone.
Maintenance: Chin and forehead rests should be wiped with alcohol between patients; the body can be dusted with a soft cloth or condensed air; adjust the eyepiece before calibration and each use; if calibration is not true, instrument must be adjusted by the manufacturer.

Equipment: Automatic keratometer
Purpose: Automated instrument used to measure the curvature of the cornea.
Maintenance: In hand-held models, clean the observation window with compressed air or an alcohol wipe; clean plastic parts by wiping with a soft dry cloth; other maintenance must be performed by the manufacturer.

Equipment: Corneal topography systems
Purpose: Used to automatically analyze and measure the shape of the cornea in fine detail.
Maintenance: Chin and forehead rests can be wiped with an alcohol wipe between patients; lightly dust the instrument if needed, but the optical cone is a sensitive component and should not be touched or routinely cleaned; a factory-trained representative should perform routine service and maintenance once a year.

Equipment: Radiuscope
Purpose: Used to objectively determine the radius of a contact lens (some can also determine lens thickness).
Maintenance: Adjust the eyepiece(s) before using; lens papers and solutions can be used to clean optical surfaces.

(continued)

Table 9-7. (continued)

Instruments Used in the Contact Lens Exam

Equipment: Lens modification systems
Purpose: Used to blend or add curves; flatten peripheral, intermediate, or secondary curves; change the lens power; reshape, thin, or blunt lens edges; clean and polish.
Maintenance: Remove and wipe splash tray; if the motor malfunctions, the entire unit can be replaced for little more than the cost of a new motor.

Equipment: Lens diameter gauge (loop)
Purpose: Used to measure the diameter of a contact lens.
Maintenance: Gauge can be wiped with a soft, damp cloth and dried.

Instruments Used in the Optical Lab (Table 9-8)

Table 9-8.

Instruments Used in the Optical Lab

Equipment: Frame warmer
Purpose: Used to heat plastic frames for glazing, adjusting, or inserting lenses.
Maintenance: The hot air frame warmer should not be placed near flammable materials or where water is used or stored; it should not be used if the air flow opening is blocked; use canned air to remove accumulated dust, especially the inside dust cover.

Equipment: Optical pliers, screwdrivers, and hex wrenches
Purpose: Used to make minor repairs on spectacles.
Maintenance: Handle with care; do not drop.

Equipment: Lens clock (Geneva lens measure)
Purpose: Used to measure the base curve of a lens.
Maintenance: Always replace the cap when the instrument is not in use; care should be taken to not drop the clock.

Equipment: Lens thickness calipers
Purpose: Used to determine the thickness of a spectacle lens.
Maintenance: Replace in a case or drawer when finished using; take care not to drop.

Equipment: Optical vernier
Purpose: Used for general measuring of inside and outside diameters of a lens.
Maintenance: Replace in a case or drawer when finished using; take care not to drop.

Equipment: Lens boxer
Purpose: Used to determine a lens' physical measurements (height and width, bifocal height and inset).
Maintenance: Replace in a case or drawer when finished using. *(continued)*

Table 9-8. (continued)

Instruments Used in the Optical Lab

Equipment: Pupilometer or pupil gauge
Purpose: Used to measure interpupillary distance.
Maintenance: The forehead and nose rest should be wiped with an alcohol wipe between patients; the outside body can be wiped with a damp cloth.

Equipment: Edger
Purpose: Used to grind uncut lens blanks to fit the size and shape of a frame.
Maintenance: The machine should be regularly checked, adjusted, and cleaned; calibration check and coolant changes can be performed on a weekly basis; clean screens and filters frequently; outside surface can be washed with a mild soapy detergent; the inside wheel and housing assembly can be wiped with a damp cloth, or debris can be blown away with a low pressure hose or canned air; a lightweight oil should be used once a week (or every other week, depending on usage) on all hinges, gears, and ball bearings; the coolant should be changed once a week; the right-hand spindle felt pad must be replaced if thin and worn; replace finger guides when the right edge has developed a curve; see manufacturer's instructions for cleaning, stoning, retruing, and rebevelling diamond wheels.

Unless otherwise noted, all text, tables, and figures are adapted or reprinted with permission from Herrin MP. Instrumentation. *Thorofare, NJ: SLACK Incorporated; 1999.*

CHAPTER 10

Special Skills and Techniques

Note: The interpretation of these tests is beyond the scope of this handbook. Please refer to *Basic Bookshelf* title *Special Skills and Techniques* for these details.

Exophthalmometry

- Exophthalmometry evaluates the forward protrusion of the eye by measuring the distance between the anterior surface of the cornea and the bony margin of the orbit.
- Proptosis can be bilateral (exophthalmos) or unilateral (proptosis), depending on the underlying cause.
- Protrusion of the eye can be caused by orbital tumors, trauma, inflammation, or disease; however, it is most commonly seen in patients who have thyroid disease.
- Protrusion can also be due to shallow orbits, in which case it is a variation of normal.
- If ocular manifestations such as exophthalmos are present in the patient with thyroid disease, the patient is said to have Graves' disease.
- Since thyroid disease and tumors are normally progressive, it is critical to measure and monitor the degree of exophthalmos or proptosis at regular intervals.

How-To: Hertel Exophthalmometry

- Wipe areas of patient contact with alcohol.
- If a previous measurement has been taken, adjust the base to the previous setting.
- Sit directly in front of the patient at eye level. Instruct the patient to fixate straight ahead.

(continued)

How-To: Hertel Exophthalmometry (continued)

- Place the small projections firmly on the lateral margin of both bony orbits. Move the right measuring device until firmly fit against the orbit.
- While checking the patient's right eye, ask the patient to fixate on your left eye. Note the reading where the cornea aligns on the scale. Without moving, view the patient's left eye with your own right eye. (Ask the patient to fixate on your right eye.) Again note the reading on the scale. In addition, the base measurement (which is the distance between the two measuring devices) is noted, recorded, and used on all subsequent measurements to ensure continued accuracy.

Pachymetry

- Normal corneal thickness ranges from 1 mm at the very periphery of the cornea to 0.5 mm at the center.
- Some individuals have thinner or thicker corneas, and some corneal diseases result in changes in corneal thickness.
- The measurement of corneal thickness can be very useful in evaluating the integrity of the cornea and is done with an instrument known as a pachymeter.
- An ultrasonic probe, somewhat similar to that of an A-scan probe, is placed directly on the cornea. Sound waves pass through the cornea, yielding a measurement of its thickness in microns.
- Always start with the central cornea, as this is the thinnest area in the normal cornea. This numeric value can be used to support peripheral corneal thickness values.

How-To: Pachymetry

- Anesthetize the eye with a local anesthetic.
- Ask the patient to look straight ahead at the fixation target.
- Start by measuring the center-most portion of the cornea. The straight probe is placed perpendicularly on the center of the cornea. Several readings should be taken and the different thicknesses should be averaged for the final reading. Accurate corneal thickness can only be obtained if the probe is perpendicular to the cornea.
- Use the angled probe to map the thickness of the peripheral cornea. Follow imaginary concentric rings around the center of the cornea. The center is measured first, then the probe is moved away from the center by about 1 mm, and a 3-mm diameter ring is measured. After that ring is successfully measured, the probe is moved out 1 additional millimeter and a second ring of about 7 mm diameter is measured.

Photokeratoscopy

- The photokeratoscope is a device used to evaluate the anterior surface of the cornea. It is a photographic unit with a cone-shaped section containing a series of concentric rings similar to that of the Placido disc.
- The resulting photograph provides a graphic representation of the anterior corneal surface.
- It is important that the central portion of the cornea is properly aligned and that the rings in this area are in focus prior to the picture being taken, since poor alignment and focus may result in erroneous findings.
- A dry cornea can appear to be irregularly shaped, but this irregularity is an artifact.
- In eyes with flat corneas, the rings will be spaced farther apart than normal.
- Steep corneas will have rings that are spaced very close together.
- In individuals with astigmatism, the rings on one axis will be spaced similarly, while the rings on the perpendicular axis will be spaced significantly different (either closer or farther apart).
- In eyes with corneal irregularities due to disease, scarring, or corneal surgery, the rings will be irregularly shaped.

How-To: Photokeratoscopy

- Wipe chin and forehead rests with alcohol.
- Position the patient and adjust the image of the rings with the focusing knob.
- Ask the patient to first close his or her eyes for a moment, then open wide. Snap the picture.

Corneal Topography

- Corneal topography creates a computerized map of the surface of the cornea.
- In corneal topography, the steep portions of the cornea are represented by dark red and red (K readings in the high 40s or low 50s), whereas the shallow areas are represented in blue and purple (K readings in the mid 30s). Corneas that are in the medium range of steepness are represented by green (K readings in the mid 40s).
- The topographic colors are not absolutely fixed to specific K readings, but represent the relative relationship of steepness and flatness of the cornea.
- A spherically shaped cornea of moderate steepness would appear almost completely green on a topographic map.

- Corneas with significant astigmatism will produce a typical hourglass shape in one color along one axis, and another color will appear along the opposite axis.
- In irregularly shaped corneas, one area of the cornea will be steep, but the area across from the steep portion may not be as steep.

How-To: Topography

- Wipe areas of patient contact with alcohol.
- Seat the patient in front of the unit and ask him or her to look straight ahead. Ask the patient to blink periodically to ensure that the cornea is moist, which results in sharper images.
- Obtain a clear and focused view of the ring-covered cornea.
- Capture the image by pressing a button on the joystick or clicking on the mouse, depending on the unit.
- The image is then analyzed by the computer. If the computer determines that the image is reliable, then it will "draw" a series of colored rings on top of the corneal image from the center of the cornea to the midperiphery. If the computer does not think that the image is reliable, then the colored image will not appear, signaling you to "try again."
- Once you have obtained an image that the computer has analyzed as reliable, a second screen appears. This gives the exact level of reliability of the image as analyzed by the computer. Reliability is presented as a confidence level, from high to low, based on such things as focus and centering of the cornea. If the level of reliability is acceptable, save the image. Patient demographics (such as age, sex, and eye) are saved as well.

Ophthalmoscopy

- Ophthalmoscopy is the examination of the internal structures of the posterior chamber of the eye through the tiny window of the pupil.
- Many systemic diseases that exhibit ocular manifestations have been diagnosed simply by the appearance of the retinal vasculature of the eye.
- Ophthalmoscopy is an integral part of the diagnosis and management of ocular diseases such as glaucoma, ocular lesions, abnormalities, and trauma.
- Two types of ophthalmoscopes may be utilized in performing the ophthalmoscopic examination. The direct ophthalmoscope and the indirect ophthalmoscope each have distinct advantages and disadvantages (Table 10-1).
- Direct ophthalmoscopy can be performed through an undilated pupil; however, dilation of the pupil is necessary for a thorough ophthalmoscopic examination utilizing either the direct or the indirect ophthalmoscope.

Table 10-1.

Comparison of Direct and Indirect Ophthalmoscopy

Direct	Indirect
Dilated or undilated pupil	Widely dilated pupil
Monocular view	Binocular stereoscopic view
Small field of view (± 10 degrees)	Larger 45 degree field of view
Approximately 14x magnification	2x to 4x depending on lens used
Upright, nonreversed view	Inverted and reversed view
Hand-held	Worn on the head of the examiner
No condensing lens necessary	Hand-held condensing lens necessary

Reprinted with permission from Van Boemel GB. Special Skills and Techniques. *Thorofare, NJ: SLACK Incorporated; 1999.*

How-To: Direct Ophthalmoscopy

- Direct the patient to look straight ahead at a distant fixation target.
- Start with the scope set on zero. From 1 foot or so away, locate the patient's red reflex.
- Move in closer, keeping the red reflex in the scope, until you are up to the patient's brow. Dial in plus or minus (depending on the refractive error) until the fundal image is clear.
- Evaluate the optic nerve. Follow each main blood vessel out from the nerve and into the periphery as far as you are able to visualize. Evaluate the macula.

How-To: Indirect Ophthalmoscopy

- Adjust the headband and binoculars for your use.
- Direct the patient to look straight ahead.
- At arm's length from the patient, hold the condensing lens about 1 inch from the patient's eye. Rest your little finger on the patient's forehead or nose to stabilize your hand. Use the other hand to gently hold the lids open. Adjust the lens to obtain the clearest view.
- Evaluate the optic nerve and macula. Evaluate the periphery by directing the patient to look in various positions of gaze. Frequently move the condensing lens briefly aside for patient comfort.

Table 10-2.
Types of Color Vision Arrangement Tests

Test Name	Features	Notes
Farnsworth-Munsell D-15	15 colored caps and one fixed reference cap	Quick Easy to administer Uses a circular score grid Also useful in low vision and children Subtle defects will not be detected
Lanthony Desaturated 15 Panel	15 pale-colored caps and one fixed reference cap	Administered and scored identically to the D-15 Good at detecting subtle defects missed by the D-15
Farnsworth-Munsell 100-Hue	85 hues divided into four boxes, one with 22 caps and three with 21 each; stationary reference cap on each end	Most popular test Time-consuming Scoring involves mathematical manipulation and then marking on a round grid or computer program May not be accurate in children or those with low vision Provides a score for evaluating progress Normals are age dependent

Color Vision: Arrangement Tests

- There are several types of arrangement tests (Table 10-2). Their common principle is that they mimic a color wheel. The patient is asked to arrange the colored caps into a graded color order that should look somewhat like a rainbow. The correct arrangement of caps reveals the patient's ability to see subtle color gradation.
- If the patient has abnormal color vision, then the cap arrangement will reveal the type of color vision mechanism that is involved (protan, deutan, or tritan defect), but generally not its severity.
- In a complete protan defect, none of the colors in the red spectrum are seen. In a deutan defect, the entire spectrum is seen, but green is seen incorrectly. A tritan defect is an abnormality in the blue color mechanism, causing confusion of blue and yellow.

- If the arrangement is abnormal, it is because the patient confuses two very distinct colors that are opposite on the color wheel.
- The test requires that the patient have sufficiently good vision to see the caps and sufficient cognitive skills in order to perform the test.
- The tests are not suitable for very young children or any others who may not be cooperative.
- The tests are qualitative in nature and reveal only the type of color mechanism involved, not its severity.

How-To: Arrangement Color Vision Tests

- The patient should be tested with his or her best spectacle correction and undilated pupils.
- Each eye is tested separately.
- The test should be conducted with a recommended light source such as the MacBeth Illuminator, which mimics sunlight.
- Mix up the colored caps (either on the desk or in the box) and then tell the patient to rearrange the caps in a graded color order. Remind the patient not to touch the colored portion of the caps, as oils from the fingers can discolor the caps.
- Record the patient's answers on the appropriate graph or form.

The Anomaloscope

- The anomaloscope (a color matching test) provides us with quantitative data on the severity of a particular defect.
- The most commonly used anomaloscope is the Nagel anomaloscope produced by Schmidt and Haensch, which is used to test red/green abnormalities.

How-To: Anomaloscope

- Test the patient one eye at a time. The patient should not be dilated and may need spectacle correction.
- Have the patient look at the white light on the base of the unit, which slightly "bleaches" the retina.
- Next, instruct the patient to look down the barrel and turn a knob on the unit to match the red/green mixture.
- "Bleach" the patient again while you change the red/green mixture dial to a new setting.

(continued)

How-To: Anomaloscope (continued)

- By doing this repeatedly, you can determine the patient's matching range. This reflects a mild, moderate, severe, or complete protan or deutan color vision defect.
- If the patient is unable to make a perfect match between the red/green mixture and the yellow, note the reason. (Typical answers may be "too much red" or "too much green" in the color presented.) Make sure that the match is a perfect match and not just close. If a close match is recorded as perfect, this will artificially widen the final matching range, and a normal individual may be given an inappropriate diagnosis of a slight color vision defect.

Dark Adaptometry

- Dark adaptometry is a psychophysical test used to determine the ability of the rod photoreceptors to increase their sensitivity in the dark.
- Dark adaptometry is a useful test for anyone complaining of night vision problems.
- Test information can supplement the results obtained from other tests, such as the ERG and EOG.
- If the patient is cooperative, the results will provide excellent information as to how well he or she sees in the dark, versus a normal population.
- There may be subtle changes in night vision that are easily detected by this test that cannot be detected by means of the ERG.

How-To: Dark Adaptometry (Goldmann-Weekers Dark Adaptometer)

- The patient is dark adapted for 2 minutes.
- After the 2-minute period, the patient places his or her head in a chin rest and is instructed to keep his or her eyes open while looking straight ahead at the illuminated bowl to light adapt for 5 minutes.
- The lights are now turned completely off. The patient is asked to look straight ahead and report when he or she first sees the test target. Increase target intensity. When the patient reports seeing the bars, mark the score sheet and turn the target light completely off again. Repeat for 5 minutes.
- Now ask the patient to fixate on a small red light that is about 2 inches above the test target. The patient is instructed to continue fixing on the red light, and report when he or she first sees the bars of the test target. Increase target intensity by rotating the knob on the side of the unit (which is calibrated in log units of light).

(continued)

How-To: Dark Adaptometry (Goldmann-Weekers Dark Adaptometer) (continued)

- When the patient reports seeing the bars, mark the score sheet and turn the light completely off. Repeat the process (increasing the target intensity, marking, and darkness) about once every 30 seconds for 30 minutes.

The Macular Photostress Test

- The macular photostress test determines how quickly vision recovers after an individual has been exposed to bright light.
- Reduced visual acuity is common to all individuals after exposure to very bright light; however, the sensation of reduced vision can be prolonged in those individuals who have macular disease.
- After exposure to a very bright light, visual recovery occurs as the visual pigments in the photoreceptors are resynthesized. In patients with macular disease, the resynthesis period is prolonged due to abnormality of the retinal pigment epithelium in the macular area.
- This test can also be quite useful in differentiating between optic nerve and macular pathology; those with optic nerve disease should have normal test results.
- The normal eye will recover in 30 to 50 seconds. In addition, the recovery rate in the two eyes should be similar.
- Each office should gather data from testing about 20 normal individuals to develop a normal response range for comparison with the tested patients.

How-To: Macular Photostress Test

- Document the patient's best vision prior to beginning the test.
- The patient should be seated in a dimly lit exam room. The eye not being tested should be covered. Set the eye chart to one line *larger* than the patient's best vision.
- Shine a bright light, either from a transilluminator or direct ophthalmoscope, into the patient's uncovered eye for 10 seconds.
- Turn off the light. Ask the patient to read the eye chart (at one line above the best vision) as soon as the vision has recovered enough to do so.
- Note the recovery time. Test the other eye.

The Potential Acuity Meter (PAM)

- The Potential Acuity Meter (Marco Ophthalmic Co, Jacksonville, Fla), commonly referred to as PAM, is a device used to estimate a patient's visual potential when his or her media is not clear.
- The PAM projects a Snellen chart directly onto the retina, bypassing any opacities in the media.
- Estimating visual potential may be very important, especially in an eye that has both opaque media and a history of such things as trauma or macular degeneration.
- Prior to cataract surgery on an eye that might not regain visual acuity, an estimate of postoperative potential is recommended.
- In some states Medicare requires a PAM test if the potential cataract surgery patient's vision is worse than 20/70.

How-To: PAM Test

- The most common PAM instrument attaches to a slit lamp. Ask the patient to place his or her forehead against the bar and chin in the chin rest.
- Dial in the patient's spherical equivalent refraction by rotating the knob on the side of the unit.
- Shine the red light into the patient's eye and ask whether or not the red light is visible. Then turn off the room light.
- Shine the white PAM light into the eye and ask whether or not the white light is seen. Make sure that the white light is over the pupil. Once the white light has been properly aligned over the patient's pupil, turn off the red light.
- Ask the patient to read the smallest figures possible. This is the PAM reading.

The Glare Test and Brightness Acuity Test (BAT)

- Individuals with early cataracts who do not have significantly reduced vision will, nonetheless, frequently complain of serious problems with glare.
- The glare test and the BAT (Marco Ophthalmic Co, Jacksonville, Fla) are methods of documenting the amount of visual debilitation resulting from glare.
- Such documentation may result in an insurance company's approval for cataract surgery in an eye with only a mild cataract.

How-To: Glare Test

- Record the patient's best-corrected vision in each eye in a darkened room. This is the "dimness" measurement.
- Record the patient's best-corrected vision in each eye in room light. This is the "room lighting" measurement.
- In room light, direct an additional light (as with a transilluminator) into the patient's eye at approximately a 20-degree angle horizontal to the pupil. Record the patient's best-corrected vision in each eye. This is the "brightness" measurement.

How-To: BAT

- Record the patient's best-corrected vision in each eye in a darkened room.
- Have the patient view the eye chart through the BAT. Cover the eye not being tested.
- Record the patient's vision through the BAT at each illumination level (low, medium, and high).

Contrast Sensitivity

- Snellen-type visual acuity charts use high-contrast black letters and shapes of specified sizes on white backgrounds.
- Many individuals with essentially normal Snellen acuity in the range of 20/40 or better may complain of poor vision. These individuals may have problems with contrast vision.
- The contrast sensitivity test comes in a variety of styles, but all consist of letters, objects, or gratings that are of graduated contrast. The patient is asked to identify the faintest object or grating on the chart.
- Contrast sensitivity function of the two eyes should be similar. If one eye has a contrast sensitivity curve that does not follow that of the other eye, the eye with the worse contrast sensitivity curve is probably abnormal.
- Contrast sensitivity testing should generally be evaluated over multiple visits.

How-To: Contrast Sensitivity Test

- The patient should wear his or her best spectacle correction (**untinted lenses**) and at the properly assigned distance. (Some tests are designed for near testing, while others are designed for distance testing.)
- Make sure that the lighting is appropriate to the test you are using. (Some contrast sensitivity tests actually come with light meters.)
- Test each eye separately. First show the patient the practice targets. Then ask the patient to identify the figure or grid direction from the most to the least possible. Encourage the patient to guess.
- Record the last correctly identified object, letter, or grating in the patient's chart.

Microbiology

- Microbiology is the study of extremely small sub-cellular, single-celled, or multi-celled organisms.
- Microorganisms are everywhere in the environment and some can cause eye disease (Tables 10-3 and 10-4).
- Proper identification of infectious ocular microorganisms is important in determining more appropriate treatment of the disease (Tables 10-5 and 10-6).
- Gram staining is used to identify bacteria. The Giemsa stain is used to detect inflammatory cells and inclusion bodies. Wright's stain also detects inflammatory cells.

How-To: Gram Stain

- Smear the specimen evenly on a clean, dry, glass microscope slide.
- Fix the smear by passing the slide through the flame of the Bunsen burner until the smear is dry, or by using a commercially available fixative.
- Cover the smear with a gentian violet solution for 1 minute, then rinse with gently running tap water.
- Cover the smear with Gram's iodine for 1 minute. After 1 minute, rinse the slide in running tap water, then decolorize with 95% ethyl alcohol (or acetone) until the color no longer bleeds off the section. (Decolorization may take about 20 seconds.)
- Wash the slide off with tap water and stain with 1% safranin for 3 minutes. Wash the slide again with tap water, blot gently, and allow to air dry. When observed under the microscope, gram-positive bacteria will stain dark blue and gram-negative bacteria will stain red.

Table 10-3.
Disease-Causing Antigens of the Eye

Viruses	Bacteria	Fungi	Chlamydia	Protozoa	Multi-Celled Parasites
Herpes simplex	*Cocci*	Candida	Inclusion conjunctivitis	Acanthamoeba	*Nematodes*
Herpes zoster	Gram-positive:	Fusarium	Trachoma	Toxoplasmosis	Toxocariasis
Adenovirus	Staphlycoccus	Aspergillus		Pneumocytosis	Onchocerciasis
	Streptococcus				Loiasis (Loa loa worm)
					Trichinosis
	Gram-negative:				Ancylostoma canimum
	Gonococcus				(possible cause of DUSN)
	(Neisseria gonorrhea)				*Cestodes*
	Meningococcus				Cysticicerosis
	(Neisseria meningitidis)				*Trematodes*
	Neisseria catarrhalis				Schistosmiasis seen
					primarily in developing countries
	Bacilli				
	Gram-positive:				
	Corynebacterium				
	Bacillus				
	Mycobacterium				
	Gram-negative:				
	Pseudomonas				
	Haemophilus				
	Moraxella				
	Spirilla				
	Treponema pallidum				
	(spirochette that causes syphilis)				

DUSN = diffuse unilateral subacute neuroretinitis

Reprinted with permission from Van Boemel GB. Special Skills and Techniques. *Thorofare, NJ: SLACK Incorporated;1999.*

Table 10-4.
Common Bacterial Ocular Infections

Organism	Microscopic Form	Gram Stain	Culture Medium	Colonies in Culture	Pathology	Potential Findings
Staphylococcus	Cocci in cluster, but may vary	+	Any nutrient	Opaque, round, smooth, raised, glistening, 1 to 2 mm diameter	Pyogenic, necrotizing	Blepharitis, hordeolum, conjunctivitis, keratitis, cellulitis
Streptococcus	Cocci in chains	+	Enriched (blood)	Pinpoint, grayish, 2 to 4 mm zone where blood in medium has been digested	Watery discharge, diffuse, spreads rapidly, often associated with injury	Cellulitis
S. pneumonia (pneumonia)	Lancet-shaped diplococci	+	Blood agar	Small, depressed in center, shiny, surrounded by zone of green	Stringy discharge, invasive, edema sudden onset	Hypopyon, keratitis, chronic dacrocystitis, conjunctivitis (acute)
Neisseria gonorrhoeae (VD)	Paired kidney-shaped intra-cellular organism	–	Chocolate or blood agar	Clear, glistening, large irregular edges	Purulent discharge, localized	Ophthalmia neonatorum, conjunctivitis, marginal corneal ulcer
Neisseria meningitidis	Small, paired	–	Chocolate or blood agar	Round, low, convex, glistening, gray or gray/blue tinge	Petechial or purpuric skin rash	Corneal ulcer
Neisseria catarrhalis	Paired	–	Chocolate or blood agar	White, smooth, and opaque	Normal throat species	Conjunctivitis
Corynebacterium	Slender rods in pairs or short chains	+	Blood agar, Tinsdale agar	Gray-black colonies with brown halo	Purulent discharge	Conjunctivitis
Bacillus	Long rods in chains	+	Blood agar	Flat & irregular, 4 to 5 mm in diameter, may have undulate margin	Associated with injury	Endophthalmitis
Mycobacterium	Typical rods	Acid fast	egg, Lowenstein-Jensen	Smooth/rough, pigmented or nonpigmented, (depends on species), generally slow-growing	Immune cell infiltrate	Conjunctivitis, corneal ulcer

(continued)

Table 10-4. (continued)
Common Bacterial Ocular Infections

Organism	Microscopic Form	Gram Stain	Culture Medium	Colonies in Culture	Pathology	Potential Findings
Pseudomonas	Single or pair, short chains or groups	–	Blood agar or fluid medium	Dark greenish-gray with zone of bluish-green Sweet hay-like odor	Purulent destructive necrosis	Severe hypopyon, keratitis, corneal abscess, cellulitis
Haemophilus	Tiny slender rod, no particular arrangement	–	Chocolate or blood agar	Pinpoint, translucent, glistening	Mucoid discharge	Conjunct-ivitis (epidemic)
Moraxella	Paired	–	Enriched blood	Small, pinpoint (less than 0.5 mm)	Subacute or chronic catarrhal	Conjunctivi-tis, endoph-thalmitis
Treponema pallidum (syphilis)	Slender, curved flagellated	Not used	No *in vitro* growth	None	3 stages	Primary: chancres Secondary: ulcerative blepharo-conjunc-tivis Tertiary: gummas

Reprinted with permission from Van Boemel GB. Special Skills and Techniques. *Thorofare, NJ: SLACK Incorporated; 1999.*

Table 10-5.
Stains

Stain	Indications	Notes
Giemsa	Cell stain, chlamydial inclusions	Takes about 1 hour
Wright	Inflammatory cells	Takes about 15 minutes
Gram	Bacteria	Gram-negative are red, gram positive are blue, all fungi are gram-positive
Methylene blue	Fungi	
Acid-fast	*Mycobacterium*	Acid-fast bacteria stain, a vivid red
India ink	*S. pneumoniae*	Viewed under dark illumination

Reprinted with permission from Ledford J. Certified Ophthalmic Medical Technologist Exam Review Manual. *Thorofare, NJ: SLACK Incorporated; 2000.*

Table 10-6.
Culture Media

Medium	Purpose
Blood agar plate	Aerobic and facultatively anaerobic bacteria; fungi
Chocolate agar plate	Aerobic and facultatively anaerobic bacteria; enhances the isolation of *Moraxella, Neissena, Hemophilus*
Sabouraud dextrose agar plate with chloramphenicol or gentamicin (50 g/mL of medium)	Fungi
Supplemented thioglycolate broth	Aerobic and anaerobic bacteria
Supplemental brain-heart infusion broth with gentamicin (50 g/mL of medium)	Fungi
Lowenstein-Jensen agar plate	*Mycobacteria, Nocardia*
Thayer-Martin agar plate	*Neisseria gonorrhoeae*

Reprinted from Nemeth SC, Shea CA. Medical Sciences for the Ophthalmic Assistant. *Thorofare, NJ: SLACK Incorporated; 1988, with permission from Sheila Nemeth and Carolyn Shea.*

How-To: Giemsa Stain

- Smear the specimen on a clean, dry slide. Let the specimen air dry.
- Fix the slide with an absolute methyl alcohol solution for 5 minutes.
- After the slide has been fixed, place it in a Coplin jar over a sink and flood it with working May-Grünwald stain. Let it stand in the stain for 6 minutes. The slide must be agitated in the solution every 30 seconds or so to ensure proper staining.
- Pour off the mixture and wash the slide in a phosphate buffer solution (6.8 pH) until no more color bleeds off.
- Place the slide in a working Giemsa stain for 13 minutes. The slide must be agitated in the solution to ensure proper staining.
- Rinse the slide again in a phosphate buffer until the slide no longer bleeds color and allow to stand in the phosphate solution for 3 minutes.
- Air dry the slide.

How-To: Wright's Stain

- Carefully place the specimen on a clean and dry slide. Allow the specimen to air dry.
- Cover the entire specimen with a small amount of Wright's stain (about 10 drops) and allow the stain to remain on the slide for 1 minute.
- After 1 minute, add the same amount of distilled water to the slide (about 10 drops) to create a stain and distilled water solution. The water and stain solution should remain on the slide for an additional 10 minutes.
- At the end of 10 minutes, drain off the solution from the slide and rinse in distilled water until the slide no longer bleeds.
- Allow the slide to air dry.

A-Scan Axial Length

- The A-scan axial eye length is a test used to measure the length of the eye.
- There are three A-scan methods used to measure the axial eye length: the immersion method, the slit lamp applanation method, and the hand-held applanation method.
- The transducer from the A-scan emits a parallel, point-like sound beam. The sound beam that is displayed on the monitor looks like a line with many spikes on it. The spikes represent different tissues in the eye.
- Inaccurate axial eye length calculations can result in an intraocluar lens (IOL) with the incorrect power being placed in the eye. This is a very serious complication of cataract surgery and may result in the patient having to undergo further surgery.
- The placement of the probe in relationship to the eye in axial eye length measurements is very important. The height of the spike is based not only on the presence of the interface, but also on how perpendicular the probe is to the tissues being examined.
- It is necessary to properly align the probe along the visual axis, because the power of the IOL is calculated so that the light is properly focused on the macula.
- The easiest way to determine if the probe alignment is accurate is to look at the echo patterns. The tissue spikes should be equally tall and sharp. The spikes behind the retinal spike will create a gradual downward slope. The space between the posterior lens and retina should be free of spikes.

How-To: A-Scan Biometry

Slit Lamp Applanation Technique:

- Anesthetize the eye and position the patient at the slit lamp.
- Instruct the patient to keep still and open the eyes wide (a fixation target helps).
- Move the probe toward the eye using the joystick.
- Gently rest the probe on the cornea without indenting it and without leaving a space between the probe tip and the cornea.
- View the patient's eye to verify correct position.
- View the monitor and adjust until appropriate echo spikes are visible.

Hand-Held Applanation Technique:

- Anesthetize the eye and position the patient at the slit lamp.
- Instruct the patient to keep still and open the eyes wide (a fixation target helps).
- Gently rest the probe on the cornea without indenting it and without leaving a space between the probe tip and the cornea. The probe must be kept perpendicular to the back of the eye, while at the same time aligning with the visual axis to the macula.
- View the monitor and adjust until appropriate echo spikes are visible.

IOL Calculations

- The eye length measurement is used in a mathematical formula to derive the power of the IOL that will be placed in the patient's eye after cataract extraction.
- There are several formulas for calculating IOL power. The formulas are available on computer programs, calculators, or the ultrasound unit itself.
- Be concerned if the axial eye length is under 22 mm or over 25 mm. Differences of more than 0.3 mm between the eyes are also suspect. If any of these situations occur, then the A-scan should be repeated.
- Be concerned (and probably repeat the reading) if the K readings are less than 40 D or greater than 47 D.
- Compare the K reading to the refractometric measurement. While some discrepancy may exist due to lenticular astigmatism, the K's and refraction should more or less agree in axis and cylinder amount.

Note: Because of the complex nature of the remaining tests, procedures will not be given.

Diagnostic A-Scan Ultrasonography

- Ocular ultrasonography is indicated for the evaluation of the eye with opacities where the view of either the anterior and posterior segments is limited, as well as in eyes with clear media where structures are apparently abnormal.
- The A-scan produces a one-dimensional view of the eye.
- Although the A-scan does not produce an image of the back of the eye, it can be quite useful in the evaluation of masses, detachments, etc.

Diagnostic B-Scan Ultrasonography

- Ocular ultrasonography is indicated for the evaluation of the eye with opacities where the view of either the anterior and posterior segments is limited, as well as in eyes with clear media where structures are apparently abnormal.
- In B-scan ultrasonography, the transducer oscillates back and forth, resulting in a two-dimensional picture that looks like a black and white photograph. The picture represents a "slice" through the portion of the eye being examined.
- In B-scan ultrasonography, the results allow for a topographic evaluation of the structures of the eye and orbit.
- Standardized echography consists of specific examination techniques that allow for the thorough evaluation of the eye.
- The probe has a specific orientation that is determined by a mark on the side of the probe. The white mark corresponds to the top of the echographic image that is displayed on the screen.
- The most common indication for B-scan ultrasonography is vitreoretinal disease.

Electrophysiology Testing

- Generally speaking, electrophysiologic tests are conducted to determine how well the visual system is functioning.
- The tests must be conducted using special computerized equipment and should be administered only by highly trained specialists.
- Electrophysiology tests are diagnostic in nature and are objective. The patient cannot fake the results of the tests since the patient cannot control electrical responses to the stimuli that are presented during the tests.
- The three main ocular electrophysiology tests are the electroretinogram, the electro-oculogram, and the visual evoked response (Table 10-7).

Table 10-7.

Electrophysiology Testing

I. Electroretinography (ERG, full field or standard)

Description	Indications	Notes
An objective test of retinal function Records a mass retinal response Records electrical responses from the retina to external stimulation by light of varying intensity A contact lens or other type of electrode is placed on the patient's eye	Detection and evaluation of hereditary and constitutional disorders of the retina: acquired color vision defects, retinitis pigmentosa, CRA occlusion, and CRV occlusion Rule out the retina as the level of blindness in cortical blindness, dyslexia, and hysteria	Individuals with focal retinal pathology will have normal full field ERG findings Use caution in epileptics Testing parameters can be modified so that either cone, rod, or cone and rod cells can be tested The test requires some cooperation on the part of the patient The ERG may not be suitable for young children who are not sedated

II. Electro-oculography (EOG)

Description	Indications	Notes
An indirect test to determine how well the retinal pigment epithelium (RPE) is functioning A qualitative test of RPE function An electrical recording of the standing potential of the eye Skin electrodes are placed at each canthi The patient watches alternating diodes Test is done in light and dark; result is an Arden (light/dark) ratio	Suspected retinal abnormalities Retinal dystrophy Retinitis pigmentosa Retinal toxicity: to medication to retained metallic foreign body Best's disease	The eye must be capable of full light adaptation Pupil must be dilated Requires good visual acuity Requires reasonable patient cooperation Useful where ERG is not sensitive enough to pick up early toxicities

III. Visual evoked response (VER)

Description	Indications	Notes
A response by the brain to a visual stimulus Skin electrodes are placed on the patient's scalp The patient is exposed to an alternating checkerboard pattern or flashing light The VER tests brain activity in the visual cortex Determines whether the visual system works well	Unexplained vision loss Evaluation of visual potential Evaluation of optic nerve disease Evaluation of visual cortex abnormality Differentiation of retinal versus visual pathway abnormalities	Does not indicate which part of the visual system is abnormal The VER pattern can only be recorded if the patient reliably watches the stimulus Use caution in epileptics

Unless otherwise noted, all text, tables, and figures are adapted or reprinted with permission from Van Boemel GB. Special Skills and Techniques. *Thorofare, NJ: SLACK Incorporated; 1999.*

CHAPTER 11

Visual Fields

Note: Because of the complexity of the subject and the format of this handbook, it is impossible to encompass the "how-to's" or finer nuances of visual field testing. We have tried to include here general guidelines, notes, and tables you might find useful.

Basics of Visual Field Testing

- Visual field refers to that portion of visual space that is visible to an individual at any given moment.
- Perimetry is the science of measuring the peripheral vision in order to determine the visual field.
- The visual field has been likened to an "island of vision in a sea of blindness." Drawing a "map" of the island of vision is the goal of perimetry.
- Automated machines may perform many aspects of perimetry, but a skilled, knowledgeable technician is still required for optimal results.
- Kinetic perimetry is a type of visual field test in which the boundaries of the visual field are determined by moving the test object while the patient's fixation is held steady.
- Static perimetry involves determining the sensitivity of a visual field point by using a test object of fixed size, keeping the stimulus on the point being tested (not moving, ie, static) and increasing its intensity until it is seen.
- Manual perimetry simply refers to the need for the perimetrist to perform all aspects of the test, including the placement and presentation of stimuli, recording of responses, and preparation of the results chart. The classic methods of manual perimetry are confrontation testing, the tangent screen, and the Goldmann perimeter.
- The incorporation of computer technology into a visual field test is known as automated perimetry.

- A moving (kinetic) test object of fixed size and intensity defines a boundary, and sensitivity within the boundary would be expected to be equal to or greater than that at the boundary. Boundaries of visual field areas of equal or greater sensitivity are known as isopters ("iso" = same). The isopters are labeled in a way that identifies the size and intensity of the object used to define them.
- Threshold for a given point is defined as that stimulus intensity (for an object of fixed size and duration of presentation) which has a 50% probability of being seen. One important consideration based on this definition is that it is possible to obtain a different answer each time threshold is determined.
- The apostilb (abbreviated as asb) is the unit used most in static threshold perimetry. The maximum stimulus intensity of the Humphrey Field Analyzer (Zeiss-Humphrey) is 10,000 asb.
- Although measured in apostilbs, it is not convenient to express threshold values in apostilbs. The scale used is the decibel (dB) scale, which measures how much the maximum available stimulus intensity was attenuated (dimmed) until threshold was determined.
- It is important to realize that the apostilb value expressed by the decibel number is relative to the maximum available stimulus intensity on a particular instrument and will thus vary from one perimeter to another if the maximum available stimulus intensities are different.

Table 11-1 relates decibels, apostilbs, and Goldmann equivalents.

Types of Visual Field Defects

Visual field loss means an alteration in the height and shape of the island of vision. Points in the field will show decreases in sensitivity from the levels they should have (alteration of height) and will not show the expected changes from neighboring points due to eccentricity (alteration of shape).

Defects can be characterized by the magnitude of their depth—those between 5 and 9 dB from expected are "shallow," 10 to 19 dB may be considered moderate, defects over 20 dB are deep, and thresholds less than the maximum available stimulus intensity are considered "absolute." It should be pointed out that the measurement of an absolute defect does not necessarily mean total loss of sensitivity—it only means that the machine was not capable of generating a stimulus bright enough to elicit a response.

Examples of focal visual field defects that could be seen in the central 30 degrees of a right eye are illustrated in Figure 11-1. Hemianopia is a special visual field term that refers to loss of one-half of the visual field in one or both eyes ("hemi" = half). Hemianopic defects are illustrated in Figure 11-2.

Table 11-1.

Decibel/Apostilb/Goldmann Equivalents

Intensity		**Actual Humphrey Test Stimulus Size**				
db	Asb	I	II	III	IV	V
0	10,000	III4e	IV4e	V4e		
1	7943	III4d	IV4d	V4d		
2	6310	III4c	III4c	V4c		
3	5012	III4b	IV4b	V4b		
4	3981	III4a	IV4a	V4a		
5	3162	II4e	III4e	IV4e	V4e	
6	2512	II4d	III4d	IV4d	V4d	
7	1995	II4c	III4c	III4c	V4c	
8	1585	II4b	III4b	IVb	V4b	
9	1259	II4a	III4a	IV4a	V4a	
10	1000	I4e	II4e	III4e	IV4e	V4e
11	794	I4d	II4d	IIi4d	IV4d	V4d
12	631	I4c	II4c	III4c	IV4c	V4c
13	501	I4b	II4b	III4b	IV4b	V4b
14	398	I4a	II4a	III4a	IV4a	V4a
15	316	I3e	II3e	III3e	IV3e	V3e
16	251	I3d	II3d	III3d	IV3d	V3d
17	200	I3c	II3c	III3c	IV3c	V3c
18	158	I3b	II3b	III3b	IV3b	V3b
19	126	I3a	II3a	III3a	IV3a	V3a
20	100	I2e	II2e	III2e	IV2e	V2e
21	79	I2d	II2d	III2d	IV2d	V2d
22	63	I2c	II2c	III2c	IV2c	V2c
23	50	I2b	II2b	III2b	IV2b	V2b
24	40	I2a	II2a	III2a	IV2a	V2a
25	32	I1e	II1e	III1e	IV1e	V1e
26	25	I1d	II1d	III1d	IV1d	V1d
27	20	I1c	II1c	III1c	IV1c	V1c
28	16	I1b	II1b	III1b	IV1b	V1b
29	13	I1a	II1a	III1a	IV1a	V1a
30	10		I1e	I2e	III1e	IV1e
31	8		I1d	I2d	III1d	IV1d
32	6		I1c	I2c	III1c	IV1c
33	5		I1b	I2b	III1b	IV1b
34	4		I1a	I2a	III1a	IV1a
35	3.2			I1e	I2e	III1e
36	2.5			I1d	I2d	III1d
37	2.0			I1c	I2c	III1c
38	1.6			I1b	I2b	III1b
39	1.3			I1a	I2a	III1a
40	1.0				I1e	I2e
41	0.8				I1d	I2d
42	0.6				I1c	I2c

(continued)

Table 11-1. (continued)

Decibel/Apostilb/Goldmann Equivalents

Intensity		Actual Humphrey Test Stimulus Size				
db	Asb	I	II	III	IV	V
43	0.5				I1b	I2b
44	0.4				I1a	I2a
45	0.32					I1e
46	0.25					I1d
47	0.20					I1c
48	0.16					I1b
49	0.13					I1a
50	0.10					I4e
51	0.08					I4d

Reprinted with permission from Choplin N, Edwards R. Visual Fields. *Thorofare, NJ: SLACK Incorporated; 1998.*

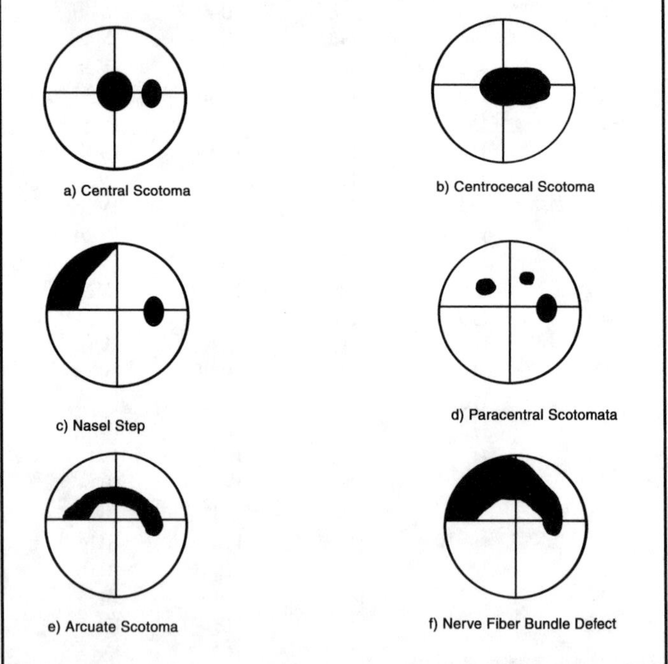

Figure 11-1. Types of monocular visual field defects (reprinted with permission from Choplin N, Edwards R. *Visual Fields*. Thorofare, NJ: SLACK Incorporated; 1998).

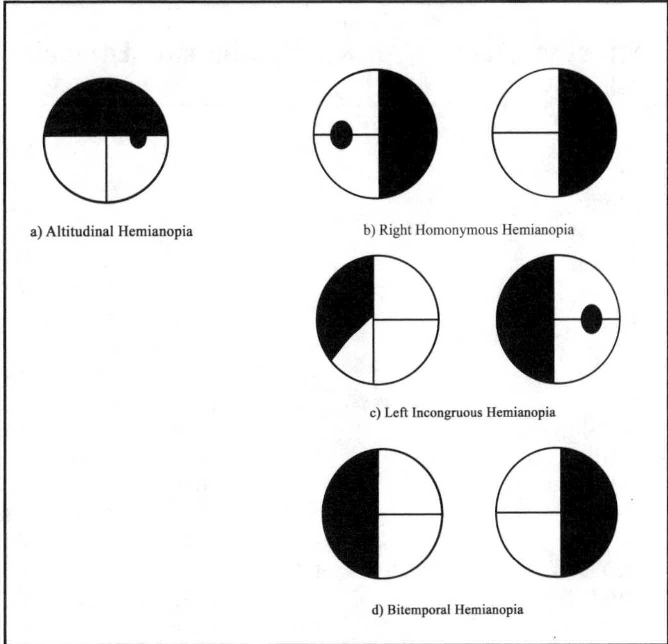

Figure 11-2. Hemianopic visual field defects (reprinted with permission from Choplin N, Edwards R. *Visual Fields*. Thorofare, NJ: SLACK Incorporated;1998).

Anatomic Basis for the Visual Field

Note: See also Chapter 1 and Figures 1-14 and 1-15.

- The anatomy of the visual system forms the basis for visual field defects.
- Since axons do not cross the horizontal raphe, lesions of the optic disc produce visual field defects that do not cross the horizontal meridian.
- Lesions in the visual pathway anterior to the optic chiasm produce monocular visual field defects; lesions of the chiasm, or posterior to it, produce visual field defects manifesting in both eyes.

Goldmann Perimetry

Table 11-2 shows the intensity values in apostilbs for all of the available Goldmann stimuli. Note that there may be more than one way to obtain a given stimulus intensity. The relative decibel scale is given in the table, with the reference (0 dB) being equal to 1000 asb. Intensity levels greater than 1000 asb are not available, as the bulb cannot be made any brighter. However, the use of stimuli larger than the size I is the same, in effect, as using a brighter bulb.

Table 11-2.

Effective Decibel/Apostilb/Goldmann Equivalents

db	Asb	0	I	II	III	IV	V
-20	100,000						V4e
-19	79,433						V4d
-18	63,096						V4c
-17	50,119						V4b
-16	39,811						V4a
-15	31,623					IV4e	V3e
-14	25,119					IV4d	V3d
-13	19,953					IV4c	V3c
-12	15,849					IV4b	V3b
-11	12,589					IV4a	V3a
-10	10,000				III4e	IV3e	V2e
-9	7943				III4d	IV3d	V2d
-8	6310				III4c	IV3c	V2c
-7	5012				III4b	IV3b	V2b
-6	3981				III4a	IV3a	V2a
-5	3162			II4e	III3e	IV2e	V1e
-4	2512			II4d	III3d	IV2d	V1d
-3	1995			II4c	III3c	IV2c	V1c
-2	1585			II4b	III3b	IV2b	V1b
-1	1259			II4a	IIi3a	IV2a	V1a
0	1000		I4e	II3e	III2e	IV1e	
1	794		I4d	II3d	III2d	IV1d	
2	631		I4c	II3c	III2c	IV1c	
3	501		I4b	II3b	III2b	IV1b	
4	398		I4a	II3a	III2a	IV1a	
5	316	04e	I3e	II2e	III1e		
6	251	04d	I3d	II2d	III1d		
7	200	04c	I3c	II2c	III1c		
8	158	04b	I3b	II2b	III1b		
9	126	04a	I3a	II2a	III1a		
10	100	03e	I2e	II1e			
11	79	03d	I2d	II1d			
12	63	03c	I2c	II1c			
13	50	03b	I2b	II1b			
14	40	03a	I2a	II1a			
15	32	02e	I1e				
16	25	02d	I1d				
17	20	02c	I1c				
18	16	02b	I1b				
19	13	02a	I1a				
20	10	01e					
21	8	01d					
22	6	01c					

(continued)

Table 11-2. (continued)

Effective Decibel/Apostilb/Goldmann Equivalents

db	Asb	0	I	II	III	IV	V
23	5	01b					
24	3	01a					

Dimmer stimuli may be obtained by use of the "bar" lever. Each bar attenuates the stimulus by two log units (reprinted with permission from Choplin N, Edwards R. Visual Fields. *Thorofare, NJ: SLACK Incorporated; 1998).*

Make sure the chart is properly positioned in its holder to ensure that the recorded points correspond to the position of the projected stimulus. The chart should be labeled with the patient's name and other identifying data, date of the examination, pupil size, distance refraction, and the near lens used for the central 30 degrees. The visual acuity and diagnosis, if known, may also be listed. Each isopter should be recorded using a different colored pencil. The standard color coding of isopters is given in Table 11-3.

The Armaly/Drance screening protocol (Figure 11-3) is excellent for visual field testing of glaucoma patients. It will elicit up to 90% of early glaucoma defects and will take 12 minutes or less in an eye with few defects, if performed properly. Although the Armaly/Drance screening was intended for glaucoma, similar techniques can be employed for patients with suspected or known neurological disease—the main difference is in the meridian explored for steps (horizontal for glaucoma, vertical for neurological).

How-To: Goldmann Perimetry

- Turn machine on and calibrate the stimulus intensity (once daily).
- Position the recording chart.
- Select the correcting lens according to the patient's distance refraction, combine with appropriate add power, and place in the lens holder.
- Instruct the patient as to the test procedures.
- Occlude the nontested eye and position the patient comfortably at the machine. Position the correcting lens as close to the eye as possible without touching the lashes.
- Calibrate the background illumination.
- Adjust the focus on the telescope so that the patient's eye is clearly seen. Note the pupil size.
- Using static techniques, determine the suprathreshold stimulus intensity at a point approximately 25 degrees temporal to fixation, slightly above or below the horizontal.

(continued)

How-To: Goldmann Perimetry (continued)

- Using this stimulus, kinetically map the blind spot and a central isopter.
- Perform static searches within the arcuate areas for scotomata.
- Map two additional kinetic isopters, one larger and one smaller than the initial.
- Verify all steps.
- Kinetically explore all missed static presentations to map any scotomata.
- Remove the correcting lens, determine a peripheral suprathreshold stimulus statically at 50 degrees, and map two to three peripheral isopters, verifying steps.
- Make sure all necessary information has been recorded on the chart.
- Test the other eye.

How-To: Patient Education for Goldmann Visual Fields

- This is a test of your side or peripheral vision.
- We test one eye at a time, so one eye will be covered.
- When we start the test, your chin will be in the cup and your forehead against this bar. Your job for the entire test is to look at this light in the middle. As you look in the center, another light will come on somewhere inside the bowl. When you first think you see the light, press this button.
- You will not see the target light all the time. Sometimes you may seem to go for a long time without seeing anything. Do not worry; just be patient until the light appears again. The main thing is not to look for the light. Always look right here in the center.
- Do not wait for the light to get all the way to you. Press the button when you first think you see it. Any areas that seem inconsistent will be rechecked.
- I have a little telescope on the other side of the machine, and I can see your eye. If I notice that you are looking around instead of at the center, I will remind you to look straight ahead.
- From time to time, you will feel your head move slightly as I keep your position adjusted.
- If you need to rest, let me know.
- Be sure not to stare. You can blink whenever you need to.
- If you are uncomfortable, let me know.

Table 11-3.
Isopter Color Coding

Isopter Name	Color
I1e	Yellow
I2e	Red
I3e	Green
I4e	Blue
II4e	Orange
III4e	Purple
IV4e	Brown
V4e	Black

Reprinted with permission from Choplin N, Edwards R. Visual Fields. *Thorofare, NJ: SLACK Incorporated; 1998.*

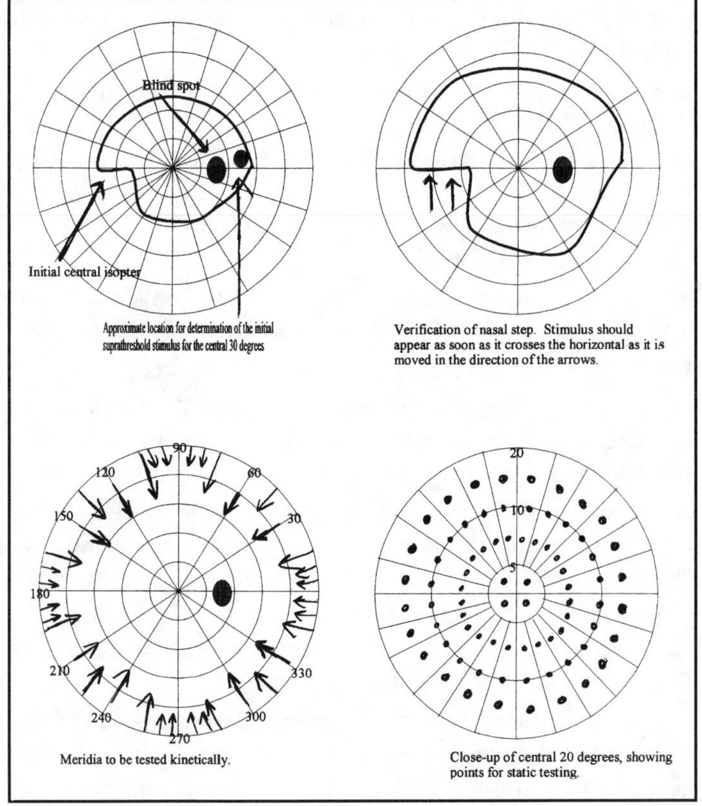

Figure 11-3. The Armaly/Drance screening technique. Top left: location of test point for initial stimulus, blindspot, and initial central isopter. Bottom left: meridia for kinetic testing. Top right: verification of nasal step. Bottom right: points for static testing within the central 20 degrees (reprinted with permission from Choplin N, Edwards R. *Visual Fields*. Thorofare, NJ: SLACK Incorporated; 1998).

Automated Perimetry

Note: Discussion pertains to the Humphrey Field Analyzer.

Most automated perimeters offer a wide variety of tests. It is recommended that the clinician review the available tests and strategies available for the machine being used and set up a user-defined menu (if that is an option) to meet the needs of the particular practice setting. Most practitioners will find that four or five examination options apply to the vast majority of clinical situations. Table 11-4 lists the type of patients commonly encountered in clinical practice and makes recommendations for appropriate tests from those available on the Humphrey Field Analyzer.

How-To: Automated Perimetry

- Pull patient's card from the file or create one if patient is new. Fill in all information.
- Check visual field order form for appropriate information, including refraction to be used.
- Set up machine for test using information on the patient data card and the order form. Place corrective lenses in holder, using age-appropriate add on top of specified distance prescription (see How-To: Select Lens Add). If dilated or aphakic, use +3.00 add.
- Position patient. Make sure table height and chin rest are adjusted properly. Ask if patient is comfortable and make appropriate corrections.
- Measure pupil size and record on the patient data screen.
- Enter patient information into machine, including refraction and pupil size. Make sure birth date and year are correct (do not enter *this* year!). Make sure patient's name is entered identically to previous tests.
- Instruct patient as to nature of test and its performance (see How-To: Patient Education for Automated Visual Fields). Read instructions to patient from machine. Make sure patient understands procedure, and answer any questions before proceeding.
- Make sure patient understands anticipated length of test and knows how to rest by holding down response button.
- Occlude untested eye, reposition patient, check position of corrective lens, recheck patient's position, make necessary adjustments, and proceed.
- Every 1 or 2 minutes, check patient fixation and position. Pause and make adjustments as necessary.

(continued)

How-To: Automated Perimetry (continued)

- **Never leave room for any reason while a test is being performed. Monitor patient and screen at all times.**
- Re-instruct patient every time a false positive or false negative response occurs, or if fixation deviation is noted. Offer periodic encouragement and reassurance. Advise when close to finished.
- **Save results.**
- Allow brief rest period and proceed with other eye. Go back to 3rd step.
- At conclusion of second eye's test, print results according to order form. Answer the questions at the bottom of the order form and make any comments deemed necessary. Place printouts and order form in the patient's chart.

Table 11-4.

Suggestions for Test Selection

Type of Patient	Test Type	Array	Strategy	Stimulus Size	Follow-Up
Routine examination, no complaints	Visual field testing not recommended	n/a	n/a	n/a	n/a
Complaints of loss of "side vision"	Screen	120 point	Three-zone or quantify defects	III	Threshold testing
Complaints of "spots" in central vision	Amsler grid	n/a	n/a	n/a	n/a
	30-2, 10-2	III	Full threshold	III	Overview, change analysis
Glaucoma—early to moderate	Threshold	30-2, 24-2	Full threshold	III	Glaucoma, change probability
Glaucoma—advanced	Threshold	30-2, 24-2	Full threshold	III, IV	Glaucoma, change probability

(continued)

Table 11-4. (continued)

Suggestions for Test Selection

Type of Patient	Test Type	Array	Strategy	Stimulus Size	Follow-Up
Glaucoma—end stage	Threshold	30-2, 24-2	Full threshold	V	Stimulus V overview
		10-2		III	Overview, change analysis
Neurologic: detection, asymptomatic patient	Screen	120 point	Quantity defects	III	Threshold test
Neurologic: detection, symptomatic patient	Threshold	30-2	Full threshold	III	Overview, change analysis
Neurologic: patient requiring serial examinations	Threshold	30-2	Full threshold	III	Overview, change analysis
Patients with Amsler grid defects	Threshold	10-2	Full threshold	III	Overview, change analysis
Monitoring patients at risk threshold for maculopathy (eg, drug toxicity)	Threshold	10-2	Full threshold	III white, red	Overview, change analysis
Any patient having difficulty with threshold test	Threshold	24-2	FASTPAC	III	Overview, change analysis
	Screen	76 point	Quantify defects	III	None available, can try threshold test next time *(continued)*

Table 11-4. (continued)

Suggestions for Test Selection

Type of Patient	Test Type	Array	Strategy	Stimulus Size	Follow-Up
Frail, infirm, disabled patients	Screen	76 point	Threshold related, three zone	III	None available

Reprinted with permission from Choplin N, Edwards R. Visual Fields. *Thorofare, NJ: SLACK Incorporated; 1998.*

How-To: Patient Education for Automated Visual Fields

- This is a test of your side or peripheral vision.
- We test one eye at a time, so one eye will be covered.
- When we start the test, your chin will be in the cup and your forehead against this bar. Your job for the entire test is to look at this light here in the middle. As you look in the center, another light will come on somewhere inside the bowl. When you first think you see this "extra" light, press this button.
- You will not see the extra light all the time. Sometimes you may seem to go for a long time without seeing anything. Do not worry; just be patient until the light appears again. The main thing is not to look for the light. Always look right here in the center.
- Do not wait and try to be sure whether you see the light or not. Press the button when you first think you see it. Any areas that seem inconsistent will be rechecked.
- I have a little screen that shows me your eye. If I notice that you are looking around instead of at the center, I will remind you to look straight ahead. If the machine catches you looking around, it will beep.
- From time to time you will feel your head move slightly as I keep your position adjusted.
- If you need to rest, hold down the response button.
- Be sure not to stare. You can blink whenever you need to.
- If you are uncomfortable, let me know.

Since a visual field test requires the patient to discern an often faint test object against a lighted background, the chances of the patient seeing the stimulus are increased if the stimulus is in focus. The simplest method for lens selection is to use the machine's automatic lens calculation feature, if available in the operating software. If the software does not allow automatic calculation, the lens must be calculated manually based on the distance prescription and the patient's age. How-To: Select Lens Add summarizes the steps used for selecting the trial lens, assuming a bowl size of 33 cm.

Save the results at the conclusion of the test, and print out the results according to clinician request. Table 11-5 lists the various printout options for central threshold tests using the Humphrey Field Analyzer.

How-To: Select Lens Add

- Ignore cylindrical powers of less than 0.25 diopters. Calculate spherical equivalent power for lenses with cylinder between 0.25 and 1.50 diopters (to calculate spherical equivalent power, add half the cylinder power to that of the sphere, then ignore the cylinder). Use the full cylinder for cylinders greater than 1.50 diopters. This determines the resultant lens.
- Determine the add required based on age or accommodation from the chart:

Patient's age	Add needed
<30	No add
30 to 39	+1.00
40 to 44	+1.50
45 to 49	+2.00
50 to 54	+2.50
>55	+3.00

aphakic, pseudophakic, or dilated (any age): +3.00

- Add the resultant distance lens to the age-required add. This is the lens to be used.

Reprinted with permission from Choplin N, Edwards R. Visual Fields. *Thorofare, NJ: SLACK Incorporated; 1998.*

Table 11-5.

Printout Options for the Humphrey Field Analyzer

Printout Types	Features
	Single Field Printouts
Value table	Numeric grid of threshold values
Defect depth (non-STATPAC)	Algebraic difference between measured threshold values and the *expected* normal values
Graytone	Graphic representation of the threshold values generated by assigning symbols of increasing darkness corresponding to decreasing sensitivity
Three-in-one (non-STATPAC)	Includes value table, defect depth, and graytone
Profile (non-STATPAC)	Static cut through a meridian specified by the operator
STATPAC (software option, two versions)	Includes standard value table and graytone, adds total deviation plot (algebraic difference between measured threshold values and an *age-corrected normal* database), pattern deviation plot (highlighting focal loss over diffuse loss), probability plots for observed deviation, visual field indices (mean deviation, pattern standard deviation, short-term fluctuation, corrected pattern standard deviation), and (in version B) the glaucoma hemifield test (designed to detect assymetric loss across the horizontal midline)
	Change Over Time Printouts (STATPAC Software Only)
Overview	Graytone, value table, total deviation probability plot, and pattern deviation probability plot displayed for up to 16 tests on a single printout printed in chronological order from earliest to most recent examination
Change analysis	Graphical representation of reduced data for all tests performed, includes "box plot" (a histogram of the total deviation plot) and plots of each of the four indices

(continued)

Table 11-5. (continued)

Printout Options for the Humphrey Field Analyzer

Printout Type	Features
Glaucoma probability plot (STATPAC II only)	Takes first two examinations as baseline and compares each subsequent examination to the baseline, showing numeric change of each point from baseline and compares the observed changes to a population of "clinically stable" glaucoma patients

Reprinted with permission from Choplin N, Edwards R. Visual Fields. *Thorofare, NJ: SLACK Incorporated; 1998.*

Errors in Visual Field Testing and How to Minimize Them (Table 11-6)

- Proper technique in visual field testing is essential to make sure that any detected defects are the result of disease and not due to an error in the performance of the test.
- Perimeters need to be calibrated on a regular basis to ensure that proper background and stimulus intensity levels are obtained.
- To avoid common errors, particular attention must be directed to the patient's pupil size, to the refractive error, and to the positioning of the correcting lens.

Table 11-6.

Errors in Visual Field Testing and How to Minimize Them

*Note: Starred items refer to automated perimetry.

Error: Miscalibration of Goldmann perimeter.
Description: The patient's sensitivity will be altered; standardization and reproducibility will be affected.
Notes: As long as the machine is set up properly, the ratio of stimulus to background will remain constant, even if the bulb is beginning to fail and the maximum intensity cannot reach 1000 asb.

*Error: Humphrey Field Analyzer bulb is no longer able to project a 10,000 asb stimulus.
Description: If the patient's sensitivities are reduced, the machine may not be capable of generating the required intensity values to test them.
Notes: This condition can be identified from a threshold test where the patient did not respond to the brightest stimulus available.

(continued)

Table 11-6. (continued)

Errors in Visual Field Testing and How to Minimize Them

*Error: Patient does not respond to brightest stimuli in automated testing.
Description: Patients with far-advanced disease may not have sufficient sensitivity remaining in their visual field to respond even to the brightest stimuli when the size is fixed at III. The nature of the loss cannot be discerned because the entire field is so depressed.
Notes: After determining that the patient is awake, alert, and understands how to perform the test, the technician should restart the test after changing to a larger stimulus size.

Error: Using the proper distance lens but forgetting to include the appropriate addition for the test distance.
Description: The undercorrection may result in apparent diffuse loss of sensitivity or in an abnormally low foveal threshold in a patient known to have good visual acuity and no macular pathology.
Notes: Always use the most recent distance refractometry measurement. Ideally, visual acuity should be checked with this measurement prior to field testing to verify.

Error: Correcting lens improperly positioned too far from patient's eye.
Description: Ring scotoma.
Notes: More common in patients requiring significant hyperopic correction.

Error: Correcting lens improperly positioned too high relative to patient's eye.
Description: Inferior visual field defect that respects the horizontal midline may be created. This defect may be distinguished by its characteristic shape (corresponding to the shape of the lens holder), its lack of connection to the blind spot, and its disappearance when the lens is positioned properly.
Notes: More common in patients requiring significant hyperopic correction.

*Error: The present year is entered in lieu of the patient's correct birth year.
Description: STATPAC compares the patient to an age-matched population of 100-year-olds.
Notes: Comparing a patient to an older population will make the deviations appear smaller, since the comparison threshold values are lower. Care must be taken when entering the patient information in the machine to avoid this sort of error.

*Error: Failing to enter the patient's name the same way every time.
Description: The computer will fail to find all of the patient's examinations for overview, change, or STATPAC analysis.
Notes: Joe Smith, Joseph Smith, and Joe E. Smith are all different patients as far as the machine is concerned. The later versions of the operating software for the perimeter allow the technician to recall patient data from disk files. This option ensures that there will be no variations in the patient's name or birth date.

(continued)

Table 11-6. (continued)

Errors in Visual Field Testing and How to Minimize Them

Error: Patient has prominent superior orbital ridges or ptotic eyelid.
Description: This will often manifest superior visual field depressions that may appear to be a superior arcuate scotoma.
Notes: This type of defect can be properly identified by its lack of connection to the horizontal midline and the blind spot, as well as by correlation with the appearance of the patient. Repeat the examination with the lid taped up or with the patient's head tilted back from the headrest in order to roll the eye down. (Taping is preferred, since rolling the eye down may result in further lowering of the upper lid.)

Error: Pupils of less than 2 mm.
Description: Small pupils result in a uniform (with regard to eccentricity) diffuse depression.
Notes: It is recommended that pupils of less than 2 mm be dilated (if safe to do so). Remember to check the distance refraction after dilation and to test with the full add (+3.00) for the test distance regardless of the patient's age, since a dilated patient has minimal or no accommodative ability.

*Error: A high rate of false positive responses.
Description: The Humphrey Field Analyzer will periodically move the projector and open the shutter without projecting a stimulus. If the patient pushes the response button to this nonprojected stimulus, it will be recorded as a false positive response.
Notes: A high false positive rate makes the measured field look better than it really is. The patient may be "button-happy," may be responding to the sound instead of the stimulus, may be worried about being blind and thus over-responding, or may not understand the test. Re-educate.

*Error: A high rate of false negative responses.
Description: Failure to respond to the brightest stimulus in an area previously determined to have some sensitivity is a false negative response.
Notes: In general, a high false negative rate (greater than 20%, although the machine defaults to 33%) makes the field look worse than it really is. High false negatives may indicate lack of attentiveness, fatigue, or "hypnosis." Pause the test if necessary to allow rest.

*Error: High fixation loss rate.
Description: During the test, stimuli are periodically projected into the center of the previously mapped blind spot. A patient response to this stimulus presentation is presumed to have resulted from a shift of fixation.
Notes: Although a high fixation loss rate may indicate poor fixation behavior and unreliability, fixation deviations should also be monitored by the technician through the telescope or video eye monitor. The loss could actually be due to a blind spot that is smaller than the stimulus, as well as incorrect location of the blind spot or a shift in the patient's position after the test has started.

Unless otherwise noted, all text, tables, and figures are adapted or reprinted with permission from Choplin N, Edwards R. Visual Fields. *Thorofare, NJ: SLACK Incorporated; 1998.*

CHAPTER 12

Motility and Strabismus

Anatomy

There are nerves from your brainstem, the part below the thinking cerebrum, called cranial nerves (CN). The 12 CNs are responsible for various duties, both motor and sensory, that help with basic functions. The CNs that are responsible for ocular movements are III (oculomotor nerve), IV (trochlear nerve), and VI (abducens nerve).

The bony orbit provides an anchor for the extraocular muscles (EOMs). The superior orbital fissure is an opening at the back of the orbit. Nerves to the EOMs and globe enter the orbit through this fissure (see Chapter 1 for more on ocular anatomy).

The annulus of Zinn is a ring of connective tissue attached to the inside of the orbital apex. The EOMs, except the inferior oblique (IO), attach and originate at the annulus of Zinn and course forward through orbital tissue to attach to the globe. Each muscle turns into a tendon that attaches to the globe (Table 12-1). The muscle fibers are in a constant state of readiness, or tonus. When the head is erect, the eye sits in the orbit with the fovea pointed straight ahead at the horizon and assumes the primary position. The visual axis is the imaginary line between the fovea and the object of regard.

Function

The sophistication of our EOMs allows for many different kinds of eye movements. Moving the eyes enables the field of view to increase and allows the fovea, the small region of best vision, to move. Our eyes can involuntarily follow a slow-moving object (smooth pursuit), or they can voluntarily jump from one object of regard to another (saccade). Once we are viewing the new object, our eyes maintain fixation by constantly readjusting so that the object remains on the foveas (microsaccades). Vergence movements allow both foveas to maintain fixation at the same time (bifoveal fixation). The rewards of maintaining bifoveal fixation are binocular vision and stereopsis.

Table 12-1.
Muscle Information

Muscle	Length	Limbus to Insertion	Muscle Plane Angle (degrees)	Innervation
MR	41 mm	5.5 mm	0	CN III
LR	40.5 mm	7.0 mm	0	CN VI
SR	42 mm	7.7 mm	23	CN III
IR	40 mm	6.5mm	23	CN III
SO	59.5 mm*	13.8/18.8 mm	54	CN IV
IO	37 mm	17 mm	51	CN III

**SO total length, 19.5 mm of it is tendon*

Adapted with permission from Hansen V. A Systematic Approach to Strabismus. *Thorofare, NJ: SLACK Incorporated; 1998.*

Table 12-2 shows the actions and testing positions for each EOM. The mnemonic "SIN RAD" will help you remember the torsional and horizontal actions of the cyclovertical muscles. "SIN" means that the Superior muscles INtort; so, by process of elimination, the two inferior muscles must extort. "RAD" means that the Recti muscles ADduct (so the obliques must ABduct).

Duction is movement of one eye. Version is movement of both eyes in the same direction. The agonist muscle is the prime mover for a desired direction of gaze. The antagonist muscle of the same eye works directly against the agonist. A muscle in the same eye that helps another muscle accomplish a particular action is called a synergist muscle. Table 12-3 shows the synergist-antagonist relationship between the six EOMs.

Yoke muscles are pairs of muscles (one in each eye) that work together to achieve a desired version movement (Figures 12-1 and 12-2). Two basic laws govern how innervation is supplied to an agonist, its antagonist, and yoke. Sherrington's law of reciprocal innervation applies to the agonist and antagonist of one eye. Every unit of innervation to the agonist is accompanied by a reciprocal amount of relaxation to the antagonist muscle. Hering's law of simultaneous innervation applies to the yoke muscles of each eye. The fixing eye determines how much innervation goes to the agonist of that eye; an equal amount of innervation then goes to its yoke in the other eye.

Examination

- Visual maturity commonly occurs at 9 years of age.
- Exam pollution is avoided by conducting the exam in a systematic order: history, fusion, alignment, and (finally) vision. (Exam protocol, history taking, and vision testing are covered in Chapter 8.)

Table 12-2.
Muscle Actions

Muscle	Actions: 1°/2°/3°	Test
MR	Only ADDucts	ADDuction
LR	Only ABDucts	ABDuction
SR	Elevation/intorsion/ADDuction	Up/out
IR	Depression/extorsion/ADDuction	Down/out
SO	Intorsion/depression/ABDuction	Down/in
IO	Extorsion/elevation/ABDuction	Up/in

Reprinted with permission from Hansen V. A Systematic Approach to Strabismus. *Thorofare, NJ: SLACK Incorporated; 1998.*

Table 12-3.
Synergists/Antagonists

Muscle	Synergists	Antagonists
MR	SR, IR	LR, SO, IO
LR	SO, IO	MR, SR, IR
SR	Elevation: IO	IR, SO
	Intorsion: SO	IR, IO
	ADDuction: MR, IR	LR, SO, IO
IR	Depression: SO	SR, IO
	Extorsion: IO	SR, SO
	ADDuction: MR, SR	LR, SO, IO
SO	Intorsion: SR	IO, IR
	Depression: IR	SR, IO
	ABDuction: LR, IO	MR, SR, IR
IO	Extorsion: IR	SO, SR
	Elevation: SR	IR, SO
	ABDuction: LR, DO	MR, SR, IR

Reprinted with permission from Hansen V. A Systematic Approach to Strabismus. *Thorofare, NJ: SLACK Incorporated; 1998.*

RSR LIO RIO LSR
RLR LMR RMR LLR
RIR LSO RSO LIR

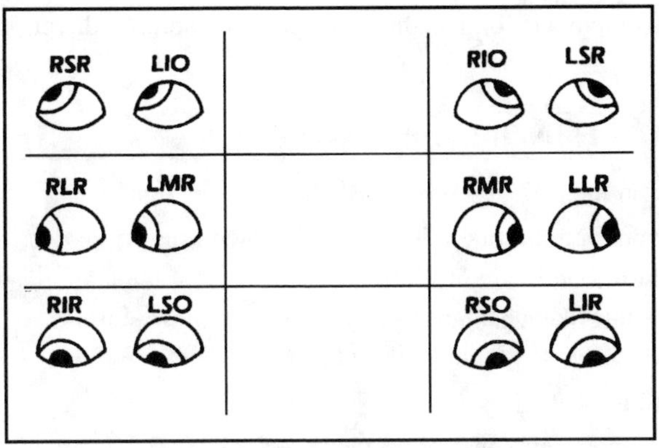

Figure 12-1. Pairs of yoke muscles responsible for moving eyes into various positions of gaze (reprinted with permission from Hansen V. *A Systematic Approach to Strabismus*. Thorofare, NJ: SLACK Incorporated; 1998).

Figure 12-2. Schematic drawing of muscles responsible for moving eyes into tertiary positions (reprinted with permission from Hansen V. *A Systematic Approach to Strabismus.* Thorofare, NJ: SLACK Incorporated; 1998).

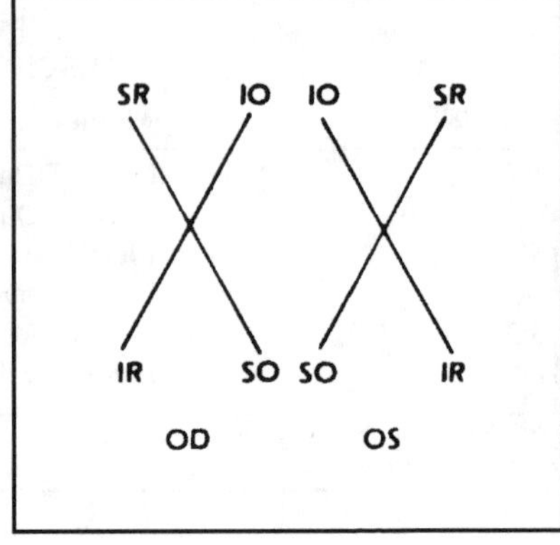

History

It is our job to narrow down the differential diagnosis by asking pertinent history questions. The pertinent questions are the ones your doctor would like you to ask. Only ask the questions you must, and be extremely specific. Use common language. Determine whether the problem is visual, symptomatic, cosmetic, or a combination of these. Symptomatic history has two categories: behavior that is observed (Table 12-4) and symptoms that the child complains about (Table 12-5). Typical questions to ask an adult are detailed in Table 12-6.

Fusion

Sensory fusion is the blending of two images, one from each eye, into a single image in the brain. Motor fusion is the effort put forth by the brain and oculomotor system to align the eyes so as to be able to achieve sensory function. There are three main methods of measuring sensory fusion: stereo tests, Worth 4 dot, and haploscopic devices such as the synoptophore and troposcope.

Alignment

A patient's strabismic deviation has three components: control, direction, and size.

How-To: Worth 4 Dot

- Place the glasses on the patient with the red lens over the right eye.
- Hold the light at near (about one-third of a meter) with the white dot at the bottom, and turn it on.
- Ask the patient to describe what he or she sees; what color the circles are, how many of each color, and their position.
- Move to 6 meters. Repeat.
- Record responses. Interpretations are provided in Table 12-7.

Table 12-4.

Observed Behavior	Potential Diagnosis
Holding objects close/sitting near the TV	Myopia
Intermittent crossing, especially at near	Hyperopia/accommodative esotropia
Tearing/discharge in infant/baby	Nasolacrimal duct obstruction
Tearing/photophobia/large eyes	Congenital glaucoma
Head positioning	Null point for nystagmus
Turning face to one side	Lateral incomitance (Duane's syndrome/VI nerve palsy)
Tilting head to one side	IV nerve palsy
Tipping chin up	Avoiding upgaze (Brown's syndrome/ double elevator palsy/A or V pattern)
Tipping chin down	Avoiding downgaze (A or V pattern)
Headache, diplopia, tires when reading	Convergence insufficiency

Reprinted with permission from Hansen V. A Systematic Approach to Strabismus. *Thorofare, NJ: SLACK Incorporated; 1998.*

Table 12-5.

Typical Childhood Complaints	Potential Cause
Blurry: distance only	Myopia
near only	Extreme hyperopia or convergence insufficiency
both	Astigmatism, malingering, or amblyopia
Headache	Any phoria with poor fusional amplitudes Convergence insufficiency
Diplopia	Any intermittent deviation with poor control Recent appreciation of physiologic diplopia
Strabismus without diplopia	Any tropic or intermittent deviation with suppression
Eyes hurt	Any of the above plus foreign body
Eyes tear while reading	Convergence insufficiency

Reprinted with permission from Hansen V. A Systematic Approach to Strabismus. *Thorofare, NJ: SLACK Incorporated; 1998.*

Table 12-6.

Adult Strabismus History Questions

Is the Patient's Complaint Visual or Cosmetic?

Visual history questions:

Diplopia: Monocular or binocular?

Ask: If you cover the right eye, does the double vision go away? If you then cover only the left eye, does the double vision go away? (Binocular diplopia exists if the patient answered *yes* to both questions. Monocular diplopia exists if the double vision persists with one eye covered.)

(continued)

Table 12-6. (continued)

Adult Strabismus History Questions

Is the Patient's Complaint Visual or Cosmetic?

If binocular diplopia, ask:

When did it start? Is it getting better or worse? Were there any precipitating factors: illness, trauma, disease? What makes it worse/better? Are the images horizontal, vertical, torsional, or combination? Are your glasses different or new? (Check for new prism or forgotten prism.)

Eye strain, pain, headache:

Ask: When? After what visual task? What job do you do with your eyes? Do you wake up with it? (Probably not visual.)

Blurry:

Ask: Same as above. Also: does the blurring come and go, like a camera going in and out of focus? Do you ever see double? What happens if you only use one eye? (May not be binocularly related.)

Reprinted with permission from Hansen V. A Systematic Approach to Strabismus. *Thorofare, NJ: SLACK Incorporated; 1998.*

Table 12-7.

Worth 4 Dot (Red Lens Over Right Eye)

Response	Means	Record as
4 lights: 1 red/3 green, 2 red/2 green	Fusion in ortho patient ARC in tropic patient	Fuse
2 red lights only	Left *green* eye suppressing	OS suppress
3 green lights only	Right *red* eye suppressing	OD suppress
2 reds, then 3 greens not at the same moment	Alternate suppression	Alt suppress
2 reds seen to the right of the 3 greens	Uncrossed (homonymous) diplopia NRC in ET patient ARC if not ET	Unc diplopia
2 reds seen to the left of the 3 greens	Crossed (heteronymous) diplopia NRC in XT patient ARC if not XT	X ed diplopia

Reprinted with permission from Hansen V. A Systematic Approach to Strabismus. *Thorofare, NJ: SLACK Incorporated;1998.*

Control is tested by the cover-uncover test. This is generally done during a routine eye exam by the single cover test, which determines the presence of a phoria, tropia, or intermittent tropia. The patient must maintain fixation on a target by attempting to identify small objects. Table 12-8 shows possible movement responses when the right eye is cover-uncovered. Table 12-9 is a similar algorithm for the left eye.

Table 12-8.

Cover-Uncover Right Eye—Test Requires Central Vision in Each Eye

If, when covering OD:	This means:	If, when uncovering OD:	This means:
1. OS doesn't move	OS was fixing	A. OD doesn't move either	Either ortho *or* R tropia
		B. OD moves *in*	OD was *out*—exophoria
		C. OD moves *out*	OD was *in*—esophoria
		D. OD moves *down*	OD was *up*—hyperphoria or DVD*
		E. OD moves *up*	OD was *down*—hypophoria
		F. Combined horizontal and vertical movement	
2. OS moves *in*	OS was *out* (LXT)	A. OD doesn't move now	Alternating XT
		B. OD moves back in to fix	LXT, prefers OD
3. OS moves *out*	OS was *in* (LET)	A. OD doesn't move now	Alternating ET
		B. OD moves back out to fix	LET, prefers OD
4. OS moves *down*	OS was *up* (LHT)	A. OD doesn't move	LHT, which alternates now
		B. OD moves back up to fix	LHT, prefers OD
5. OS moves *up*	OS was *down* (LhyptoT)	A. OD doesn't move	RHT, which alternates now
		B. OD moves back down to fix	RHT, prefers OD
6. Combination of moves	Combined horizontal/vertical	A. Combination	
7. OS has unsteady fixation	Latent nystagmus		

**Dissociated vertical deviation.*

Reprinted with permission from Hansen V. A Systematic Approach to Strabismus. *Thorofare, NJ: SLACK Incorporated; 1998.*

Table 12-9.

Cover-Uncover Left Eye—Test Requires Central Vision in Each Eye

If, when covering OS:	This means:	If, when uncovering OS:	This means:
1. OD doesn't move	OD was fixing	A. OS doesn't move either	Either ortho *or* L tropia
		B. OS moves *in*	OS was *out*—exophoria
		C. OS moves *out*	OS was *in*—esophoria
		D. OS moves *down*	OS was *up*—hyperphoria or DVD*
		E. OS moves *up*	OS was *down*—hypophoria
		F. Combined horizontal and vertical movement	
2. OD moves *in*	OD was *out* (RXT)	A. OS doesn't move now	Alternating XT
		B. OS moves back in to fix	RXT, prefers OS
3. OD moves *out*	OD was *in* (RET)	A. OS doesn't move now	Alternating ET
		B. OS moves back out to fix	RET, prefers OS
4. OD moves *down*	OD was *up* (RHT)	A. OS doesn't move	RHT, which alternates now
		B. OS moves back up to fix	RHT, prefers OS
5. OD moves *up*	OD was *down* (RhyptoT)	A. OS doesn't move	LHT, which alternates now
		B. OS moves back down to fix	LHT, prefers OS
6. Combination of moves	Combined horizontal/vertical	A. Combination	
7. OD has unsteady fixation	Latent nystagmus		

**Dissociated vertical deviation.*

Reprinted with permission from Hansen V. A Systematic Approach to Strabismus. *Thorofare, NJ: SLACK Incorporated; 1998.*

Table 12-10.
Strabismus Abbreviations

Tropia	T
Intermittent tropia, add ()	(T)
Phoria, drop T	
Esodeviation	E
Exodeviation	X
Hyperdeviation, add R or L eyeH	RH or LH
Hypodeviation, add R or L hypo	R hypo or L hypo
Dissociated vertical deviation,	DVD
add R or L eye	R DVD or L DVD
Near, add prime'	ET'
Examples:	
Left exotropia	LXT
Right hypertropia	RHT
Left dissociated vertical deviation	L DVD
Esophoria at near	E'
Right hypotropia at distance	R hypoT
Intermittent exotropia at near	X (T)'

Reprinted with permission from Hansen V. A Systematic Approach to Strabismus. *Thorofare, NJ: SLACK Incorporated; 1998.*

Direction of the strabismus is determined by the direction of movement of the eye during cover measurements. An eye that moves out to fixate must have been in (eso) under the cover. An eye that moves in must have been out (exo), up must have been down (hypo), and down must have been up (hyper). Useful abbreviations are shown in Table 12-10.

The most accurate means of measuring the *size* of the deviation is with prisms. Table 12-11 gives useful details about various measuring tests. While it is the least sophisticated, one may use the Hirschberg test to evaluate the deviation without prisms by viewing the light reflex from both eyes. The position of the reflex can also be measured with prisms via the Krimsky technique. (How-To's for Hirschberg and Krimsky are found in Chapter 8.)

How-To: Prism and Cover Measurements

- Direct patient to look at 20/40 or smaller size targets. During the test, direct the patient to read different lines of letters so that accommodation continues.
- Select a prism that is the estimated size of the deviation. Hold it over one eye with the *apex* pointing in the direction of the deviation.
- Place the cover alternately over each eye, never allowing the eyes to fuse together, and watch for movement. *(continued)*

How-To: Prism and Cover Measurements (continued)

- If there is no movement, record this prism power as the measurement of the deviation.
- If the deviation is smaller but still present, select a stronger prism. If the deviation has changed to the opposite direction (ie, an eso has now become an exo), select a weaker prism. Continue until there is no movement.
- If a horizontal deviation has been neutralized but vertical movement remains, add base up or down prism to the horizontal prism and neutralize the vertical deviation.

Notes:

- If the eyes make an extra back and forth movement—a redress movement—each time the cover is moved, neutralization is estimated to be when the movement is equal in each direction.
- Split prisms rather than stacking them.
- This test requires steady fixation with either eye and cannot be used on infants or some very young children.
- If one eye is restricted, the test may be modified by placing the prism over the restricted "frozen" eye.

Table 12-11.
Measurement Requirements

Test	Vision	Retinal Correspondence	Patient Cooperation	Fixation Distance	Target
Hirschberg	In one eye	Not required	Needs to fixate	Near test	Accommodative
Krimsky	In one eye	Not required	Fixate, prism near face	Near test and distance estimate	Accommodative
Prism and cover	In each eye	Not required	Fixate, prism and cover near face	Near test and distance test	Accommodative
Maddox rod	In each eye	Normal	Fixate, prism near test and Maddox rod near face, comprehension	Distance test awkward	Non-accommodative

Reprinted with permission from Hansen V. A Systematic Approach to Strabismus. *Thorofare, NJ: SLACK Incorporated; 1998.*

Table 12-12.
Fusion Tests

Tests for sensory fusion:
- Stereo tests
- Worth 4 dot
- Haploscopic devices (synoptophore, troposcope, amblyoscope)
- Red filter

Tests for stereo acuity:
- Titmus
- Randot
- Random dot E
- Lang

Exclusive motor fusion tests:
- Vergence amplitudes (convergence or divergence)
- 4 diopter base-out prism

Binocularity

Binocularity is a broad term that refers to the use of the two eyes together, either correctly (normally) or incorrectly (abnormally or anomalously). Normal binocularity results in comfortable three-dimensional vision, or stereopsis. True stereopsis is the three-dimensional vision that you can have only with normal binocularity and normal vision. Fusion is a type of binocularity in which the blending of two images, one from each eye, creates a single image in the brain.

There are two types of fusion—sensory and motor. Sensory fusion is the fusion that occurs in your brain. Motor fusion is the coordinated eye movements that are performed in order to maintain sensory fusion. Existence of good motor fusion generally means that there is good sensory fusion. The converse is not true—excellent sensory fusion does not automatically mean excellent (or even adequate) motor fusion. Table 12-12 lists tests for sensory fusion (some of which are also stereo tests), tests for stereo acuity, and tests used exclusively for evaluating motor fusion. Stereo testing is covered in Chapter 8.

Differential Diagnosis

A working differential diagnosis begins with a thought process that leads an examiner through the exam to a final diagnosis. The patient's history, appearance, and age provide the first clues. Tables 12-13 through 12-26 address the different types of strabismus by listing a tentative diagnosis, and the additional history that will be helpful to secure the diagnosis, along with the appropriate tests (and their results) that will clinch the diagnosis. Types of strabismus surgery are detailed in Table 18-7.

Table 12-13.

Esodeviations

Tentative diagnosis:	
1. Infantile ET	
a. Additional history:	
Onset before 6 months	
Fixates with either eye	
Constant ET	
b. Test:	Indicates:
ABDuction	Reluctant but intact
Measurements	Large ET, frequent V pattern
Cross-fixates	Equal vision
Cycloplegic refraction	Small refractive error
Versions	Possible inferior oblique (IO) overaction
Cover-uncover	Possible DVD
2. Accommodative ET	
a. Additional history:	
E(T), N>D	
Eye preference	
Worse when tired, concentrating	
Typical age of onset 18 months to 3 years	
Range of onset 7 months to 10 years	
b. Test:	Indicates:
P + C, cc + sc	Accommodative component
Cycloplegic refraction	< 4 D hyperopia, usually high AC/A
	>4 D hyperopia, usually normal AC/A
Fusion, cc	Usually excellent
Vision	Frequent amblyopia
3. LR palsy (CN VI)	
a. Additional history:	
Severe head and neck trauma	
ET greater to right gaze, left gaze, or both sides	
Head position to left or right	
Variable horizontal diplopia, worse at distance	
Sudden onset of ET/diplopia	
Present since birth if congenital	
Associated with facial nerve palsy (Moebius or brainstem tumor)	
Associated with ear pain (Gradenigo)	
Worsens with fatigue (myasthenia gravis)	
b. Test:	Indicates:
Fusion using head position	Recent onset
Measurements	ET > right and/or left gaze
	ET D > N, slight A tendency

(continued)

Table 12-13. (continued)
Esodeviations

Measure with OD, OS fix	Primary/secondary deviation
Versions/ductions, saccades	Decreased LR function
Diplopia testing	Horizontal, incomitant Young child may suppress
Vision	Possible amblyopia if early onset
Forced ductions	Negative unless very longstanding with resultant MR contracture
4. Duane's retraction syndrome type I	
a. Additional history:	
No trauma	
Lid fissure changes with gaze	
Abnormal head position	
Present since birth	
b. Test:	Indicates:
Versions/ductions	No ABDuction, lid fissure narrows during ADDuction
Fusion with head position	Frequently fuses
Vision	Possible amblyopia
5. Consecutive ET	
a. Additional history:	
Previous surgery for XT	
b. Test:	Indicates:
Fusion with ET corrected	Usually fuses if X or X(T) preop
6. Nystagmus compensation syndrome	
a. Additional history:	
Nystagmus during ABDuction	
Large ET present since birth	
Cross fixates, turns head to see	
b. Test:	Indicates:
Krimsky	Overconverges with correcting prism
Versions/ductions	Jerk nystagmus in ABDuction, both eyes
Cross-fixation	Does not move fixing eye out of ADDucted position to midline
7. Cyclic ET	
a. Additional history:	
24-, 48-, or 96-hour schedule or alternation between ET one cycle and straight next cycle	
Fairly sudden onset during childhood	
b. Test:	Indicates:
ET day: Fusion	Initially may have diplopia, then suppression/ARC
P + C	Large ET, usually comitant

(continued)

Table 12-13. (continued)

Esodeviations

Straight day: Fusion	Excellent
P + C	Ortho or small esophoria
Vision	May have amblyopia eventually
8. Strabismus fixus	
a. Additional history:	
Longstanding ET	
b. Test:	Indicates:
Forced ductions	Positive MR tightening
Measurements	Large ET, greater in R and L gaze
Versions/ductions	Decreased ABDuction, fixed ADDuction
Vision	Must cross-fixate and turn head to see
9. Divergence paralysis	
a. Additional history:	
General health: Normal intracranial pressure	
Infections, parasites, and travel abroad	
Possible trauma	
b. Test:	Indicates:
Divergence amplitudes	Nearly nonexistent
Version/ductions	Full, ABDuction okay
Diplopia testing	Uncrossed, worse at distance
Measurements	Comitant esodeviation D > N
Fusion	May fuse at near
Vision	Equal
10. Accommodative effort syndrome	
a. Additional history:	
Near asthenopia, blurring, or diplopia	
b. Test:	Indicates:
NPA	Normal
P + C	E', possible E(T)'
Divergence amplitudes	Poor
Plus lenses for near	Helps relieve symptoms
11. Pseudo ET	
a. Additional history:	
Onset: usually since birth	
Appears incomitant	
b. Test:	Indicates:
Hirschberg/cover-uncover/cross-cover	No deviation
External	Frequently has epicanthal folds
Angle kappa	Negative
Fusion	Excellent, no suppression
Versions/ductions	Appears to have increasing ET to right and left gaze

Reprinted with permission from Hansen V. A Systematic Approach to Strabismus. *Thorofare, NJ: SLACK Incorporated; 1998.*

Table 12-14.
Decreased ABDuction

1. Duane's retraction syndrome type 1—see Table 12-12
2. CN VI palsy—see Table 12-13
3. Infantile ET—see Table 12-13
4. Nystagmus compensation syndrome—see Table 12-13
5. Strabismus fixus—see Table 12-13
6. Moebius syndrome—see Table 12-13
7. Duane's retraction syndrome type 3—see Table 12-20
8. Myasthenia gravis—see Table 12-13

Reprinted with permission from Hansen V. A Systematic Approach to Strabismus. *Thorofare, NJ: SLACK Incorporated; 1998.*

Table 12-15.
Exodeviations

1. Basic, divergence excess type, convergence insufficiency type	
a. Additional history:	
Intermittency	
Worse at distance or near	
Worse with fatigue, illness	
b. Test:	Indicates:
Fusion	Usually excellent
Measurements	Exodeviation, usually comitant
Vision	Equal
Convergence amplitudes	Poor fusional convergence amps
2. Infantile XT	
a. Additional history:	
Present since birth	
Eye preference	
b. Test:	Indicates:
Vision	Decreased in nonpreferred eye
Health of eyes	No specific ocular disease
Measurements	Usually large comitant XT
3. MR palsy/CN III palsy	
a. Additional history:	
Present since birth if congenital	
Severe trauma	
General health: possible headaches, myasthenia gravis	
Other signs: ipsilateral ptosis, mydriasis, cycloplegia, hypodeviation, contralateral body paralysis (syndrome of Benedikt)	
b. Test:	Indicates:
Versions/ductions	Decreased ADDuction
Measurements	Incomitant exodeviation, greater in ADDuction
Measure with OD, OS fix	Primary and secondary deviation

(continued)

Table 12-15. (continued)

Exodeviations

Vision	Possible amyblopia, cycloplegia
Head position	Present if to attain fusion
4. Duane's retraction syndrome type 2	
a. Additional history:	
No trauma	
Lid fissure changes with gaze	
Abnormal head position	
Present since birth	
b. Test:	Indicates:
Versions/ductions	Decreased ADDuction with lid narrowing, ABDuction okay
Head position	Needed to achieve fusion
Fusion with head position	Often present
Vision	Possible amblyopia
5. Blind eye	
a. Additional history:	
Age of blindness in one eye (if over 7, likely to drift exo)	
Constant alternating XT	
b. Test:	Indicates:
Vision	Blind eye
Krimsky measurements	Fairly comitant XT
6. Consecutive XT	
a. Additional history:	
Previous surgery for ET	
b. Test:	Indicates:
Measurements	XT
Fusion	Diplopia or suppression/ARC
7. Cranial-facial anomalies	
a. Additional history:	
Apert's syndrome	
Crouzon syndrome	
b. Test:	Indicates:
Measurements	Large VXT, RHT in left gaze, LHT in right gaze
Versions/ductions	IO overaction, SO underaction
External	Bilateral exophthalmos (Crouzon)
Refraction	Astigmatism (Apert's) Progressive hyperopia (Crouzon)
8. Convergence paralysis	
a. Additional history:	
Trauma	
General health: possible recent neurological condition	
b. Test:	Indicates:
Convergence amplitudes	Nearly nonexistent
Measurements	Comitant exodeviation N > D

(continued)

Table 12-15. (continued)

Exodeviations

Versions/ductions	Full
Diplopia	Crossed, worse at near
Fusion	Distance only
Vision	Equal

9. Internuclear ophthalmoplegia (INO)
   a. Additional history:
      Bilateral: systemic multiple sclerosis
      Unilateral: vascular accident, inflammation, infection, tumor in brainstem, possible myasthenia gravis

b. Test:	Indicates:
Versions/ductions	Decreased ADDuction with jerk nystagmus in ABDucted eye
Convergence amplitudes	Intact convergence

10. Pseudo XT
   a. Additional history:
      Constant

b. Test:	Indicates:
Krimsky/Cover-uncover	No eye deviation
Fusion	Excellent, no suppression
Angle kappa	Positive
Funduscopy	May have retinopathy of prematurity with temporally dragged fovea

Reprinted with permission from Hansen V. A Systematic Approach to Strabismus. *Thorofare, NJ: SLACK Incorporated; 1998.*

Table 12-16.

Decreased ADDuction

1. Duane's retraction syndrome type 2—see Table 12-15
2. CN III palsy, MR palsy—see Tables 12-15, 12-19
3. Internuclear ophthalmoplegia (INO)—see Table 12-15
4. Myasthenia gravis—see Table 12-13

Reprinted with permission from Hansen V. A Systematic Approach to Strabismus. *Thorofare, NJ: SLACK Incorporated; 1998.*

Table 12-17.

Hyperdeviations

1. Isolated CN IV palsy (SO most common)
   a. Additional history:
      Trauma, may be mild
      Head tilt
      Combined horizontal and vertical diplopia
      Diplopia/asthenopia worse to right and left

(continued)

Table 12-17. (continued)

Hyperdeviations

Myasthenia gravis	Indicates:
Old photographs	Old head tilt if congenital/long-standing
External inspection	Facial slant if congenital/long-standing (horizontal lines of brows and lips are not parallel)
b. Test:	Indicates:
Fusion with head position	Usually fuses
P + C, 9 positions	Incomitant HT
3ST	Isolates EOM palsy
Versions/ductions	SO—May show underactive SO, overactive IO, inhibitional palsy of contralateral (IPC) SR IO—May show underactive IO, overactive SO, IPC IR SR—May show underactive SR, overactive IR, IPC SO IR—May show underactive IR, overactive SR, IPC IO
Vertical amplitudes	May exist if congenital/long-standing No vertical amps if recent onset May exist if recent onset
Subjective torsion	No torsion if congenital/long-standing SO, SR—extorsion IO, IR—intorsion
2. DVD	
a. Additional history:	
Associated with congenital/infantile ET	
One or both eyes go up, neither eye ever goes hypotropic	
Intermittent HT, either eye	
b. Test:	Indicates:
Cover-uncover	Either eye elevates under cover without associated hypodeviation of the fellow eye
P + C	Difficult to measure, variable
Versions/ductions	Rule out IO overaction as "cause"
3. Brown's syndrome	
a. Additional history:	
Trauma to trochlear region of globe	
Sinus, orbital surgery	
Juvenile rheumatoid arthritis	
Present since birth if congenital	

(continued)

Table 12-17. (continued)

Hyperdeviations

b. Test:	Indicates:
Version/ductions	No elevation of globe in ADDuction Eye elevates easily in ABDuction
Forced ductions	Restriction of globe up and in
Fusion	Often fuses in downgaze
Vision	Possible amblyopia
Krimsky	Hypotropia of affected eye when up and in
4. Blowout fracture	
a. Additional history:	
Blunt trauma—orbital fracture	
Diplopia/discomfort often worse in upgaze	
b. Test:	Indicates:
Ductions/versions	Hypotropia worsens toward upgaze Restrictions of ductions: upgaze may be down, right, or left gaze
Forced ductions	Restriction of globe, usually upgaze
X-ray/CT scan	Orbital fracture, frequently floor or nasal wall
Diplopia field	Often has region of single binocular vision
Exophthalmometry	Affected eye often enophthalmic
5. Double elevator palsy (DEP)	
a. Additional history:	
Present since birth	
Ptosis on affected side	
Chin up head position	
No trauma	
b. Test:	Indicates:
Fusion with chin up	Possible fusion
Versions/ductions	Constant hypotropia of affected eye
Forced ductions	No restrictions of elevation unless very longstanding
External	Pseudoptosis on affected side
6. Graves' ophthalmopathy	
a. Additional history:	
Thyroid dysfunction in past or present	
b. Test:	Indicates:
Ductions/versions	Restriction of upgaze (IR), lateral gaze (MR), or any EOM
Forced ductions	Positive for restriction
Fusion with head position	Usually has fusion
Diplopia	Variable, vertical > horizontal

(continued)

Table 12-17. (continued)

Hyperdeviations

7. Pseudo HT
   a. Additional history:
      Previous EOM or lid surgery
   b. Test:

Test	Indicates:
Cover-uncover	No deviation
Lift lid	Appearance of HT disappears
Assess pupils	Possible assymetry
External photography	No deviation by light reflex

Reprinted with permission from Hansen V. A Systematic Approach to Strabismus. *Thorofare, NJ: SLACK Incorporated; 1998.*

Table 12-18.

True Hypodeviations

1. Brown's syndrome—see Table 12-17
2. Double elevator palsy—see Table 12-17
3. Blowout floor fracture—see Table 12-17
4. Restrictive thyroid eye disease (Graves' disease)—see Table 12-17

Reprinted with permission from Hansen V. A Systematic Approach to Strabismus. *Thorofare, NJ: SLACK Incorporated; 1998.*

Table 12-19.

Decreased Elevation

1. Thyroid ophthalmopathy—see Table 12-17
2. Brown's syndrome—see Table 12-17
3. Blowout floor fracture—see Table 12-17
4. Double elevator palsy—see Table 12-17
5. Myasthenia gravis—see Table 12-13
6. CN III palsy
   a. Additional history:
      Ptosis, mydriasis, decreased elevation and ADDuction
      Trauma possible
      Present since birth if congenital
      Diabetes in adult
   b. Test:

Test	Indicates:
Versions/ductions	Absent elevation and ADDuction
Forced ductions	No restrictions unless very longstanding
Lid assessment	Ptosis, may be complete
Pupil assessment	No reaction to light or accommodation, unless diabetic
Vision/refraction	Cyclopleged, unless diabetic
Krimsky	Incomitance, often never ortho

(continued)

Table 12-19. (continued)
Decreased Elevation

ABDuction (LR)	Intact
Depression, intorsion (SO)	Intact

Reprinted with permission from Hansen V. A Systematic Approach to Strabismus. *Thorofare, NJ: SLACK Incorporated; 1998.*

Table 12-20.
Decreased Ductions

1. Duane's retraction syndrome type 1—see Table 12-13
2. Duane's retraction syndrome type 2—see Table 12-15
3. Duane's retraction syndrome type 3
   a. Additional history:
      No trauma
      Lid fissure changes with gaze
      Present since birth
   b. Test:

Test	Indicates:
Versions/ductions	Absent ABDuction and ADDuction Enophthalmos during attempted ADDuction with narrowing of lid issure

4. Cyclovertical muscle palsy—see Table 12-17
5. Brown's syndrome—see Table 12-17
6. Blowout fracture—see Table 12-17
7. Thyroid ophthalmopathy—see Table 12-17
8. Strabismus fixus—see Table 12-13
9. Double elevator palsy—see Table 12-17

Reprinted with permission from Hansen V. A Systematic Approach to Strabismus. *Thorofare, NJ: SLACK Incorporated; 1998.*

Table 12-21.
Abnormal Head Position

1. Congenital torticollis
   a. Additional history:
      Present since able to hold head up unassisted (approximately 6 months of age)
      No eye turn ever seen, no nystagmus ever seen
   b. Test:

Test	Results:
Prolonged occlusion	Head position persists
EOM exam	No motility disturbance
Force head tilt to opposite side	No hyperdeviation seen (no SO palsy)

(continued)

Table 12-21. (continued)
Abnormal Head Position

2. Congenital nystagmus
   a. Additional history:
      Horizontal jerk nystagmus seen without head position
      Nystagmus dampens during near fixation
      Present since birth
   b. Test: / Results:

Test:	Results:
Binocular, monocular vision	Usually better binocularly
Versions/ductions	Nystagmus worse away from null point
Assess nystagmus, D + N	Usually less at near

3. CN IV palsy—see Table 12-17
4. Duane's retraction syndrome types 1, 2, 3—see Tables 12-13, 12-15, 12-20
5. Nystagmus compensation syndrome—see Table 12-13
6. Strabismus fixus—see Table 12-13
7. Graves' ophthalmopathy—see Table 12-17
8. Uncorrected refractive error

Reprinted with permission from Hansen V. A Systematic Approach to Strabismus. *Thorofare, NJ: SLACK Incorporated; 1998.*

Table 12-22.
Diplopia

1. Uncorrected refractive error causing blur
   a. Additional history:
      Images very close together
      Possibly more than two images per eye
   b. Test:

Test:	Results:
Refraction	Frequent astigmatism, blur disappears with proper refractive correction
Pinhole	Second image disappears

2. Monocular diplopia
   a. Additional history:
      Diplopia persists in one or both eyes with occlusion
      Extra image(s) may be blurred or smeared
      Injury to cornea/lens causing scarring
      Retinal injury, laser
      Bifocal line obstructing visual axis
   b. Test:

Test:	Results:
Monocular occlusion	Diplopia persists
Health of eye	Organic cause of diplopia Rule out cataract or corneal opacity

(continued)

Table 12-22. (continued)

Diplopia

True Binocular Diplopias	
3. Decompensated phoria not tropic	
a. Additional history:	
Previous intermittent tropia with diplopia	
b. Test:	Results:
Fusion with deviation corrected	Usually fuses
P + C	Often comitant, usually XT or HT
Fusion potential	Usually excellent
4. EOM palsy—see Tables 12-13, 12-15, 12-17	
5. Newly noticed diplopia from long-standing condition	
a. Additional history:	
Brown's syndrome—see Table 12-17	
Duane's retraction syndrome types 1, 2, 3—see Tables 12-13, 12-15, 12-20	
Thyroid ophthalmopathy—see Table 12-17	
Blowout fracture—see Table 12-17	
Have they ever looked into that field of gaze before? (Probably not)	
6. Secondary to restrictive strabismus	
a. Additional history:	
Thyroid ophthalmopathy—see Table 12-17	
Brown's syndrome—see Table 12-17	
Duane's retraction syndrome types 1, 2, 3—see Tables 12-13, 12-15, 12-20	
If the strabismus had been present since childhood, have they ever looked into that field of gaze before? (Probably not)	
7. Divergence paralysis—see Table 12-13	
8. Convergence paralysis—see Table 12-15	
9. Intractable diplopia	
a. Additional history:	
Previous antisuppression exercises	
Trauma	
Previous strabismus surgery	
b. Test:	Results:
Fusion potential	None
Occlusion	No diplopia
Retinal correspondence	Often abnormal, paradoxical
10. Paradoxical diplopia	
a. Additional history:	
Previous strabismus surgery	
Consecutive tropia	
b. Test:	Results:
Retinal correspondence	ARC
11. Glasses-induced	
a. Additional history:	
New glasses	
New bifocals	
Aphakic correction	

(continued)

Table 12-22. (continued)

Diplopia

Glasses recently adjusted
Diplopia disappears with glasses removed
Diplopia is typically vertical, but may be uncrossed

b. Test:	Results:
Check for prism in glasses	Optical center misalignment creating prism, typically vertical or base-in
Check height of bifocal	May be asymmetric

Reprinted with permission from Hansen V. A Systematic Approach to Strabismus. *Thorofare, NJ: SLACK Incorporated; 1998.*

Table 12-23.

Near Vision Problems

1. Convergence insufficiency
   a. Additional history:
      Blurring while reading/near work or prolonged distance fixation
      Occasional horizontal diplopia
      Difficulty changing from N to D or D to N fixation
      Headaches after using eyes; never upon awakening

b. Test:	Results:
Fusion	Normal steropsis
P + C	May have small to large exo, eso, or may be ortho Often has congenital SO palsy
Fusional amplitudes	Poor fusional amplitudes for visual demands, uses accommodative convergence, poor recovery/jump point
Prolonged occlusion	Symptoms completely disappear

2. Presbyopia
   a. Additional history:
      40+ years old
      Previous hyperopic correction
      Older myope who was recently fit with contact lenses for the first time
      Older hyperope who was recently switched from contact lenses to full-time glasses

b. Test:	Results:
Cycloplegic refraction	Possibly over-minused or has latent hyperopia
NPA, cc	Should be normal for age

(continued)

Table 12-23. (continued)

Near Vision Problems

3. Systemic convergence insufficiency
   a. Additional history:
      Trauma
      Illness: encephalitis, drug intoxication, mononucleosis
      Increasing diplopia and blurring with near vision
   b. Test: — Results:
      Convergence — Convergence insufficiency
      NPA — Severely decreased and often fixed
      Plus lenses — Improves near vision
      Near P + C — Constant XT at N requiring BI prism for fusion
4. Convergence paralysis—see Table 12-15
5. Divergence paralysis—see Table 12-13
6. Accommodative spasm
   a. Additional history:
      Possible psychogenesis
      Severe distance blurring after near fixation
   b. Test: — Results:
      Distance VA — Usually worse than 20/200
      Manifest refraction — Up to 8 to 10 D myopia
      Cycloplegic refraction — High myopia disappears
7. Accommodative effort syndrome—see Table12-13
8. Juvenile presbyopia
   a. Additional history:
      Drug use
      History of hysteria
      Symptoms of presbyopia, except age is much younger
   b. Test: — Results:
      Near vision — Decreased
      P + C — Insignificant eye turn
      NPA — Decreased for age
      Plus lenses for near — Relieves symptoms
9. CN IV palsy (SO palsy)—see Table 12-17
   a. Additional history:
      Asthenopia, diplopia increases in reading position

Reprinted with permission from Hansen V. A Systematic Approach to Strabismus. *Thorofare, NJ: SLACK Incorporated; 1998.*

Table 12-24.

Pseudostrabismus

1. Prominent epicanthal folds (ET)—see Table 12-13
2. Narrow lateral canthi (XT)
3. Angle kappa: Positive (XT)—see Table 12-15
   Negative (ET)—see Table 12-13
4. Ectopic macula
   a. Additional history:
      Previous retinal problems or surgery
   b. Test: | Results:
      Funduscopy | Displaced macula
5. Anisocoria
   a. Additional history:
      May be associated with mild ptosis with miotic pupil (Horner's syndrome)
      May or may not have heterochromia (congenital Horner's syndrome has heterochromia)
      May or may not have facial anhydrosis (absence of perspiration)
      Trauma
      CN III palsy
   b. Test: | Results:
      Pupil evaluation | Anisocoria
      Cover-uncover | No eye deviation
      Fusion | Normal
6. Exophthalmos—see Table 12-25

Reprinted with permission from Hansen V. A Systematic Approach to Strabismus. *Thorofare, NJ: SLACK Incorporated; 1998.*

Table 12-25.

Exophthalmos

1. Graves' ophthalmopathy
   a. Additional history:
      Proptosis not present years ago
      Thyroid disease
      Diplopia, particularly in up gaze
      May be both eyes, but asymmetrical
   b. Test: | Results:
      Exophthalmometry | Either greater than 22 mm or difference between eyes > 2 mm
      Lid fissure height | May be greater on side of proptosis
2. Orbital tumors: lymphoma, malignant melanoma, rhabdomyosarcoma, retinoblastoma, neurofibroma, glioma, dermoid, lacrimal gland tumor, carcinoma, mucocele
   a. Additional history:
      May be sudden onset
      May be any age, frequently children

(continued)

Table 12-25. (continued)

Exophthalmos

b. Test:	Results:
Exophthalmometry	Exophthalmos
CT scan, B scan	Orbital mass
3. Inflammations: pseudotumor, myositis	
a. Additional history:	
Pain	
Ophthalmoplegia	
4. Infections: orbital cellulitis	
a. Additional history:	
Sudden onset, worsens quickly	
Hot eye	
Monocular	
Usually young child	
b. Test:	Results:
CT scan	Orbital involvement
General health	Sick child/fever/malaise
5. Vascular disorders: orbital varix, cavernous sinus thrombosis, pulsating exophthalmos	
a. Additional history:	
Eye bulges when baby cries (varix)	
Previous orbital infection (thrombosis)	
Neurofibromatosis	
b. Test:	Results:
Orbital venography	A-V malformation
View patient from side	Pulsating exophthalmos visible
6. Orbital anomalies: Crouzon syndrome, Apert's syndrome	
7. Enophthalmos of contralateral eye	
a. Additional history:	
Blowout fracture	
Blind, phthisical eye	
b. Test:	Results:
Exophthalmometry	Enophthalmos of contralateral eye
8. Pseudoexophthalmos	
a. Additional history:	
Old photographs	
Unilateral lid retraction or ptosis	
Large eye due to buphthalmos (juvenile glaucoma), axial myopia, or staphyloma	
True enophthalmos of contralateral eye	
b. Test:	Results:
Exophthalmometry	Normal

Reprinted with permission from Hansen V. A Systematic Approach to Strabismus. *Thorofare, NJ: SLACK Incorporated; 1998.*

Table 12-26.
Enophthalmos

1. Blowout fracture—see Table 12-17, item 4
2. Phthisis bulbi—see Table 12-25, item 7
3. Pseudoreal exophthalmos of contralateral eye—see Table 12-25, item 8

Reprinted with permission from Hansen V. A Systematic Approach to Strabismus. *Thorofare, NJ: SLACK Incorporated; 1998.*

Syndromes with Ocular Manifestations

A syndrome is a constellation of characteristic findings. Once the syndrome is identified, the characteristics of it can be found in the patient. Early diagnosis of a syndrome helps initiate proper treatment and, in some cases, can help other clinicians identify additional problems in the patient's health. The most common will be discussed here.

Duane's retraction syndrome is a horizontal deviation that is present at birth and varies in primary, right, and left gazes (Table 12-27). It is thought to be caused by a misfiring, or true cofiring, of the medial rectus (MR) and lateral rectus (LR). The patient is often ortho near or at the primary position, may fuse, and may have equal vision in each eye. There are three types, all of which result in both narrowing of the lid fissure and globe retraction when ADDuction is attempted. Table 12-28 lists the tests that should be done on a patient with Duane's syndrome.

Brown's syndrome is a mechanical restriction preventing free passage of the superior oblique (SO) through its trochlea when the eye looks up and in. There appears to be decreased elevation in ADDuction by duction testing (the inferior oblique [IO] appears weak). In Brown's syndrome the eyes are often straight in the primary position, so fusion is often present and amblyopia is uncommon. Table 12-29 lists the tests that should be performed on a patient with Brown's syndrome.

Monofixational syndrome is characterized by mild amblyopia (as little as a half line difference) and by foveal/central suppression of the affected eye on fusion tests such as the stereo test, Worth 4 dot, or the 4 diopter base-out test. Table 12-30 lists tests and typical findings in a patient with monofixational syndrome.

Table 12-27.

Duane's Syndrome: All three types have narrowing of lid fissure with globe retraction during attempted ADDuction.

Type 1:	Decreased ABDuction
Type 2:	Decreased ADDuction
Type 3:	Decreased ABDuction and ADDuction

Reprinted with permission from Hansen V. A Systematic Approach to Strabismus. *Thorofare, NJ: SLACK Incorporated; 1998.*

Table 12-28.

Tests for Duane's Syndrome	Results
Stereopsis/fusion:	Usually intact with head position
P + C: In primary position	Small tropia, often ET
and secondary positions	Incomitance
Versions:	Decreased ABDuction (type 1), ADDuction (type 2), or both (type 3)
	Lid fissure narrowing in ADDuction
Vision:	Rule out amblyopia
Other:	Note any head position; look at old pictures

Reprinted with permission from Hansen V. A Systematic Approach to Strabismus. *Thorofare, NJ: SLACK Incorporated; 1998.*

Table 12-29.

Tests for Brown's Syndrome		Results
P + C:	Primary position	May be ortho
	Secondary positions	Hypodeviation in upgaze
	Tertiary positions	Hypotropia in ADDuction only
	Head tilts	No EOM palsy
Versions:		Limited elevation in ADDuction
Ductions:		Limited elevation in ADDuction
Vision:		Rule out amblyopia
Stereopsis/fusion:		Often intact

Reprinted with permission from Hansen V. A Systematic Approach to Strabismus. *Thorofare, NJ: SLACK Incorporated; 1998.*

Table 12-30.

Tests for Monfixational System	**Results**
Stereopsis:	Less than 67 seconds of arc
Simultaneous P + C:	Small constant esotropia (may be XT or vertical)
P + C:	Larger phoria
Vision:	Mild amblyopia
Refraction:	Often anisometropic
4 D base-out test:	Monocular suppression
Worth 4 dot:	Fusion at near Monocular suppression at distance
Bagolini lenses:	Cross (fusion) with central scotoma

Reprinted with permission from Hansen V. A Systematic Approach to Strabismus. *Thorofare, NJ: SLACK Incorporated; 1998.*

Unless otherwise noted, all text, tables, and figures are adapted or reprinted with permission from Hansen V. A Systematic Approach to Strabismus. *Thorofare, NJ: SLACK Incorporated; 1998.*

CHAPTER 13

Low Vision

Introductory Thoughts

- Low vision is not defined by specific acuity limits. It includes any functional visual loss after the correction of refractive error and presbyopia.
- Low vision aids are defined as devices that improve the efficiency of remaining vision.
- Complete low vision care includes rehabilitation as well as optical aids.
- Legal blindness is defined as best visual acuity (BVA) of 20/200 or less in the better seeing eye, or a visual field loss such that the maximum diameter of the visual field is 20 degrees or less (even if the measurable acuity is good).
- "Visual efficiency" refers to an individual's functional visual ability in spite of loss.
- A low vision aid is only useful if the patient is educated properly in its use.

Optical Low Vision Aids

- Optical low vision aids use magnification to enlarge retinal image size (Table 13-1).
- The power of a lens is measured in diopters. One diopter (D) is defined as the optical power needed to focus parallel rays of light at 1 meter. In practical terms for low vision, to focus the image of an object held at 1 meter, a 1 D lens is needed (Table 13-2).
- When discussing magnification, "X" refers to the number of times the retinal image is enlarged in size. 1X means there is no change in the size, 2X means the image is twice the "normal" size, etc. For common low vision notation, 40 cm is considered to be the standard reference distance (Table 13-3).
- Spectacles require an eye-to-print distance equal to the focal length of the lens.

Table 13-1.

Magnification Types

Type	Action	Examples	Notes
Relative size	Object is made larger	Large print Enlarged phone pads	No change in optical correction is needed
Relative distance	Retinal image is enlarged by bringing object closer	N/A	Necessary to focus the image by lenses or accommodation
Angular magnification	A system of lenses is used to make distant objects appear closer	Telescopes Binoculars	
Projection magnification	Print or images are enlarged by projection	Overhead projector Closed circuit television (CCTV)	

Table 13-2.

Diopter/Distance Chart

Distance to Object	Power Needed to Focus Image
5 cm (1/20 m)	20 D
10 cm (1/10 m)	10 D
12.5 cm (1/8 m)	8 D
20 cm (1/5 m)	5 D
25 cm (1/4 m)	4 D
33.3 cm (1/3 m)	3 D
40 cm (1/2.5 m)	2.5 D
100 cm (1 m)	1 D
200 cm (2 m)	0.5 D

Reprinted with permission from Brown B. The Low Vision Handbook. *Thorofare, NJ: SLACK Incorporated; 1997.*

Table 13-3.
Magnification Power Equivalencies

Magnification (X)	Dioptric Equivalent (40 cm Reference)	Dioptric Equivalent (25 cm Reference)
1	+2.50	+4.00
2	+5.00	+8.00
3	+7.50	+12.00
4	+10.00	+16.00
5	+12.50	+20.00
6	+15.00	+24.00
10	+25.00	+40.00

Reprinted with permission from Brown B. The Low Vision Handbook. *Thorofare, NJ: SLACK Incorporated; 1997.*

- Hand magnifiers require a lens-to-print distance equal to the focal length of the lens. Distance correction should be worn when using hand magnifiers.
- Stand magnifiers require either reading correction or sufficient accommodative ability.
- Telescopes can be used by children, adults, and patients with nystagmus or visual field loss. They are the only low vision aid used at distance.

How-To: Patient Education for Low Vision Optical Aids

- When using spectacles, reading material must be held at the focusing distance of the lenses, which is *closer* to the eyes than normal. Touch the reading material to your nose and *slowly* move it away until it is in clear focus. Maintain that distance while reading.
- It may help to move reading material from side to side, keeping the eyes still, instead of scanning material in the normal way by moving your eyes from the beginning to the end of a line of print.
- The distance from a hand magnifier to the printed page must be kept constant. To find this distance, start with the lens on the page and *slowly* pull it away from the print until optimal focus is reached.
- Hand magnifiers should be used with distance glasses.
- If the magnifier is brought closer to your eye to increase the field of view, bring the reading material closer as well. The distance from print to lens must always be kept constant to maintain focus.
- Wear your bifocals, reading glasses, or other near correction when using a stand magnifier. You will feel a "pull" on your eyes if you try to use the portion of your glasses that is for driving and watching television.

(continued)

How-To: Patient Education for Low Vision Optical Aids (continued)

- Always keep the distance from your eyes to the magnifier constant. Do not pull the magnifier up to your eye or the focus will be lost.
- Telescopes must be balanced and held steady by resting your hand against your face and your arm against your body or other support.
- To locate an object, first view it with your naked eye before lifting the telescope and spotting through it.
- Do not walk or move when viewing through a telescope.
- Objects seen through a telescope appear to be closer than they are.

Nonoptical and Electronic Low Vision Aids

- Nonoptical aids are available for reading, writing, medical use, and household use, as well as for hobbies and games.
- Lighting is the most important nonoptical aid.
- Electronic aids include closed circuit television (CCTV), computer programs, and synthesized speech devices. Before using any of these, personal assessment and training should be undertaken in order to allow efficiency with the appliance.

How-To: Patient Education for Low Vision Lighting

- Brighter lightbulbs are not the only answer to help you read better. Sometimes a lower watt bulb is better. In either case, the illumination should shine directly on the subject matter.
- Light can be placed in any location that provides optimal contrast of the print. It is not necessarily best if it comes over your shoulder from behind.
- Bright light on a page of print will not harm your eyes.
- If glare is a problem for you, it is okay to move your reading light further away or wear sunglasses indoors.

History Taking (Table 13-4)

- A low vision history should address rehabilitation as well as optical concerns.
- A low vision exam and history should not be attempted until the patient has reached a level of acceptance of his or her visual loss.
- A well-informed patient experiences more success with low vision aids.
- Teacher input should be solicited for the history of school-age patients.

Table 13-4.
History Taking

Questions to Narrow a Patient's Needs
Chief Complaint What is the main problem you have related to your visual loss? What visual struggle affects you the most in your daily life? If we can restore one task for you with the help of aids, what do you most want it to be?
Vocational What is your job? What difficulties have you been experiencing in your work because of your eye problem? What size print do you most often encounter in your work? Do you have distance limitations, such as working at a computer screen or a large drafting table? Have you measured this viewing distance?
General Have you used magnifiers in the past? Were they helpful? Why or why not? How do you think we could improve on them for your use? What kind of light do you use for reading? What light is best for you? Do you experience glare outdoors or difficulty adjusting to light changes?
Hobbies Have you had to give up any hobbies or sports specifically because of your visual loss? Does your vision prevent you from trying some sport or hobby you would like to try?
Activities of Daily Living How do you shop for groceries? Can you see the labels and price tags? Do you cook your own food? What is your biggest difficulty in preparing meals? Has your menu changed since your vision has become poorer? Do you feel you can keep your house clean and handle the laundry, or are you having trouble with household chores? Can you read your own mail? Do you write your own checks and balance your checkbook, or do you find it an impossible task?
Questions to Evaluate Acceptance
What is medically wrong with your eyes? Is your vision going to get better? Worse? Is your doctor still considering any treatments? Do you feel that your vision problem has been thoroughly explained to you? Do you understand it?
Questions to Determine Support Level
Who brought you to the exam today? Are they friends or relatives? Who do you call if you need help with shopping or other chores? Do you have people whom you can trust and rely on for personal needs, such as balancing your accounts?

(continued)

Table 13-4. (continued)

History Taking

Do you live with or near people who can help you? (Do not ask if he or she lives alone, for security reasons.)

Questions for the Pediatric Low Vision History

How far does the child sit from the board or other distant objects in the classroom (such as the clock)?

Is he or she able to read the appropriate size of printed material without much difficulty? What print size generally is used in his or her grade?

Is there a vision resource room or itinerant vision teacher available at the school?

Does he or she engage in any sports or extracurricular activities that require better vision?

Has he or she wanted to participate in any of these activities, but felt limited visually?

How does he or she get to and from school? Can the child move freely about the school without assistance?

How close does he or she hold material when reading?

What type of lighting is used for reading?

Are current glasses made with polycarbonate lenses? Even if there is no distance refractive error, are safety glasses worn?

Has a telescope or other magnifier ever been tried?

Assessment of Visual Function

- Move the test chart closer to allow the patient to experience success in reading more letters, and for a more precise evaluation of distance acuity. Record the actual testing distance.
- Always verify the refractometric measurement before beginning low vision testing. Optimal refractive correction is imperative.
- Near vision should be tested using continuous text cards and selecting the smallest size of print that can be read fluently.

How-To: Vision Assessment in Low Vision

- Measure acuity monocularly at 10 ft or 5 ft with a hand-held low vision distance test chart.
- Record the vision appropriately to reflect the testing distance. For example, 50-size optotypes seen at 10 ft would be recorded as 10/50.
- Measure near acuity with both eyes open in preferred conditions.
- Verify refractive error using a trial frame and full field trial lenses, holding the chart at the same distance at which the acuity was recorded. Correct to infinity.

(continued)

How-To: Vision Assessment in Low Vision (continued)

- Remeasure distance acuity monocularly with the new optimum distance correction. This should still be done at 5 ft or 10 ft.
- Put +2.50 lenses over the distance correction in the trial frame.
- Hold a near-vision reading card at a distance of 40 cm and remeasure near reading ability with this combination of lenses. The reading card should have print in continuous text rather than as isolated symbols. Test each eye monocularly. Record the size of type in M units as the denominator and 40 cm as the numerator. For example: The patient reads 4 M print at 40 cm. Record as 40/4M.
- Convert the reading ability in M units to a near acuity level. Do this by multiplying the M units by 100 to convert to centimeters. Divide the M units in centimeters by 40 to determine the power in diopters of the reading add that will most likely allow reading of 1 M print. For example: Near vision is 4 M.

  4 M x 100 = 400 cm

  400/40 = 10

  Use a 10 D reading add
- Try the calculated power as a reading add in the trial frame if possible. The same power can be used to try a hand magnifier while the patient looks through his or her distance refractive correction. If a stand magnifier is tried, the magnifier power should be slightly higher and a standard reading add should be used along with it.
- Perform contrast sensitivity, visual fields, or other testing as indicated before giving official trials with any aid or making final recommendations.

Selecting Aids for Individuals

- Aid selection is determined by the patient's needs and goals as indicated by the history.
- The power of the near aid is determined by the patient's reading ability at a 40 cm testing distance.
- After several trials with a chosen aid, the final determination of whether it is appropriate and affordable will be made by the patient. Follow-up care is always necessary.

How-To: Select an Aid

- Consider the primary goal of the patient. Must the hands be kept free?
- Convert the near reading ability from M units to diopters to determine power, adjusting to allow for refractive error or accommodative ability if indicated.
- Determine the focal distance of the chosen magnifier considering the power before adjustments were made.
- Teach the patient to hold the magnifier or reading material at the proper focal distance. Use a reading stand, optimum lighting, and the desired size of printed material.
- Allow the patient to try the aid while left alone for a few minutes with other sizes and choices of printed material on hand.
- Make adjustments in power or style as necessary, considering the patient's financial situation when making decisions.
- Send the patient home for 1 to 2 weeks to try the selected aid in the home setting. Supply the patient with a trial aid from your loan library as well as preprinted information on how to correctly use the aid. If possible, provide the information to a family member as well.
- On follow-up, listen carefully to the patient's difficulties and successes, making adjustments or recommending additional aids as necessary.

Other Notes

- State-run and private agencies are available to help your patients. Check with your state government for local details.
- Professionals who provide assistance to blind or low vision patients include rehabilitation teachers, rehabilitation counselors, teachers of the visually impaired, orientation and mobility specialists, and occupational therapists.
- People who experience loss of vision undergo a grieving period for the "death" of both their previous identity and their independence.
- When partial vision is lost, there is always a fear that total blindness will occur next.
- It is far better for eyecare professionals to be honest than to offer insincere encouragement about prognosis. We should educate and not avoid discussing the realities of visual loss.
- Be careful not to "pigeonhole" your patients into particular groups. Each patient, even among those with the same diagnosis, will have unique needs. The low vision provider's challenge is to understand each of these needs and offer as much assistance and support as possible.

- Offer, but do not force, suggestions on patients who are resistant to them. Remember that success or failure depends largely on an individual's personality.

Unless otherwise noted, all text, tables, and figures are adapted or reprinted with permission from Brown B. The Low Vision Handbook. *Thorofare, NJ: SLACK Incorporated; 1997.*

CHAPTER 14

Slit Lamp

The Basic Slit Lamp Exam

- Patient education is an important aspect of the slit lamp exam.
- A comfortable patient is a more cooperative patient.
- Before beginning, adjust the ocular power and pupillary distance.
- Using lower voltage settings preserves bulb life.
- Manipulate the microscope with one hand on the light source and the other hand on the joystick.
- Developing and following an examination protocol will help ensure quality patient care.
- Accurate, legible documentation is the last step of any slit lamp examination.

Protocol and Documentation

It is important to develop your own slit lamp examination protocol. Performing the exam the same way, in the same order, on every patient, will increase the quality of your examination by ensuring that nothing is missed. Table 14-1 is a typical protocol. This protocol might be modified depending on the patient and the situation. For example, if the patient may be uncooperative, select the structures that are most vital and examine them first. In addition, each examiner may modify this plan to suit him- or herself. For example, some might prefer to completely examine the right eye before moving to the left rather than the method suggested here.

Documentation is the last step of the slit lamp exam. It is not enough to look at the eye; you must write down what you see... even if it is normal. Never underestimate the importance of accurate, legible notations in the patient's chart. (Remember these axioms: "If it is not in the chart, it was not done. If it is not readable, it is not in the chart.") Such notes may be the only thing that keeps you and/or your physician/employer from being sued.

Table 14-1.
Slit Lamp Examination

Suggested Power	
6X or 10X	External (lids, conjunctiva), contact lenses
16X	Angles, cornea, lens, foreign bodies, corneal abrasions
40X	Corneal endothelium
Beam Width	
1. Narrowest	Angles, cornea, anterior chamber
2. A bit wider	Cornea, lens, etc
3. A bit wider yet	External, contact lenses
4. Full width	External, applanation tension (with blue filter)
Beam Height	
Full	Most areas and structures
Short	Checking anterior chamber for cells and flare
Color/Filter	
White	Most areas and structures
Blue	(Use fluorescein dye) applanation tensions, corneal staining, tear film, staining patterns of rigid contact lenses
Green (red-free)	Evaluating blood vessels, iron lines
Position (of light source)	
R = right	
L = left	
C = center	
Degrees (given; indicated at base of illumination arm)	
Stage (position)	
R = right	
L = left	
Abbreviations	
OD	Right eye
OS	Left eye
SCH	Subconjunctival hemorrhage
AC	Anterior chamber
SPK	Superficial punctate keratitis
PEE	Punctate epithelial erosions
PSC	Posterior subcapsular cataract
AT	Applanation tension

Notes: Unless contraindicated, fluorescein is instilled before the slit lamp exam begins.

(continued)

Table 14-1. (continued)

Slit Lamp Examination

Settings	Area/Structure	Observe for
	OD lids	
Power: 10X		Blepharospasm
Width: 2 to 4		Collarettes
Height: full		Coloboma
Color: white		Crusting/matting
Position: R, sweep to L		Discharge
Stage: L		Edema (swelling)
		Erythema
		Growths
		Lash loss
		Lid closure
		Lid lag
		Lid position
		Notching
		Reflux
		Trauma
	OS lids	
Position: R, sweep to L		
Stage: R		
	OD conjunctiva, episclera, sclera	
Power: 10 to 16 X		Ciliary flush
Width: 2		Color
Position: L, sweep to R		Dryness
Stage: L		Edema (chemosis)
		Follicles
		Foreign body
		Growths
		Injection
		Leash vessels
		Papillae
		Pinguecula
		Scleral show
		Scleral thinning
		SCH
		Trauma
	OD tear film	
Power: 10 to 16X		Break-up time
Width: 2		Debris
Position: L, sweep to R		Discharge
Stage: L		Epiphora

(continued)

Table 14-1. (continued)

Slit Lamp Examination

Settings		Findings
	OD cornea	
Width: 2 Position: L, sweeping to R		Abrasion Arcus senilis Dellen Dystrophy Edema Filaments Foreign body Ghost vessels Guttata Infiltrates Iron lines Keratitic precipitates Keratitis Keratopathy Krukenberg spindles Opacities Pannus Phlyctenule Pterygium Rust ring Scar Stria/folds Ulcer Vascularization
	OD corneal staining	
Color: blue Position: L, sweeping to R		Abrasion Bullae Dendrites Dry spots PEE/SPK Stained areas Tear film Ulcer
	OD temporal angle	
Power: 16X Width: 1 Color: white Position: L, ~45 degrees		AC depth Angle grade
	OD nasal angle	
Position: R, ~45 degrees		

(continued)

Table 14-1. (continued)

Slit Lamp Examination

	OD AC	
Width: 1 to 2 Position: L, sweeping to R		Hyphema Hypopyon Vitreous
Width: 1 Height: small Position: L, sweeping to R with vertical searching motions		Cells Flare
	OD iris/pupil	
Width: 2 Height: full Position: L, sweeping to R		Atrophy Coloboma Iris detachment Iris movement Iris nevus Iris strands Laser iridotomy Normal iris vessels Peripheral iridectomy Pigment dispersion Pupil reaction Pupil shape Rubeosis Sector iridectomy Synechiae
	OD lens	
		Cortical spoking Nuclear sclerosis Opacities PSC Pseudoexfoliation Subluxation Vacuoles
	OD IOL	
		Capsule opacity Capsulotomy Location Position Precipitates
	OD anterior vitreous	
Position: L, sweeping to R		Clarity Opacities

(continued)

Table 14-1. (continued)

Slit Lamp Examination

OS conjunctiva and globe

(Repeat process using opposite directions)

AT, OD

Power: 6 or 10X
Height: full
Width: full
Color: blue
Position: L, ~60 degrees
Stage: L

AT, OS

Position: R
Stage: R

Reprinted with permission from Ledford JK, Sanders VN. The Slit Lamp Primer. *Thorofare, NJ: SLACK Incorporated; 1998.*

It is important to note findings, not diagnoses. For example, write "3+ lash crusting, 2+ lid edema, 2+ lash loss" instead of "blepharitis." Blepharitis is a diagnosis, which belongs in the physician's assessment.

In cases where abnormalities are expected (or likely) yet are not found, you may record negative information. For example, the patient has diabetes, so you carefully examine the iris for abnormal blood vessels (rubeosis). Finding none, you record "No iris rubeosis."

If abbreviations are used, they should be standardized and written down for the office. This small bit of effort might also save you in court. Documentation advocates are fond of saying that the abbreviation WNL (which is supposed to mean "within normal limits") may actually mean "we never looked." Do not fall into sloppy documentation habits. It is better to write out the words "clear" or "normal." Do not neglect to note a normal finding just because it is normal.

Illumination Techniques (Table 14-2)

- The slit lamp exam is dynamic; the observer uses multiple types of illumination simultaneously.
- The three main categories of illumination are diffuse, direct, and indirect.
- Diffuse illumination provides an even light over the entire ocular surface.
- With direct illumination techniques, the light is shone directly onto the area or structure of interest.
- With indirect illumination methods, the object of interest is illuminated by light that is reflected off of another structure.

Table 14-2.
Illumination Techniques

I. Diffuse
Description: Light is spread evenly over the entire observed surface.
Procedure: Beam is opened all the way. Direct light at 45 degree angle, microscope directed straight ahead. Use diffuser and lowest magnification.
Observe: Eyelids, lashes, conjunctiva, sclera, pattern of redness, iris, pupil, gross pathology, and media opacities.

II. Direct
A. Beam
Description: Beam is shone directly on area of interest.
Procedure: Use a narrow, full length beam to sweep the structures. Microscope is usually directed straight ahead. The greater the angle between the illuminator and the microscope, the greater the width of the illuminated section.
Observe: Cornea, iris, lens, vitreous.
B. Tangential
Description: Beam is directed at object of interest from an oblique angle to highlight surface irregularities.
Procedure: Using a medium-side beam of moderate height, swing the slit lamp arm to the side at an oblique angle (almost parallel to the structure being viewed). The microscope is pointing straight ahead. Magnifications of 10, 16, or 25X are used.
Observe: Anterior and posterior cornea, anterior iris, anterior lens (especially useful for viewing pseudoexfoliation).
C. Pinpoint
Description: Single round beam of light is used to detect suspended particles in aqueous.
Procedure: Lower beam height to a single round beam, using highest intensity. Direct the beam to enter the cornea temporal to the pupil. Use 16 or 25X magnification.
Observe: Cells, flare.
D. Specular reflection
Description: Beam reflection is used to visualize the integrity of the corneal and lens surfaces.
Procedure: Position the illuminator about 30 degrees to one side and the microscope 30 degrees to the other side. To view the endothelium, start at 10 to 16X magnification. Direct a relatively narrow beam onto the cornea so that the reflection dazzles you. Then move the light a little to the side and look adjacent to it. Switch to high magnification and use only one ocular.
Observe: Corneal epithelium and endothelium, endothelial mosaic, lens surfaces.

III. Indirect
A. Proximal
Description: Reflected light is used to observe internal detail, depth, and density.
Procedure: Use a short, fairly narrow slit beam. Place the beam at the border of the structure or pathology. This creates a light background that highlights the edges of the abnormality.
Observe: Corneal opacities (edema, infiltrates, vessels, foreign bodies), lens, iris.

(continued)

Table 14-2. (continued)

Illumination Techniques

B. Sclerotic scatter

Description: Reflected light is used to view the distribution of corneal pathology.
Procedure: Shine a tall, wide beam onto the limbal area. Use a moderate angle, and offset the illuminator. A ring of light will appear around the cornea, highlighting pathology. Use 10X magnification, and aim the microscope straight ahead.
Observe: General pattern of corneal opacities.

C. Retroillumination

Description: Reflected light is used to evaluate the optical qualities of a structure.

1. Direct retroillumination from the iris:

Description: Light reflected from the iris illuminates the back of the cornea.
Procedure: Aim a moderately wide slit beam toward the iris directly behind the corneal abnormality. Use 16 to 25X magnification, direct the beam from 45 degrees, and keep the microscope straight.
Observe: Cornea.

2. Indirect retroillumination from the iris:

Description: Light is indirectly reflected from the iris, providing a dark background and better contrast for viewing corneal opacities.
Procedure: Aim a moderately wide slit beam toward the iris bordering the portion of the iris behind the pathology. Use 16 to 25X magnification, direct the beam from 45 degrees, and keep the microscope straight.
Observe: Cornea, angles.

3. Retroillumination from the fundus:

Description: Light reflected from the fundus creates a glow behind any media abnormalities.
Procedure: Project a moderate beam through a dilated pupil, with the illuminator and microscope nearly coaxial. Direct the illumination proximally to 2 to 4 degrees. Shorten the beam to fit inside the pupil. Focus directly on the pathology, using 10 to 16X magnification.
Observe: Cornea, lens, vitreous.

D. Transillumination

Description: The iris is illuminated from behind by light reflected off the fundus.
Procedure: The illuminator and microscope are directly in line. Use a full circle beam equal to the size of the pupil (3 to 4 mm when light stimulated). Project light through pupil, focus on iris with 10 to 25X.
Observe: Iris defects (they will glow with the orange light reflected from the fundus).

The Subjective Grading System

An important, but confusing, part of documenting abnormalities is the subjective grading system. Even the term "subjective" causes confusion, because such grading occurs during the objective examination. Some clarification seems to be in order.

First, many of the patient's symptoms are subjective. These are symptoms that the patient tells us about but that we cannot see, such as pain. Other findings are objective. That is, they do not involve the patient's ability to report them...we can see them ourselves when we examine the patient. Cell and flare in the anterior chamber is an objective finding; the patient did not (and cannot) tell us about it, but we can see it. Other findings fall into both realms. The patient may say, "My right eye is red," which is subjective. We can also see the injection through the slit lamp whether the patient has reported it or not, which is objective. The slit lamp exam is an objective test.

Grading pathology and other findings, although they are discovered during the objective examination, are subjective on the part of the examiner. By subjective we here mean that the assignment of a rating to a finding is dependent on the observer's opinion. You may look at the patient and grade her lid edema as 2+. Another clinician may rate the same finding (same patient, same day, and same time) as 1+ or 3+. The best we can advise you is that if you are auxiliary personnel, try to learn the grading system of your employer. As you examine more and more eyes, you will get a feel for how marked a finding is. If you are a physician, do your best to teach your grading philosophy to your staff.

With that said, we would like to offer our own opinion about how to grade your findings (Tables 14-3 through 14-11). Some prefer a numbered grading system. If you use this, then 0+ means that a finding is absent. 1+ would indicate that a finding is just barely perceptible. 4+ would refer to a full-blown case. Using this schematic, 2+ and 3+ would fall somewhere in between. Interjecting half steps in between, such as 2.5+ sometimes complicates this system. We will leave it up to you as to whether this practice is truly necessary or not.

Instead of numbers, specific terms can be used, including "none, absent, bare trace, trace, slight, moderate, marked, severe," and other such words. This is even more subjective than the numbering system. If everyone uses a scale of 0 to 4, then we have a better chance of understanding what 2+ means. Who is to say what the difference really is between "bare trace" and "trace"? (Alas, perhaps it is that nebulous 0.5 half-step!) The dilemma of subjective grading is not likely to be solved.

Table 14-3.
Grading Injection

Feature	Grade
No injection present	0
Slight limbal (mild segmented), bulbar (mild regional), and/or palpebral injection	1
Mild limbal (mild circumcorneal), bulbar (mild diffuse), and/or palpebral injection	2
Significant limbal (marked segmented), bulbar (marked regional or diffuse), or palpebral injection	3
Severe limbal (marked circumcorneal), bulbar (diffuse episcleral or scleral), or palpebral injection	4

Adapted from FDA document Premarket Notification Guidance Document for Daily Wear Contact Lenses. *Reprinted with permission from Ledford JK, Sanders VN.* The Slit Lamp Primer. *Thorofare, NJ: SLACK Incorporated; 1998.*

Table 14-4.
Grading Corneal Haze

Feature	Grade
Clear	0
Between clear and trace; barely perceptible	0.5+
Trace; easily seen with slit lamp	1+
Mild haze	2+
Moderate haze, pronounced, iris details still visible, AC reaction not visible	3+
Marked haze, scarring, iris details obscured	4+

Adapted from Stein HA, Cheskes AT, Stein RM. The Excimer: Fundamentals & Clinical Use. *Thorofare, NJ: SLACK Incorporated; 1995.*

Table 14-5.
Grading Corneal Vascularization

Features	Grade
No vascular changes	0
Congestion and dilation of the limbal vessels; single vessel extension <1.5 mm	1
Extension of multiple vessels <1.5 mm	2
Extension of multiple limbal vessels 1.5 mm to 2.5 mm	3
Segmented or circumscribed extension of limbal vessels >2.5 mm or to within 3.0 mm of corneal apex	4

Adapted from FDA document Premarket Notification Guidance Document for Daily Wear Contact Lenses. *Reprinted with permission from Ledford JK, Sanders VN.* The Slit Lamp Primer. *Thorofare, NJ: SLACK Incorporated; 1998.*

Table 14-6.
Grading Corneal Staining

Feature	Grade
No staining	0
Minimal superficial staining or stippling	1
Regional or diffuse punctate staining	2
Significant dense coalesced staining, corneal abrasion, or foreign body tracks	3
Severe abrasions >2 mm diameter, ulcerations, epithelial loss, or full thickness abrasion	4

Adapted from FDA document Premarket Notification Guidance Document for Daily Wear Contact Lenses. *Reprinted with permission from Ledford JK, Sanders VN.* The Slit Lamp Primer. *Thorofare, NJ: SLACK Incorporated; 1998.*

Table 14-7.
Grading Angles

Features	Grade
Closed angle	0
Angle extremely narrow, probable closure	1+
Angle moderately narrow, possible closure	2+
Angle moderately open, closure not possible	3+
Angle wide open, closure not possible	4+

Reprinted with permission from Ledford JK, Sanders VN. The Slit Lamp Primer. *Thorofare, NJ: SLACK Incorporated; 1998.*

Table 14-8.
Grading Cell (1 mm Conical Beam)

Cell #	Grade
1 to 10	Trace
10 to 20	1+
20 to 30	2+
30 to 40	3+
40 up to hypopyon	4+

Reprinted with permission from Ledford JK, Sanders VN. The Slit Lamp Primer. *Thorofare, NJ: SLACK Incorporated; 1998.*

Table 14-9.
Grading Cortical Cataracts

Feature	Grade
Gray lines, dots, and flakes aligned along the cortical fibers in periphery; visible in oblique direct illumination	1+ (early or incipient)
Opaque spokes, anterior chamber may be shallower than normal for patient	2+ (immature or intumescent)
Cortex opaque up to capsule, anterior chamber may again be normal depth	3+ (mature)
Lens is smaller, wrinkly capsule, nucleus may float in liquified cortex	4+ (hypermature)

Reprinted with permission from Ledford JK, Sanders VN. The Slit Lamp Primer. *Thorofare, NJ: SLACK Incorporated; 1998.*

Table 14-10.
Grading Nuclear Sclerotic Cataracts

Lens Color	Grade
Gray-blue (normal)	0
Yellow overtone	1+
Light amber	2+
Reddish brown	3+
Brown or black, opaque; no fundus reflection	4+

Reprinted with permission from Ledford JK, Sanders VN. The Slit Lamp Primer. *Thorofare, NJ: SLACK Incorporated; 1998.*

Table 14-11.
Grading Posterior Subcapsular Cataracts

Feature	Grade
Optical irregularity on posterior capsule; visible only on retroillumination	1+
Small, white fleck	2+ (early)
Enlarged plaque; round or irregular borders	3+ (moderate)
Opaque plaque	4+ (advanced)

Reprinted with permission from Ledford JK, Sanders VN. The Slit Lamp Primer. *Thorofare, NJ: SLACK Incorporated; 1998.*

The Postoperative Eye (Table 14-12)

One of the key purposes in the slit lamp examination following any type of ocular surgery is to detect the presence of infection... as early as possible. Signs of infection (in any structure or tissue) are redness (injection), swelling (edema), and purulent discharge. The patient may complain of tenderness and pain. External tissue may be warm to the touch.

Endophthalmitis is the most serious complication of infection following any penetrating surgery or injury. This condition is an infection of the internal ocular tissues and can destroy the eye in a short period of time. Worse yet, endophthalmitis can trigger sympathetic ophthalmia, a situation in which the other eye may also be lost. Slit lamp signs of endophthalmitis include postoperative inflammation that is exaggerated beyond what would normally be expected. In addition, watch for lid edema and spasms, redness, conjunctival chemosis, corneal edema, and a marked anterior chamber reaction that may include a hypopyon. The patient may complain of intense discomfort and light sensitivity.

Contact Lens Evaluation for Nonfitters

Soft Contact Lenses (Table 14-13)

One of the first things you will notice about a soft contact lens is its surface. Build up of film and deposits generally (but not always) indicate how well the patient is complying with cleaning regimens.

Compare the diameter of the lens to the diameter of the cornea. A soft lens should overlap the limbus by 1.0 mm on all sides.

A lens of standard thickness should move 1.0 to 2.0 mm with every blink and on upgaze. Less movement may be seen in an ultrathin lens (0.5 mm).

Table 14-12.

Postoperative Slit Lamp Examination Notes

I. Lid Surgery

External	Globe
Lid swelling	Tearing
Lid bruising	Corneal abrasion
Lid redness	Corneal dry spots
Skin sloughing	
Lid position	
Lash position	
Presence of a discharge	
Broken or missing sutures	
Wound gape	
Recurrence of lesion(s)	
Excessive, irregular scarring (keloids)	

II. Lacrimal Surgery

External	Globe
Lid swelling	Tearing
Lid redness	Discharge
Sutures	Silicone tube position
	Corneal abrasion

III. Enucleation

External	Socket
Lid swelling	Conformer in place
	Conjunctival edema (2+ edema would be expected at first)
	Conjunctival injection (conjunctiva may look like a piece of raw meat at first)
	Presence of conjunctival prolapse (abnormal)
	Presence of discharge (a mild mucus discharge is normal)
	Sutures

IV. Extraocular Muscles

Globe
Discharge
Injection
Subconjunctival hemorrhage
Conjunctival wound gape
Exposed sutures
Visible choroidal pigment
Corneal abrasion

(continued)

Table 14-12. (continued)

Postoperative Slit Lamp Examination Notes

V. Corneal Transplant

Globe
Wound leak (Seidel's sign)
Ciliary flush
Corneal staining (of any kind)
Corneal edema
Corneal haze
Corneal opacities
Striae
Graft swelling
Rejection line
Vascularization at suture sites
Keratitic precipitates
Broken sutures
Wound leak
Wound dehiscence (gape)
Healing
Anterior chamber reaction
Anterior chamber depth

VI. Pterygium

Globe
Injection
Graft placement
Corneal dry spots
Corneal staining
Corneal edema
Striae
Presence of sutures
AC reaction
Corneal scarring
Presence of new vessels at limbus
Dellen formation

VII. Radial or Astigmatic Keratotomy

Globe
Conjunctival injection
Conjunctival edema
Superficial keratitis
Staining of incision sites
Corneal edema
Corneal infiltrates
AC reaction

(continued)

Table 14-12. (continued)

Postoperative Slit Lamp Examination Notes

VIII. Excimer Laser

Globe

Bandage contact lens
- Coverage
- Movement

Re-epithelialization
Corneal haze
Corneal infiltrates
Recurrent corneal erosion

IX. Surgical Trabeculectomy

Globe

Conjunctival injection
Subconjunctival hemorrhage
Appearance of drainage bleb
Corneal edema
Corneal striae
AC depth
AC reaction
Hyphema
Pupil shape and size
Anterior synechiae
Posterior synechiae
Cataract formation

X. Laser Trabeculoplasty

Globe

Conjunctival injection
Corneal staining (keratitis most common)
AC reaction
Hyphema
Pupil size and shape
Peripheral anterior synechiae

XI. Laser Iridotomy

Globe

Conjunctival injection
Corneal staining (keratitis most common)
AC reaction
Hyphema
Evaluate iridotomy opening
Anterior synechiae

(continued)

Table 14-12. (continued)

Postoperative Slit Lamp Examination Notes

XII. Cataract

External	Globe
Lid swelling	Conjunctival injection
Ptosis	Conjunctival chemosis
	Wound location
	Wound size
	Wound gape
	Wound leak
	Broken sutures
	Keratitis
	Corneal edema
	Corneal striae
	Endothelial detachment
	AC reaction
	AC depth
	Vitreous in AC
	Hyphema
	Pupil size
	Pupil shape
	Location of IOL
	Position of IOL
	IOL precipitates
	Posterior capsule opacity

XIII. Scleral Buckle for Retinal Detachment

External	Globe
Lid swelling	Conjunctival sutures
	Conjunctival injection
	Conjunctival edema
	Subconjunctival hemorrhage
	Epithelial staining (exposure keratitis most common)
	AC reaction
	Hyphema
	Cataract

XIV. Vitrectomy or Fluid/Gas Exchange

Globe

Conjunctival sutures
Conjunctival edema
Conjunctival injection
Subconjunctival hemorrhage
Corneal staining/epithelial defects (exposure keratitis most common)
AC reaction
Cataract

(continued)

Table 14-12. (continued)

Postoperative Slit Lamp Examination Notes

XV. Laser Photocoagulation

Globe
Corneal edema
Corneal staining (keratitis most common)
AC reaction
Iris atrophy
Pupil shape
Posterior synechiae
Cataract

Reprinted with permission from Ledford JK, Sanders VN. The Slit Lamp Primer. *Thorofare, NJ: SLACK Incorporated; 1998.*

Table 14-13.

Soft Contact Lens (SCL) Evaluation

- **Hygiene/cleanliness:** deposits, film.
  Doc: note, describe, grade 1+ to 4+
- **Coverage:** generally a SCL will extend beyond the limbus in every direction, the edge will not be on the cornea.
  Doc: note, describe ("limbal touch nasally," etc)
- **Movement:** a soft lens will generally move about 1 mm with a blink. If it does not, have the patient look up; you should see a 1 mm slide of the lens downward. If it still does not move, have the patient blink while looking up; there should now be 1 mm movement.
  Doc: note ("good," "excessive," "none," etc)
- **Centration:** ideally the optical center of the lens will align with the patient's visual axis. If the lens is off-center, this should be noted.
  Doc: describe ("good," "centers temporally," etc)
- **Alignment:** an astigmatic lens has marks to evaluate lens alignment.
  Doc: describe location of mark(s) as if the eye were a clock ("astig rides at 6:00," "astig rides at 7:00," etc)
- **Integrity:** look for tears, holes, etc
  Doc: note, give location if possible ("edge," "center," etc)
- **Corneal staining:** the healthy cornea will not stain. Stain indicates a broken epithelial layer.
  Doc: note, draw or describe giving location and extent ("cornea clear," "3+ central staining," etc)
- **Other:** look for bubbles, puckers, anything else unusual
  Doc: note, describe

Reprinted with permission from Ledford JK, Sanders VN. The Slit Lamp Primer. *Thorofare, NJ: SLACK Incorporated; 1998.*

Also, have the patient look left and right, watching how the lens follows the eye. If movement is adequate, the lens will lag 0.5 to 1.0 mm in the lateral gazes.

Notice where the lens settles after blinking. Ideally the optic center of the lens should be in line with the patient's visual axis.

Lens centration is of critical importance when fitting soft astigmatic lenses. Typically, these lenses are marked with dots or lines to aid in evaluation. Depending on the type of lens, the mark should ride at 6:00 or on the horizontal meridian. Have the patient blink while you watch the mark. Alignment is also key in bifocal contacts. These lenses may be truncated (flattened on the bottom edge) or prism ballasted (thicker on the bottom edge for weight) to assist in positioning.

Rigid Contact Lenses (Table 14-14)

Deposits can also plague rigid lenses. Because of the lens material, these deposits may manifest more as a waxy coating on the lens. Each time the patient blinks, a smooth sheet of tears should be swabbed over the lens. This may be best observed after fluorescein dye has been instilled.

A rigid lens is smaller than a soft lens, and thus will not cover the cornea. The old polymethylmethacrylate (PMMA) hard contact lenses were designed to have an interpalpebral fit. That is, the centered lens lies entirely between the lids. The more modern method of fitting gas permeable lenses (which are larger than PMMA contacts) is the alignment fit, where the upper third of the lens stays under the upper lid.

The movement of a rigid lens is much different from that of a soft lens. The rigid lens will move slightly upward with each blink (about 1 to 2 mm), then smoothly drift down and resettle. It should not "drop" down. Normally the lens should not bump into the lower lid margin. When the patient looks left or right, the contact may lag 1 to 2 mm behind, but it should not move past the limbus.

Ideally the lens will center so that the optic zone of the contact falls in front of the patient's visual axis.

Rigid lenses can be left in place when fluorescein dye is instilled. In fact, observing the pattern of the dye under and around the lens provides the fitter with valuable information about the lens fit. If you, as a nonfitter, are asked to evaluate the fluorescein pattern, the general rule is to note areas where the dye pools and areas where the dye is absent. Be sure to use the cobalt blue filter.

Table 14-14.

Rigid Contact Lens Evaluation

- **Hygiene/cleanliness:** deposits, film.
  Doc: note, grade 1+ to 4+, describe
- **Ride/centration:** ideally the center of the lens should come to rest over the optic zone of the pupil.
  Doc: note, describe decentration ("nasal ride," "superior ride," etc)
- **Movement:** a rigid lens will usually be drawn up by a blink, then slide down into place right after the blink.
  Doc: note ("good," "excessive," "none," etc) or grade 1+ to 4+
- **Fluorescein dye pattern:** a properly fit lens will generally have a thin, even layer of dye under it with slight pooling in the periphery.
  Doc: describe ("good dye pattern," "pooling under central lens," etc)
- **Lens surface:** an even coat of tears should be swabbed over the lens with every blink.
  Doc: describe ("good wetting," several dry spots," "poor wetting")
- **Integrity:** look for chips, crazing, scratches.
  Doc: note, describe, grade scratches 1+ to 4+
- **Bifocal segments:** alignment is critical with these lenses.
  Doc: describe ("seg well aligned," "lower seg rocks temporally," etc)
- **Corneal staining:** the healthy cornea will not stain. Stain indicates a broken epithelial layer.
  Doc: note, draw, or describe giving location and extent ("cornea clear," "3+ central staining," etc)
- **Bubbles under lens:** in the average fit, there should not be any bubbles under the lens.
  Doc: note location

Reprinted with permission from Ledford JK, Sanders VN. The Slit Lamp Primer. *Thorofare, NJ: SLACK Incorporated; 1998.*

Unless otherwise noted, all text, tables, and figures are adapted or reprinted with permission from Ledford JK, Sanders VN. The Slit Lamp Primer. *Thorofare, NJ: SLACK Incorporated; 1998.*

CHAPTER 15

Clinical Ocular Photography

Scientific Photography

- Standardize your photographic technique to ensure reproducibility.
- Use metric measurements for precision (Table 15-1).
- Magnification is how large or small an object is on film.
- The hand-held positive lenses used in patient examinations are generally referred to by their dioptric designation, while camera lenses are customarily described by their focal length in millimeters. Magnifying lenses are labeled by how many times they enlarge their subject. Despite the variation in nomenclature, when using a simple single-element lens, all of these lens types can be converted to and classified by their dioptric power, focal length in millimeters, and their power to magnify (Table 15-2).
- Patients are people, not diseases.

Basic Photography

- The 35 mm single lens reflex (SLR) camera is preferred in scientific photography.
- Flash illumination is recommended for patient photography.
- Focusing is the procedure of adjusting a camera lens to obtain the sharpest image of an object.

How-To: Focus a 35 mm SLR

- Rotate the focusing ring of the lens until the image in the view finder appears sharp.
- Measure the distance between you and your subject and preset it on the lens by using the distance scale.
- If your subject must be recorded on film at a specific magnification (eg, 1:10) and your camera has a reproduction ratio scale, once the magnification ratio has been set, focusing is accomplished by moving the camera toward or away from the subject until it appears sharp.

Table 15-1.

Metric Measurements of Length

Unit Name	Symbol	Number	Scientific Notation	Fraction	Meaning
Kilometer	km	1000 m	1 x 10^{3} m	1000/1m	1000 meters
Hectometer	hm	100 m	1 x 10^{2} m	100/1 m	100 meters
Decameter	dam	10 m	1 x 10^{1} m	10/1 m	10 meters
Meter	m	1 m	1 x 10^{0} m	1/1 m	1 meter
Decimeter	dm	0.1 m	1 x 10^{-1} m	1/10 m	One tenth of a meter
Centimeter	cm	0.01 m	1 x 10^{-2} m	1/100 m	One hundredth of a meter
Millimeter	mm	0.001 m	1 x 10^{-3} m	1/1,000 m	One thousandth of a meter
Micrometer	µm	0.000001 m	1 x 10^{-6} m	1/1,000,000 m	One millionth of a meter
Nanometer	nm	0.000000001 m	1 x 10^{-9} m	1/1,000,000,000 m	One billionth of a meter

Reprinted with permission from Cunningham D. Clinical Ocular Photography. *Thorofare, NJ: SLACK Incorporated; 1998.*

Table 15-2.

The Simple Lens

Dioptric Power (D) =	Focal Length (mm) =	Magnification (X)
+1	1000	.25
+2	500	.50
+3	333.33	.75
+4	250	1
+5	200	1.25
+6	166.66	1.50
+7	142.86	1.75
+8	125	2
+9	111.11	2.25

(continued)

Table 15-2. (continued)

The Simple Lens

Dioptric Power (D) =	Focal Length (mm) =	Magnification (X)
+10	100	2.50
+20	50	5
+28	35.71	7
+60	16.66	15
+78	12.82	19.50
+90	11.11	22.50

Reprinted with permission from Cunningham D. Clinical Ocular Photography. *Thorofare, NJ: SLACK Incorporated; 1998.*

- The aperture of an ordinary 35 mm SLR camera, located in the lens assembly, can be adjusted by rotating a click stop mechanism, which moves the overlapping metal leaves of the diaphragm. The opening is designated by size as a standard scale of numbers called f-stops. If maximum sharpness is required, selecting the smallest aperture possible is recommended.
- Relative aperture, or "speed" of a lens, is a measure of the maximum capacity of a lens to transmit light. It depends on the focal length of the lens and its largest effective diameter. The largest effective diameter of a lens is obtained when the iris diaphragm is opened to its widest f-stop setting. Regardless of the number of f-stops on a given lens, its speed is a designation of its largest opening only. A very "fast" lens will have a larger opening than a "slow" lens, although the faster lens will have a smaller f-number.
- The area in front of your camera within which all objects appear to be in acceptable focus is called the "depth of field." The size of this zone varies with numerous factors including focal length, f-number, and object distance.
- A lens with a short focal length will provide more depth of field than a longer lens when a picture is taken from the same camera position.
- Selecting the smallest f-stop will also increase depth of field.
- The length of time that the shutter is open is called shutter speed. A numbered dial, located on the camera body or lens, is set to the desired speed. Although these times are listed as whole numbers (1, 2, 4, 8, 15, 30, 60, 125, etc), they actually represent time in fractions of seconds.
- A lens with a focal length of 50 mm is considered "normal" for a 35 mm camera because it provides an angle of view similar to that of the macula. If a 15 mm lens were substituted and a photograph were taken from the same camera position, a much larger area of interest would be recorded, with the increased coverage obtained with its wider 110 degree angle of view. If, however, a very long 500 mm telephoto lens was used instead, a much smaller area would be covered by its narrower 8 degree field of view.

Table 15-3.

Film Speed Chart

	Slow	Medium	Fast
ISO	10	64	400
	12	80	500
	16	100	640
	20	125	800
	25	160	1000
	32	200	1250
	40	250	1600
	50	320	2000

Reprinted with permission from Cunningham D. Clinical Ocular Photography. *Thorofare, NJ: SLACK Incorporated; 1998.*

- The common characteristics of film are type, size, speed, graininess, resolution, sharpness, and color balance.
- The lower the ISO number, the slower the film and the less sensitive it is to light (Table 15-3). In ophthalmic photography, the 64 or 100 speed color film routinely used during fundus photography is considered to have a medium speed, while the ISO 400 black and white film used in fluorescein angiography is classified as being fast.
- Exposure is controlled by the aperture and shutter on a 35 mm SLR camera. When a flash is used, it also plays an important role in determining the amount of light that will reach the film. To ensure that the film is correctly exposed, select the appropriate f-stop, shutter speed, and flash output for the subject and the film in use.

The Darkroom

- Develop your film as soon as possible after taking the photographs.
- A data sheet suggesting solutions, dilutions, times, and temperatures is usually included with every roll of film and serves as a recipe for developing film shot under ordinary conditions (ie, except fluorescein angiography).
- Developing chemicals include developer, stop bath, and fixer. The film is then washed and allowed to dry in a clean and dust-free environment.

How-To: Develop Black and White Film

- On the dry side of the darkroom (in the dark or in the changing bag), remove the film from its cassette and wind it onto the film reel.
- Place the reel in the tank, and cover the tank with the lid. You may now turn on the room lights and proceed to the designated wet area of the darkroom.
- Consult film data sheet. After deciding which developer and development recipe to use, gather and assemble all the ingredients and necessary utensils. A watch or clock is needed to measure time, a thermometer to check the temperature, and graduated cylinders for accurately measuring the volume of the solutions.
- Arrange the solution-filled graduates from left to right in the following order: developer, stop bath, fixer, water (or some other washing agent).
- Check to be sure that the developer is the proper temperature.
- With the tank slightly tilted, pour the developer into its spout as quickly as possible without spilling. Start the timer when the tank is full of developer, tap the tank once or twice (to eliminate air bubble formation), place the cap on the lid, and agitate as recommended on the data sheet.
- When the required time for development has elapsed, pour out the exhausted solution.
- Pour the contents of the second graduate quickly into the tank and agitate continuously.
- When the required time is up, pour out the stop bath and discard, unless a reusable type is being used.
- Fill the tank with the fixer contained in the third graduate. It, too, usually requires constant agitation for optimum results and is usually reusable. After fixing, film can be safely exposed to light.
- To ensure its permanence, film must be washed properly and allowed to dry in a clean and dust-free environment.
- Once dry, the roll of film should be cut into strips and placed in protective pages, sleeves, or envelopes.

External Eye Photography

- Establish standard photographic views to eliminate the guesswork in external eye photography (Table 15-4).
- The "nine positions of gaze" best demonstrate a deviation from normal position, and may be chosen for a patient with strabismus (Figure 15-1).

External Eye Photography Standard Series

☐ **Eye Plastic Series** Head Shot (1:10) Both Eyes (1:4) • Primary Position • Upgaze • Downgaze Each Eye (1:2) • Primary Position	☐ **Motility Series** Head Shot (1:10) Both Eyes (1:4) • Primary Position • Upgaze • Downgaze • Looking Left • Looking Right
☐ **Orbital Series** Eye Plastic Series Worm's Eye View (1:4)	☐ **Ptosis Series** Both Eyes (1:4) • Primary Position • Upgaze • Downgaze
☐ **Nine Positions of Gaze**	☐ **Other** ________________

Table 15-4. A sample external eye photography standard series (reprinted with permission from Cunningham D. *Clinical Ocular Photography*. Thorofare, NJ: SLACK Incorporated; 1998).

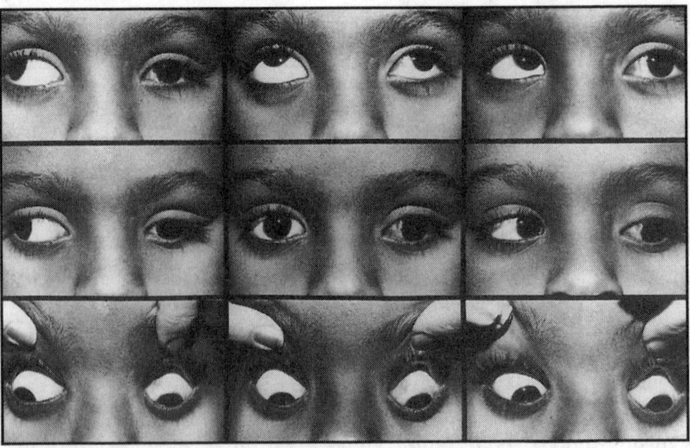

Figure 15-1. The nine positions of gaze (reprinted with permission from Cunningham D. *Clinical Ocular Photography*. Thorofare, NJ: SLACK Incorporated; 1998).

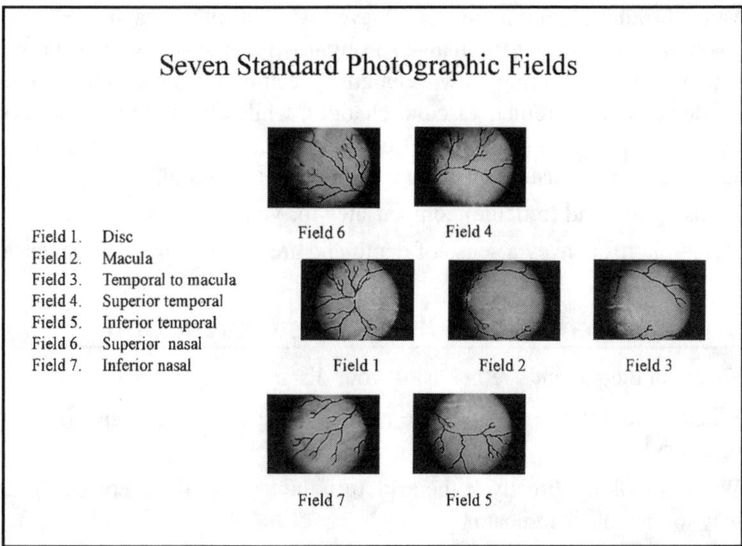

Figure 15-2. The seven standard photographic fields encompass overlapping views of the fundus (model eye) (reprinted with permission from Cunningham D. *Clinical Ocular Photography.* Thorofare, NJ: SLACK Incorporated; 1998).

- A simple arrangement, consisting of a hand-held 35 mm camera, long lens, and portable flash is recommended for external ocular photography.
- The ability of color slide film to provide an accurate and detailed representation of the eye and adjacent structures, make it an ideal film for external eye photography.

Fundus Photography

- The "seven standard photographic fields" have been incorporated as part of many studies of retinal disease and should be familiar to all those who perform fundus photography (Figure 15-2).
- If the camera is too far from or too close to the eye, or not centered on the pupil, unwanted light reflections will appear in the picture.
- For ordinary documentation of intraocular conditions, daylight color positive transparency (slide) film is chosen for fundus photography. The white light of the flash tube is balanced for use with this film. In general, a medium speed film (ISO 64 to 100) is utilized, although slower film may be used if the flash unit is powerful enough.
- Some intraocular structures (such as the choroid, retinal vasculature, and nerve fiber layer) are better appreciated when photographed with black and white film.

- Monochromatic illumination is achieved when a filter of a single (mono) color (chrom) is used to change the light (illumination) shining into the patient's eye by altering its wavelength. Green light is an excellent choice for demonstrating retinal vascular changes, while blue light provides optimal visualization of vitreoretinal interface abnormalities. If a red filter is added, choroidal disturbances may be highlighted as well.
- Focusing the grid (reticule) compensates for your refractive error.
- Stereo photos convey a sense of depth and are usually taken in sequence.

How-To: Focus the Fundus Camera Grid

- Focus on the patient's retina using your distance vision.
- While continuing to focus on the retina, notice whether the grid is sharp or blurry.
- Without looking directly at the grid, turn the knob of the eyepiece all the way to the "plus" indicator.
- Slowly turn the knob toward the "minus" side until the grid appears sharp. Stop. Do not go beyond this point or you will stimulate accommodation.
- When both the grid and the retina are clearly focused, you may take a picture.

How-To: Stereoscopic Fundus Photography

- Center the illumination donut on the patient's pupil with the joystick vertically oriented, and take the first picture.
- Move the camera at least 1 mm laterally to the left or the right and take the second picture. A good 3-D representation of the subject will result if the eye remained stationary.

Fluorescein Angiography

- Use a requisition form to eliminate confusion by enhancing communication.
- Advocate and document informed consent. Patient education is also key.
- Have an emergency medical kit readily available, and inspect its contents on a regular schedule.
- It is necessary to use a "fast" black and white film (ISO 400) with most cameras to record the small amount of fluorescence emitted from the inner eye. If you are recording onto a computer chip rather than onto a piece of photographic film, your video camera must have the sensitivity to pick up the very low level of light available in fundus fluorescein angiography.

- The necessary fluorescein angiography materials include a tourniquet, butterfly needle, vial of fluorescein dye, syringe, alcohol wipe, gauze pad, adhesive bandage, patient, and person to inject the dye.
- The filling stages of a fluorescein angiogram are choroidal flush, arterial, early venous, full venous, and late.

How-To: Educate the Patient for Fluorescein Angiography

- These pictures will be taken using ordinary colored light, not x-radiation or laser light.
- It takes approximately ____ minutes to complete this test.
- Your permission is required to perform this test. You will be informed about the procedure before giving your written consent. Please ask questions about anything you do not understand.
- Although most patients tolerate this procedure well, a few experience nausea following the injection of the dye. Since this passes quickly, try to remain at the camera. On rare occasions, someone may react to the dye by vomiting.
- Your urine and skin may be temporarily discolored because of the dye.
- For the results of your test, contact your doctor in approximately ___ hours/days.

How-To: Fluorescein Angiography

- Educate the patient and obtain informed consent.
- Gather equipment.
- Perform color photography as usual, then prepare for angiography by loading the appropriate camera with black and white film.
- Shoot an ID tag of the patient's name.
- Position the patient in front of the camera, and take monochromatic views of both eyes with the green filter.
- With the fluorescein filters in place, take a control photograph of the eye to be studied, and set the timer to zero.
- After a suitable site has been found to inject the dye, the photographer should first signal the injector to push the fluorescein into the vein, then start the camera's timer.
- The transit of dye through the eye of primary interest is then photographed in rapid sequence, followed by representative views of the other eye. The needle can then be removed.
- A short while later, late views of both eyes should be obtained.
- Rewind, unload, and process the film.

Slit Lamp Photography

- Slit lamp photos are useful in documenting structural abnormalities and pathological processes.
- Slit lamp illumination (see Table 14-2) can be classified as diffuse, direct, or indirect.
- Illumination techniques may be used alone or in combination.
- The slit lamp camera is usually loaded with color transparency film. Depending on the output of the flash, a slow, medium, or high speed may be chosen. If your slit lamp has adjustable f-stops, select a film that allows you to use the smaller apertures in order to take advantage of the increased depth of field.

How-To: Slit Lamp Photography

- Take a photograph of the patient's ID tag.
- For purposes of orientation, first take an overall view of the subject using diffuse illumination and a low magnification. This is important for differentiating between the right and left eye, particularly when the subject is very small or lacks normal landmarks.
- Isolate the area of interest by selecting an appropriate magnification and lighting technique (see Table 14-2). It is customary to position the light source on the temporal side of the eye being photographed.

Photographic Organization

- Data on every patient who is photographed should be recorded in a photography log.
- Patient ID can be recorded on film by photographing an area of the requisition form, using an internal ID tag, or using film check tabs.
- Photos and slides should be labeled to indicate which eye appears in the photograph, as well as what direction is up.
- The position and appearance of the macula, optic nerve, and blood vessels can be used to orient the viewer of retinal photographs (Figure 15-3).
- No matter how perfect a photograph, if it cannot be located, it is worthless.

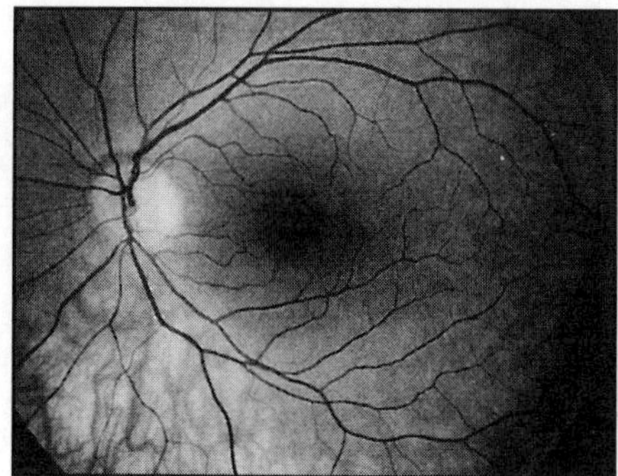

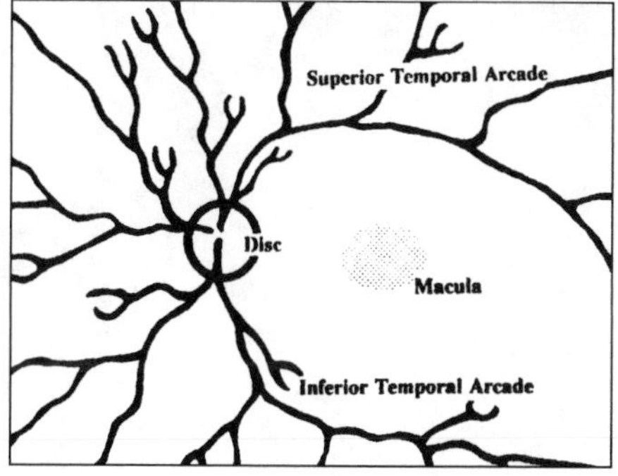

Figure 15-3. The landmarks of the ocular fundus include the disc, macula, and temporal arcades. Upper left: A monochromatic fundus photograph of a normal left eye. Lower left: A graphic representation of the landmarks of a left fundus (reprinted with permission from Cunningham D. *Clinical Ocular Photography*. Thorofare, NJ: SLACK Incorporated; 1998).

Unless otherwise noted, all text, tables, and figures are adapted or reprinted with permission from Cunningham D. Clinical Ocular Photography. *Thorofare, NJ: SLACK Incorporated; 1998.*

Chapter 16

Contact Lenses

Contact Lens Parameters

- The base curve establishes the core fit of the contact lens and acts as the template for the peripheral curve system.
- Rigid and hydrophilic lenses are designed as "ultra thin" to enhance oxygen permeability (referred to as the dK/L) to the central cornea.
- The contour of the lens edge will have a direct interaction with the lid, cornea, and conjunctiva to stabilize the lens on the eye, assist with lens movement, and optimize tear exchange.
- The optic zone diameter (OZD) has a major influence on the lens power, overall dimensions, and central fit.
- The general rule is that smaller optic zone diameters will act flatter, and larger diameters will act steeper.

Safety, comfort, and vision are accomplished by understanding contact lens parameters and their relation to anterior segment anatomy. Contact lens parameters establish a blueprint for lens design. There are a multitude of parameters for hard, rigid, and soft (hydrophilic) contact lenses (Table 16-1). Each individual parameter can have a dramatic effect on the final contact lens-corneal relationship.

Patient Selection

It is a rarity that a patient cannot be fit with contact lenses (Table 16-2). Patient selection for contact lenses is largely based on motivation. If the motivation exists, then the door is open. Once the door is open, the clinician must identify the variety of contact lens options that will best meet the needs of the patient. Such needs involve vision, health, and desired use of contact lenses.

Table 16-1.
Contact Lens Parameters

Parameter	Corneal/Contact Lens Relation
Base curve (BC) or central posterior curve (CPC) in diopters or millimeters	Primary curve of the contact to match the central corneal contour and shape. The BC establishes the core fit of the contact lens and establishes the base for the peripheral curve (PCR) system.
Power (P) or diopters of sphere (DS), diopters of cylinder (DC), and axis (x)	The vertex-corrected dioptric value of the contact lens. $F = \{F_1 - (L_c F_1/n)\} + F_2$ F_1 = back vertex power = $(1 - n)/r_1$ F_2 = front surface power = $(1 - n)/r_2$ r_1 = radius of front focal r_2 = radius of back focal (or F = power) L_c = lens thickness n = index of refraction for the material
Overall diameter (D) in millimeters	Linear measure from lens edge to lens edge, respecting the overall corneal diameter in the horizontal, vertical, and oblique.
Center thickness (L or CT) in millimeters	The thickness in the geometric center of the contact lens, which will determine the stability or prevention of flexure and the oxygen permeability of the material.
Edge thickness/profile (ET) in millimeters	Thickness/profile at the edge of the lens that will affect lid and conjunctival relationships.
Optical zone diameter (OZD) in millimeters	The optical portion of the lens surrounding the geometric center. This area influences power and fit. It establishes the base measure for overall diameter and the PCR widths.
Posterior PCR system in millimeters	Additional paracentral curves that will establish the proper alignment to the peripheral cornea and conjunctiva, provide tear reservoir, and allow for the proper lens movement in relation to lid interaction.
Transition zones or blends	Point of juncture between each posterior curve, CPC, and posterior PCR system.
Central anterior curve (CAC)	Establishes the front vertex power of the lens.
Anterior optical zone (AOZ) or optical cap	Encompasses the front surface of the contact. It may incorporate a toric (astigmatic) correction.
Lens mass	Weight of the contact lens in milligrams.

(continued)

Table 16-1. (continued)
Contact Lens Parameters

Parameter	Corneal/Contact Lens Relation
Aspheric (nonspherical surface) = eccentricity (e)	Deviation from a circular path established by a series of conical sections, such as an ellipse, parabola, hyperbola. Establishes a front and back surface curvature to contour the corneal surface center to periphery.
Material	Hard (PMMA), rigid gas permeable, hydrophilic—hydrogel.
Fenestration	Holes drilled through the lens surface to increase tear fluid exchange.
Lenticulation or carrier	Added or reduced peripheral mass to assist in lens positioning and lid interaction.
Chord	The distance from edge to edge of the contact lens or the diameter of the optic zone.
Sagitta	The distance between a point on the lens surface and the midpoint of the chord.

Reprinted with permission from Daniels K. Contact Lenses. *Thorofare, NJ: SLACK Incorporated; 1999.*

Table 16-2.
Indications and Contraindications for Contact Lenses

Indications for Contact Lenses
Cosmesis
Refractive
Improvement of visual quality (ie, high refractive errors, aphakia, irregular astigmatism, postoperative)
Corneal disease (ie, keratoconus, pellucid, dystrophies, scar, trauma)
Binocular vision (ie, anisometropia, nystagmus, amblyopia, aniseikonia)
Occupational requirements
Sports activity: enhanced peripheral field of vision
Social activity: cosmetics
Therapeutic (ie, drug delivery, bandage, exposure protection)
Low vision aid (ie, telescope or microscope—contact lens systems)

Contraindications of Contact Lenses
Age
Hygiene problems
Hypersensitivity reactions (care product concern)

(continued)

Table 16-2. (continued)

Indications and Contraindications for Contact Lenses

Contraindications of Contact Lenses
Aphakia and/or glaucoma with blebs
Moderate to severe dry eye (circumvented with punctal occlusion or lubricant therapy)
Immunosuppression
Thyroid disease (hypothyroidism: dryness, tear insufficiency; hyperthyroidism: exophthalmos—exposure)
Diabetes mellitus (healing problems—cellular fragility)
Skin disorders (increased risk of ocular infection)
Neurological or retinal disease (ie, CN 5/7 with related corneal hypothesia injury risk; however, may need a lens for therapeutic protection)

Reprinted with permission from Daniels K. Contact Lenses. *Thorofare, NJ: SLACK Incorporated; 1999.*

Soft Contact Lenses

- Conventional or durable lenses are replaced after 6 months (or longer). Frequent replacement lenses have a life span of 1 to 3 months. Disposable lenses are worn either 1 day or 1 to 2 weeks (Table 16-3).
- Daily wear lenses are removed each night; flexible wear are removed alternate nights; extended wear are removed after 6 nights (see Table 16-3).
- The water content of a material is classified as low to moderate (50% or less) or high (50% or higher).
- Hydrophilic lens diameters range from 12.5 to 16 mm, averaging between 13.8 and 14.5 mm.
- Spherical equivalency is calculated as half of the cylinder added to the spherical component of the prescription (with appropriate vertex correction).
- A lens evaluation is performed on lens insertion and after 5 minute settling time. During the time of equilibration, the lens will start to dehydrate and steepen on the eye.
- A subjective survey of lens handling (including insertion and removal plus recognition of an inverted lens) and visual quality increases the potential success of the contact lens fit.
- The goal of a "best fit scenario" is to find the best fit, which is complemented by subjective acceptability for a variety of lens characteristics (Table 16-4).

An efficient diagnostic lens fitting method will expedite the process and decrease chair time at aftercare visits (see Table 16-4). There are two methods of diagnostic lens fits: a bilateral same lens and a bilateral comparative lens fit.

Table 16-3.
Classification of Hydrogel Lenses According to Wear and Replacement Schedule

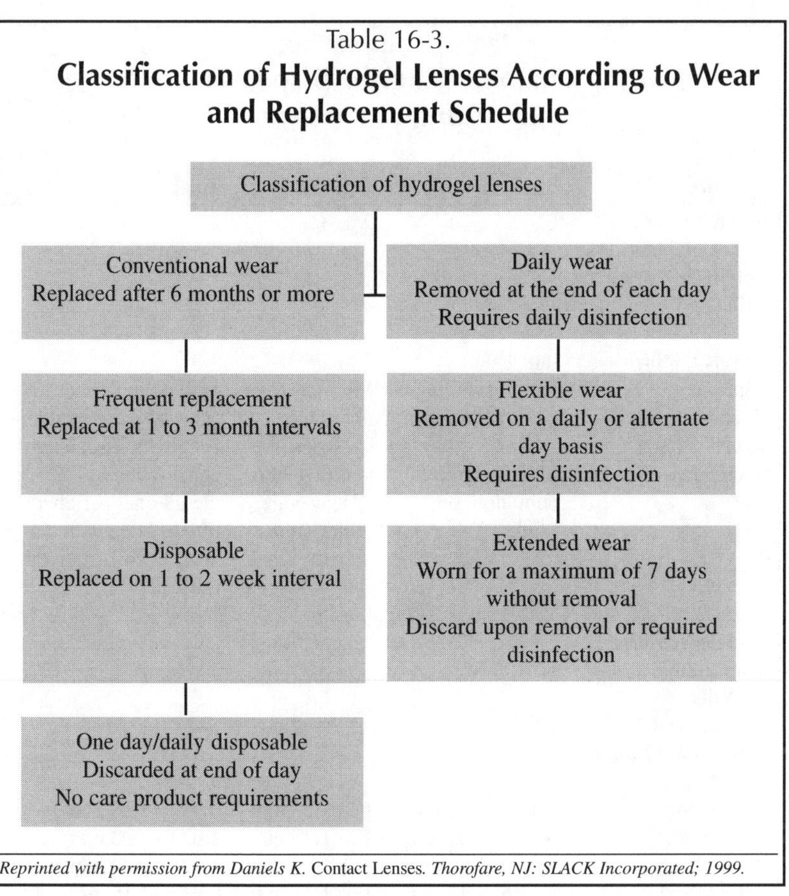

Reprinted with permission from Daniels K. Contact Lenses. *Thorofare, NJ: SLACK Incorporated; 1999.*

Table 16-4.
Fitting Characteristics of Disposable Hydrogel Contact Lenses

Characteristic/ Measure	Flat	Optimal	Steep
Primary gaze	0.51 mm >	0.15 to 0.50 mm	< 0.14 mm
Upgaze	0.65 mm >	0.45 to 0.60 mm	< 0.4 mm
Lateral gaze	0.65 mm >	0.45 to 0.60 mm	< 0.4 mm
Tightness percentage (subj.)	< 40%	45% to 55%	60% >

(continued)

Table 16-4. (continued)

Fitting Characteristics of Disposable Hydrogel Contact Lenses

Characteristic/ Measure	Flat	Optimal	Steep
Tear reservoir = edge accumulation with macromolecular NaFl (0 to 4 scale)	0 to 1	2 to 3	4
Vessels impingement = compression of lens edge onto superficial conjunctival vessels	0 to 1 No vessel dilation or constriction to either side of lens edge, no conj. drag on blink	2 to 3 Minimal vessel dilation or constriction to either side of lens edge, minor conj. drag on blink	4 Vessel dilation to external peripheral lens edge with associated constriction of the internal periphery of lens edge with significant conj. drag on blink
Lens decentration estim. limbus to lens edge (avg. corneal diameter = 12 mm)			
Superior	1.17 to 1.42 mm	1 to 1.25 mm	0.93 to 1.15 mm
Inferior	0.83 to 1.02 mm	1 to 1.25 mm	1.07 to 1.32 mm
Nasal	0.83 to 1.02 mm	1 to 1.25 mm	1.07 to 1.32 mm
Temporal	1.17 to 1.42 mm	1 to 1.25 mm	0.93 to 1.15 mm
Edge fluting	Yes (inf. nasal)	None	None
Coverage	Potential corneal exposure inf. nasal	Complete	Potential corneal exposure superior temporal
Additional characteristics to be evaluated	Lid tension (0 to 4)	Tear meniscus (0 to 0.4)	Iris diameter

(continued)

Table 16-4. (continued)

Fitting Characteristics of Disposable Hydrogel Contact Lenses

Characteristic/ Measure	Flat	Optimal	Steep
Evaluation of fit	Optimal: A fit that demonstrates proper movement, centration, physiological and physical comfort, and visual quality. On lens movement, there is complete coverage of the cornea without limbal exposure.	Marginal: A fit that demonstrates proper movement, centration, physiological and physical comfort, and visual quality. Movement may allow the lens to come into close proximity of the limbus but still maintains complete coverage of the cornea without limbal exposure.	Unacceptable: A fit that demonstrates improper movement; poor centration; potentially decreases physiological or physical comfort, and visual quality. Movement allows the lens to translate onto the corneal surface or forbids translation due to tightness.

*LD = lens diameter, VID = visible iris diameter, PGM = primary gaze movement

Reprinted with permission from Daniels K. Contact Lenses. *Thorofare, NJ: SLACK Incorporated; 1999.*

The "same lens" diagnostic fit is used in the majority of cases when there is clinical confidence in the lens design to complement the visual, comfort, and physiological needs of the patient. In this case, the same lens (ie, same lens type and parameters) is placed on both eyes.

The "bilateral comparative" method is a forced choice comparison between two different lens designs. In this method, the examiner should ask the patient which lens feels better on the eye (physical comfort, not visual). If one lens feels significantly better, or if there is less lens awareness of one versus the other, it suggests that the lens with lesser awareness is probably tighter. In contrast, an *excessive* amount of lens awareness would imply that that lens is fit more loosely (ie, flatter). In either case, it will tell the fitter what to expect on slit lamp examination.

With either method, the lens should be observed immediately on insertion in order to monitor its initial "on eye" fitting characteristics. The lens should then be allowed to settle on the eye, and observed again. (Examiners vary in their opinion as to how long the lens should be allowed to settle, from 2 to 30 minutes. This author [Daniels] prefers an immediate lens evaluation on lens insertion and once again after a 5 minute settlement time.)

Rigid Gas Permeable Lenses

- The basic rule of lens design is to create a synergistic relationship between the anterior surface of the cornea and the back surface of the contact lens.
- There should be an even distribution of the lens mass over the paracentral (3 to 4 mm) cornea.
- The base curve is designed to conform to the corneal cap, establishing an alignment.
- Any residual lacrimal lens effect will manifest in either a plus or minus and/or toric over-refraction. The over-refraction can either be incorporated into the contact lens power or minimized by flattening the base curve and/or decreasing the optic zone diameter.
- A bearing ("negative tear layer") effect of the lens onto the corneal surface will create pressure on the corneal cap while forcing tear fluids to the periphery of the lens.
- Alignment ("plano tear layer") is a method of designing the base curve and optic zone diameter in order to support the lens evenly across the corneal cap without bearing.
- Clearance ("positive tear layer") implies that the lens is fit steep, as compared to the curvature of the central cornea.

The base curve selection should be biased to the amount of corneal astigmatism (Table 16-5). If there is a low corneal cylinder power, a "flatter than flat K" or "on flat K" curve is selected. The goal of an "on flat K" fit is to align the back surface of the contact to the cornea and negate the corneal cylinder-lacrimal lens effect.

The diagnostic fit and aftercare evaluations should be repeated (Table 16-6). The examination should always start with visual acuity. The lens should be viewed grossly on lens insertion and then allowed to settle. This should be followed by a spherocylinder over-refraction. Judgment of centration, movement, and the NaFl pattern must be documented. Lens centration is graded based on its vertical and horizontal positioning on the cornea. Vertical positioning of the lens may be noted numerically as follows: 1 = superior, 2 = superior-central, 3 = central, 4 = central-inferior, or 5 = inferior. Horizontal positioning of the lens may be noted as 1 = nasal, 2 = temporal, and 3 = central. Additionally, the lens-lid relation can be noted as lid attachment, partial lid attachment, or no lid attachment.

Table 16-5.
BC Selection Based on Corneal Cylinder

Corneal Cylinder	BC Selection for Minus Lenses: 9.2 Lens Diameter	BC Selection for Minus Lenses: 9.2 Lens Diameter
Plano to -0.50 DC	0.50 D flatter	0.75 D flatter
0.75 DC to 1.25 DC	0.25 D flatter	0.50 D flatter
1.50 DC to 2.00 DC	On K	0.25 D flatter
2.25 DC to 2.75 DC	0.25 D steeper	On K
3.00 DC to 3.50 DC	0.50 D steeper	0.25 D steeper

For plus lenses, fit the BC 0.25 to 0.50 steeper than recommended for minus lenses.

Adapted from Morgan BW. RGP Material Selection and Design. Eyequest. *1994;4:49-58.*

Table 16-6.
Fitting Characteristics of Rigid Gas Permeable Contact Lenses

Characteristic/Measure			
Overall NaFl: Optic zone of lens (central 7 to 8 mm)	Bearing -2 (excessively flat) -1 (slightly flat < 10 μm)	Alignment = 0 10 to 20 μm	Clearance +1 (slightly steep 20 to 40 μm) +2 (excessively steep 40 μm <)
Overall NaFl: Mid-periphery of lens (8 to 9.4 mm, 9.6 mm)	Bearing: -2 (excessively flat) -1 (slightly flat <10 μm)	Alignment = 0 10 to 20 μm	Clearance +1 (slightly steep 20 to 40 μm) +2 (excessively steep 40 μm <)
Options: Documentation for NaFl relations	Bearing: -2 (excessively flat) -1 (slightly flat <10 μm)	Alignment = 0 10 to 20 μm	Clearance +1 (slightly steep 20 to 40 μm) +2 (excessively steep 40 μm <)
Overall NaFl: PCR system of lens	-2 (extremely narrow < 0.1 μm) -1 (slightly narrow 0.10 to 0.20 μm)	Optimal = 0 0.20 to 0.30 μm	-2 extremely wide >0.40 μm -1 slightly narrow 0.30 to 0.40 μm

(continued)

Table 16-6. (continued)

Fitting Characteristics of Rigid Gas Permeable Contact Lenses

Characteristic/Measure			
Tear reservoir (microns) or axial edge clearance (AEC): accumulation of NaFl beneath the furthest extent of the lens edge	-2 insufficient < 40 mm -1 less than optimal ~60 μm	Optimal ~80 μm	+2 insufficient ~120 μm +1 less than optimal ~100 μm
Post-blink position: Vertical	1 = Superior 2 = Superior/central	3 = Central	4 = Central/inferior 5 = Inferior
Post-blink position: Horizontal	1 = Nasal	3 = Central	2 = Temporal
Lid relationship: related to vertical position	Complete lid attachment (noted as position 1)	Partial lid attachment (noted as position 2)	No lid interaction (noted as position 3, 4, or 5)
Pattern	With-the-rule	Against-the-rule	Oblique
Observable Patterns of Astigmatism (area in gray implies clearance)	With-the-rule (x180)	Against-the-rule (x 90)	Oblique (x 45) (x 135)

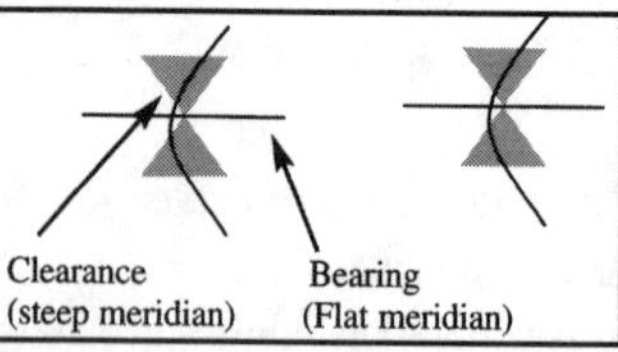

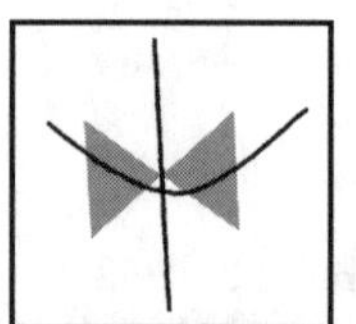

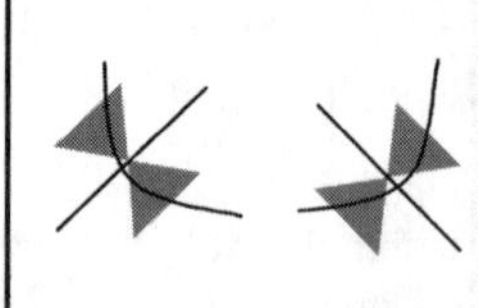

Note: Micron (μm) measurements are estimated.

(continued)

Table 16-6. (continued)

Fitting Characteristics of Rigid Gas Permeable Contact Lenses

Documentation of Lens Position

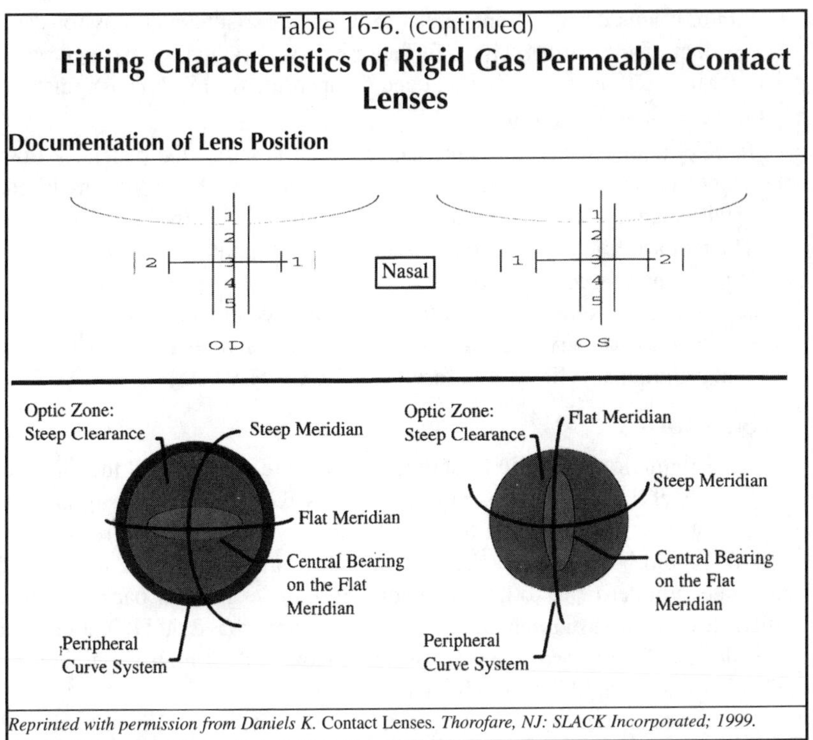

Reprinted with permission from Daniels K. Contact Lenses. *Thorofare, NJ: SLACK Incorporated; 1999.*

Astigmatic Lenses

- Be conservative in toric correction; most patients can tolerate an astigmatic under-correction with complete satisfaction.
- The lid will force a soft toric lens to rotate nasally on lid closure and temporally on opening.
- Transient blur implies that the soft toric lens may have a flat base curve, which is easily remedied by using a steeper base curve.
- Constant blurred vision with soft toric lenses implies that there is either an uncorrected refractive error or a constant misalignment of the lens axis.
- A back surface toric rigid lens is designed so that the posterior lens surface matches the cornea. It is used in cases where the cylinder induced by the lens equals the uncorrected subjective cylinder.
- Saddle fit rigid lenses are designed based on a full alignment to the two principle meridians of power.
- A low toric simulation rigid lens is fit "flatter than K" for the flat meridian, and undercorrects the steep meridian by approximately one-third.

- A bitoric lens design is analogous to designing a spherical lens for each meridian of the cornea with a fit factor that will flatten the base curve in order to avoid the tear lens effect and compensate for residual astigmatism on the front surface of the lens.

In determining which toric alternative would best suit the patient, a flow chart approach is recommended. The patient's needs and other factors are listed, along with the type of lens(es) that fit those criteria (Tables 16-7 and 16-8).

The major refractive question is whether the astigmatism is corneal and/or lenticular. This is ascertained by subtracting the corneal astigmatism (CA), as measured with the keratometer, from the manifest astigmatism (MA), as measured via refractometry. The resulting difference is referred to as internal residual astigmatism (IRA). The formula is IRA = MA-CA.

Soft Torics

An astigmatic diagnostic fit should not be more complicated than a standard hydrogel fit. The lens design should be based on the type of astigmatism. A keratometric reading equal to the refractive cylinder and no greater than 0.67 DC could be fit with a spherical equivalent or masking lens. In cases of moderate cylinder (0.75 to 2.25), a hydrogel of either front or back design is satisfactory. If the astigmatism is significantly higher (> 2.50 DC), a custom toric design would need to be fabricated. However, in higher cylinders, a hybrid or bitoric rigid is properly more appropriate.

All hydrogel toric lenses have markings to indicate the position of axis and ballasting (prism weight at the bottom of the lens). These orientation marks assist the examiner in predicting the possible misalignment of the toric axis. The left, add; right, subtract (LARS) principle implies that if the lens rotates left, the compensation would be to add the estimated number of degrees to the subjective axis. If the lens turns right, then one should subtract the number of degrees from the subjective axis. (The LARS principle applies to both hydrogel and rigid front toric designs.)

The most common problems associated with soft toric lenses are usually related to vision and comfort (Figures 16-1 and 16-2). Comfort complaints are primarily due to an increased lens awareness related to increased lens mass and thickness. This may also cause lens displacement, leading to reduced visual acuity. Proper use of wetting drops will prevent lens steepening and maintain a proper lens-cornea alignment, thus enhancing comfort and visual stability.

Rigid Gas Permeable Torics

There are numerous methods for correcting astigmatism with rigid gas permeable lenses. The main problem in rigid lens fitting is the presumed difficulty in lens design. However, rigid lenses allow the clinician to become a "contact lens tailor." Keep it simple. Design the lens with respect to the corneal topography and refractive error (Table 16-9).

Table 16-7.
Lens Design Options

Flourosilicone Acrylate	Hybrid Design*	Hydrogel
a. Moderate to high Dk	a. Limited to low Dk	a. High water, toric
b. Back or bitoric design	b. Satisfies corneal cylinder only	b. Back or front toric
c. Distance vision only	c. Distance vision only	c. Distance vision only
d. Monovision	d. Monovision	d. Monovision
e. Bifocal	e. Overcorrection for uncorrected astigmatism	

**Hybrid implies a soft/gas permeable lens, such as Softperm. Hybrid lens designs are limited to correcting corneal cylinder only.*

Reprinted with permission from Daniels K. Contact Lenses. *Thorofare, NJ: SLACK Incorporated; 1999.*

Table 16-8.
Corneal/Refractive Astigmatism and Lens Selection

Amount of Refractive Corneal Cylinder	Lens Choice
Low (< 0.67 DC)	Spherical equivalent or masking lens (masking: high rigidity or prism base-down)
Moderate (0.75 to 2.50 DC)	Front or back toric prism ballast or double thin zone (consider frequent replacement)
High (> 2.75 DC)	Front or back toric, custom, or rigid bitoric
Low (< 0.67 DC)	Spherical equivalent
Moderate (0.75 to 2.50 DC)	Front or back toric with ancillary spectacles; rigid bitoric more appropriate
High (> 2.75 DC)	Front or back toric with ancillary spectacles; rigid bitoric more appropriate

Reprinted with permission from Daniels K. Contact Lenses. *Thorofare, NJ: SLACK Incorporated; 1999.*

Spherocylinder Over-Refraction (SCO)
Unexpected power or visual acuity (VA) response
Variable VA
Poor VA with accurate SCO
Verify contact lens power
Recheck SCO
Check subjective Rx
Lens rotation
Toricheck
Lensometer verification
Apply cross cylinder
Estimation method
Trial frame mount
Change BC
Re-evaluate fit (BC)

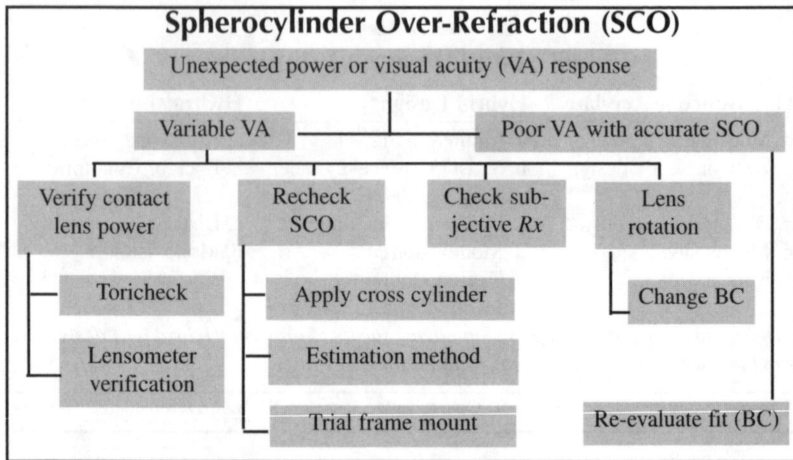

Figure 16-1. Flow chart for poor visual acuity with hydrogel torics (adapted from Myers RI, et al. Using over-refraction for soft toric fitting. *International Contact Lens Clinic*. 1990;17[9/10]:233).

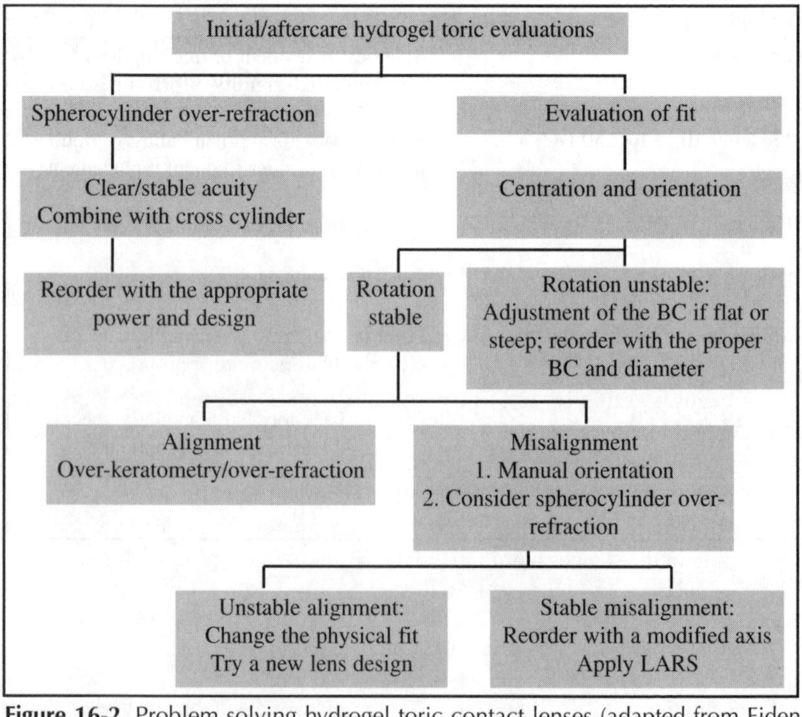

Initial/aftercare hydrogel toric evaluations
Spherocylinder over-refraction
Evaluation of fit
Clear/stable acuity
Combine with cross cylinder
Centration and orientation
Reorder with the appropriate power and design
Rotation stable
Rotation unstable:
Adjustment of the BC if flat or steep; reorder with the proper BC and diameter
Alignment
Over-keratometry/over-refraction
Misalignment
1. Manual orientation
2. Consider spherocylinder over-refraction
Unstable alignment:
Change the physical fit
Try a new lens design
Stable misalignment:
Reorder with a modified axis
Apply LARS

Figure 16-2. Problem solving hydrogel toric contact lenses (adapted from Eiden SB. Precision management of high astigmats with toric hydrogel contact lenses. *Contact Lens Spectrum*. 1992; June: 43-49).

Table 16-9.
Base Curve Selection Based on Corneal Cylinder

	Corneal Cylinder	BC Selection (for minus lenses)
Low cylinder	Plano to -0.50 DC	0.50 to 0.75 D flatter
	0.75 to 1.00 DC	0.25 to 0.50 D flatter
Moderate cylinder	1.25 to 1.50 DC	On K to 0.25 D flatter
	1.75 to 2.00 DC	0.25 D steeper
	2.25 to 2.50 DC	0.50 D steeper
High cylinder	2.75 to 3.00 DC	0.50 to 0.75 D steeper

For plus lenses, fit the BC 0.25 to 0.50 steeper than recommended for minus lenses.

Adapted from Morgan BW. RGP material selection and design. EyeQuest. *1994;2:49-58.*

When the corneal toricity is low (-0.25 to –0.75 DC), a spherical lens design can be used. The base curve should match the flat keratometric reading. This will create an alignment with the flat meridian and allow the tear lens to act as a cylindrical lens, correcting the majority of the corneal cylinder.

When corneal toricity becomes significantly greater than 2.00 DC, various toric lens design alternatives should be considered. These include back toric, saddle fit, low toric simulation, and bitoric lenses; bitoric will be discussed here.

The bitoric lens design is highly favorable in many cases of moderate to high amounts of corneal astigmatism, particularly if there is lenticular astigmatism. The bitoric lens is essentially a back surface toric designed to be flatter in each meridian with additional compensating front toric correction

Mandell and Moore[1] have developed a simple guideline in designing bitoric lenses (Table 16-10). The premise to a bitoric design is to simply think of each meridian separately. A spherical lens will be designed for each meridian with a fit factor that will flatten the BC in order to avoid the tear lens effect. Generally, the flat meridian is fit 0.25 D flatter than K while the steeper meridian is fit 0.50 to 1.25 D flatter, based on the amount of corneal cylinder. The flattening in the steeper meridian will be 0/50 to 1/25 D progressing from 2.00 corneal cylinder and up, respectively.

Patient Instructions and Care

The patient's eye will need to adapt to lens wear. An abbreviated lens wear schedule should be prepared for the patient based on the type of lens. There are two lens adaptation schedules that are recommended (Table 16-11).

Table 16-10.
Fit Factor

Corneal Cylinder	Steep Meridian	Flat Meridian
2.00	0.50 flatter	on K
2.50	0.50 flatter	0.25 flatter
3.00	0.75 flatter	0.25 flatter
3.50	0.75 flatter	0.25 flatter
4.00	1.00 flatter	0.25 flatter
5.00	1.25 flatter	0.25 flatter

Adapted from Mandell RB, Moore CF. A bitoric lens guide that really is simple. *Contact Lens Spectrum. 1988; November: 4(11).*

Table 16-11.
Adaptive Lens Wearing Schedule

Schedule One		Schedule Two	
Day 1	4 to 5 hrs on	Day 1	3 hrs on—3 hrs off—4 hrs on
Day 2	5 to 6 hrs on	Day 2	4 hrs on—3 hrs off—4 hrs on
Day 3	6 to 7 hrs on	Day 3	5 hrs on—2 hrs off—5 hrs on
Day 4	7 to 8 hrs on	Day 4	5 hrs on—1 hr off—5 hrs on
Day 5	8 to 10 hrs on	Day 5	10 hrs on
Day 6	8 to 10 hrs on	Day 6	10 hrs on
Day 7	8 to 10 hrs on	Day 7	10 hrs on

Reprinted with permission from Daniels K. Contact Lenses. *Thorofare, NJ: SLACK Incorporated; 1999.*

How-To: Educate Patients with Contact Lenses

- Washing the hands is the most important aspect of lens handling and lens care.
- Do not use lotions, creams, deodorant soaps, or oils that may coat the lens.
- Never expose your contact lenses to saliva or tap water.
- Use the specified care products only.
- Avoid touching the contact lens with the fingernails.
- Before placing the lens on the eye, inspect it for defects and tears.
- Rehydration of a dried-out soft lens will not sufficiently restore the lens. The lens should be discarded.
- If the lens becomes dislodged or dislocated, examine the eye in a mirror to locate the lens. If the lens cannot be located (and if the lens was not dropped or lost), report to your doctor.

(continued)

How-To: Educate Patients with Contact Lenses (continued)

- If the lens is difficult to remove or if there is an increased sensitivity on lens removal, your lens may be too tight. This should be reported to your doctor.
- If the eye becomes red, swollen, or uncomfortable, or if your vision is blurred or there is a discharge, remove the lens immediately and report to the doctor right away.
- Do not use aerosol products when wearing contact lenses. If you are in the area of an aerosol product, shield your eyes or wear safety eyewear.
- Avoid wearing lenses in the area of fumes, irritating vapors, dust, or smoke.
- If you work in a laboratory, check OSHA (Occupational Safety and Health Association) regulations to determine if contact lenses are forbidden.
- Do not wear lenses in swimming pools, hot tubs, or steam rooms, or during water sport activities.
- If you are hospitalized, contact lens use should be discontinued.
- Lenses should be discontinued if you are undergoing immunosuppression treatment.
- Do not use eyedrops (except for approved rewetting drops) with the contact lens on the eye. Eye medications should be administered *prior to* or *after* the removal of contact lenses.
- Apply makeup *after* inserting your lenses.
- Remove your lenses *before* removing makeup.
- Cover your eyes when using any type of hair spray.
- If daily wear lenses are prescribed, do not sleep with the lenses inserted over night. (Short naps may be safe if you use wetting drops when you wake up… ask your doctor.)
- Maintain a regular aftercare schedule with your eye doctor at the suggested intervals.

The various care product systems presently available on the market are heat (thermal), chemical, multipurpose, and peroxide. All of the products incorporate a rinsing agent, a daily cleaner, and a disinfectant product. The ultimate goal of a system design is to promote compliance by making the care product system safe and easy to use, while maintaining a high level of effectiveness (Table 16-12).

Contact Lens Complications

- The majority of contact lens-related complications of the cornea and conjunctiva are directly related to chronic hypoxia (lack of oxygen).

Table 16-12.

Adverse Reactions and Lens Changes Associated with Care Products

Complications	Cause/Etiology
Corneal staining	1. Improper combination of products 2. Thimerosal products used concurrently with tetracycline 3. Insufficient rinsing of daily cleaner 4. Insufficient removal of enzymatic cleaner 5. Insufficient neutralization of peroxide 6. Storage in benzalkonium chloride
Acute red eye	1. Preservative hypersensitivity 2. Insufficient neutralization of peroxide 3. Inadvertent mixing of sorbate or chlorohexidine with quaternary ammoniums
Ocular irritation	1. Insufficient rinsing of daily cleaner 2. Insufficient neutralization of peroxide 3. Hypersensitivity to preservative agents 4. Acidic or alkaline shift in care product pH 5. Use of nonbuffered agents 6. Debris on lens surface on insertion 7. Insufficient removal or rinsing of enzymatic residue
Lens parameter changes	1. Excessive peroxide exposure 2. Heating lenses in chemical disinfectants
Lens discoloration	1. Gray/black: thimerosal used with thermal units 2. Yellowish/brown: a) Use of sorbate-containing products b) Excessive proteinaceous coating 3. Yellow/green: use of standard sodium fluorescein 4. Opaque: a) Use of chlorohexidine with thermal disinfection b) Use of expired care products c) Switching from chemical to thermal disinfection without purging d) Heating with products of high viscosity
Fading of tinted lenses	1. Use of solvent-based products 2. Use of benzoyl peroxide (ie, acne preparations)
Incompatibilities	1. Generic hydrogen peroxide 2. Mismatching of products leading to instability and ineffective disinfection 3. High water content parameter changes using thermal disinfection

(continued)

Table 16-12. (continued)

Adverse Reactions and Lens Changes Associated with Care Products

Complications	Cause/Etiology
Incompatibilities	4. Polyquad not compatible with sorbic buffers
Lens dryness	1. Improper digital cleaning 2. Improper use of enzymatic cleaner 3. Improper use of oil- and/or lanolin-based hand cleaners and lotions
Rigid gas permeable surface defects	1. Exposure to alcohol cleaners 2. Excessive polishing at high speeds 3. Excessive digital pressure, inducing lens warping

Adapted from Wesibarth RE, Ghormley NR. Hydrogel lens care regimens and patient education. In: Bennett E, Weissman BA, eds. Clinical Contact Lens Practice. *Philadelphia, Pa: JB Lippincott; 1991.*

- The most common contact lens complication is due to difficult insertion and removal, poor lens conditions (such as scratched lens surfaces or deposits), and the presence of debris on the back surface of the lens.
- Vascularization is the formation and extension of capillaries that had not previously existed.
- Subepithelial infiltrates (SEI) are secondary to an inflammatory reaction associated with chronic hypoxia, causing the aggregation of cellular components in the tissue.
- Corneal edema is due to the leakage of fluid into the cornea secondary to a change in the endothelial pump mechanism (which leads to fluid influx into the stromal layer). Fluid leakage into the stroma results in central corneal clouding, striae, or folds.
- In giant papillary conjunctivitis (GPC), the surface of the palpebral conjunctiva, notably the upper lid, is covered with papillae. It is primarily an allergic reaction.

A corneal ulcer is a form of severe microbial infiltration of the corneal tissue. The ulcer will progressively destroy the underlying stroma, leading to possible perforation. Extended wear soft lenses have the greatest incidence of corneal ulcers. Patients who are immunocompromised (ie, HIV, chemotherapy, or long-term steroid use), have healing problems (such as diabetics), or have severe dry eye may be more susceptible to either lens-related or nonlens-related ulcers. Table 16-13 shows the differential diagnosis of ulcerative keratitis versus subepithelial infiltrates.

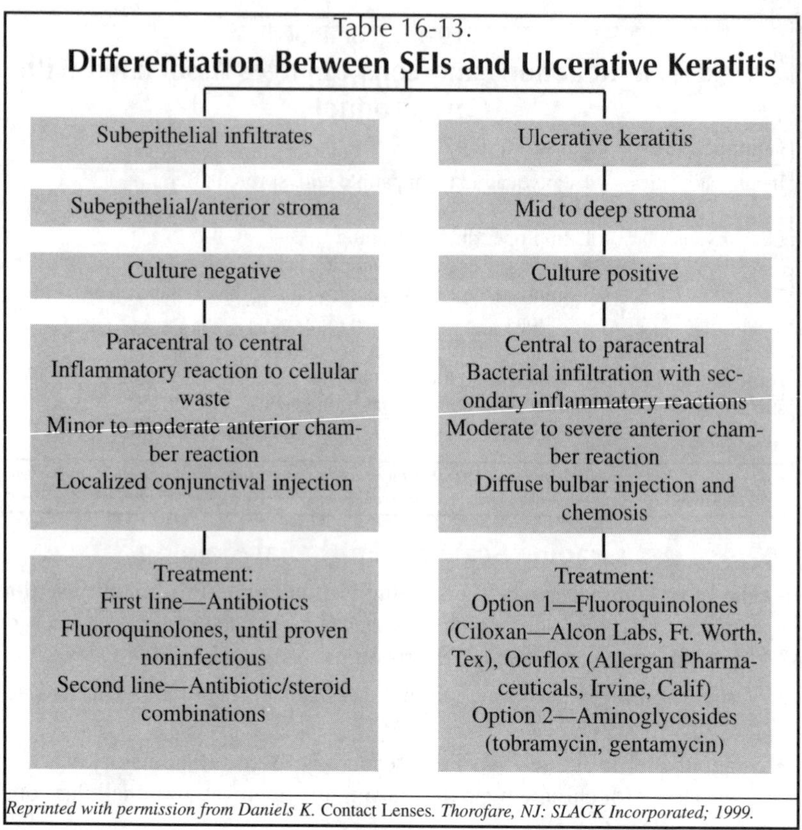

Table 16-13.
Differentiation Between SEIs and Ulcerative Keratitis

Subepithelial infiltrates	Ulcerative keratitis
Subepithelial/anterior stroma	Mid to deep stroma
Culture negative	Culture positive
Paracentral to central Inflammatory reaction to cellular waste Minor to moderate anterior chamber reaction Localized conjunctival injection	Central to paracentral Bacterial infiltration with secondary inflammatory reactions Moderate to severe anterior chamber reaction Diffuse bulbar injection and chemosis
Treatment: First line—Antibiotics Fluoroquinolones, until proven noninfectious Second line—Antibiotic/steroid combinations	Treatment: Option 1—Fluoroquinolones (Ciloxan—Alcon Labs, Ft. Worth, Tex), Ocuflox (Allergan Pharmaceuticals, Irvine, Calif) Option 2—Aminoglycosides (tobramycin, gentamycin)

Reprinted with permission from Daniels K. Contact Lenses. *Thorofare, NJ: SLACK Incorporated; 1999.*

When corneal edema occurs, fluid also leaks into the stromal layer. This may lead to striae or folds in the stroma, along with a central haze (Table 16-14).

Corneal abrasions and foreign body tracking is the chafing or drying of the epithelium created by lens fracture or defect, lens deposits, foreign bodies, or blunt trauma as demonstrated by a distinct path or pattern of corneal staining (Table 16-15).

Contact Lenses for Presbyopes

- Patient selection is premised on motivation, realistic expectations, and the ability to accept minor visual compromise.
- When refining monovision, leave the patient with a subtle blur of approximately 20/25 at distance and near.
- Multifocal contact lenses can be described as "simultaneous view designs" due to their position over the pupil.

Table 16-14.
Corneal Edema Levels

Corneal Swelling	Signs	Relationships	Level
< 2%	Undetectable edema	Unknown	Benign
2% to 5%	Early stages of striae	Implies chronic hypoxia	Safe
5%	Vertical striae observed	Chronic hypoxia	Caution
8%	Posterior folds and striae	Acute edema	Danger
20%	Loss of corneal transparency, folds, striae	Pathological	Pathological

Adapted from Grant TJ, Terry R, Holden BA. Extended wear of hydrogel lenses: clinical problems and their management. In: London R, ed. Problems in Optometry: Contact Lenses and Ocular Disease. *Philadelphia, PA; JB Lippincott Co;1990.*

Table 16-15.
Grading Scale for Epithelial Staining

Grade	Extent	Depth
0 (None)	Absent	Absent
1 (Trace)	1% to 15% surface involvement	Superficial epithelial
2 (Mild)	16% to 30% surface involvement	Stromal glow within 30 seconds after NaFl instillation
3 (Moderate)	31% to 45% surface involvement	Immediate, localized stromal glow
4 (Severe)	46% or greater surface involvement	Immediate, diffuse stromal glow

Adapted from Grant TJ, Terry R, Holden BA. Soft lens extended wear. In: Harris MG, ed. Contact Lenses: Treatment Options for Ocular Disease. *New York, NY: Mosby Publishing; 1996.*

- The annular or concentric design multifocal lens utilizes a near, center/distance, peripheral or distance, center/near, peripheral design.
- Aspheric multifocals utilize a pseudoannular design and are generally referred to as progressive power lenses.
- Translating or alternating bifocal lens designs are essentially "miniature" executive, flat top, or crescent style bifocals, which are position-dependent.
- The patient should be educated that a translating lens design will be "low riding," which can cause easier dislodgement and loss of the lens.
- In all forms of presbyopic fitting, the dominant eye will need to be selected in order to bias one eye for distance and the other for near.

How-To: Eye Dominance

- Hole in the hand (demonstrates visual dominance and alignment): The patient is asked to fully extend the arms and place the hands together, making an opening the approximate size of a quarter. The patient is asked to view an isolated letter on an acuity chart through the opening. The fitter covers one eye and then the other. The eye that sees the target through the "hole" is the dominant eye.
- Plus lens test (demonstrates ocular dominance and level of "blur toleration"): Place the best distance refraction into a trial frame. Place a +1.50 lens in front of each eye in an alternating fashion as the patient views the distance acuity chart. (Note: The test should be performed with an add power +0.25 to +0.50 less than the patient's spectacle add.) Ask the patient: "When the lens is held over your eye, which eye is least disturbed or appreciates the least amount of blur?" The eye that appreciates the least amount of blur is the eye that should be selected for distance dominance. (Less add power is required due to the vertex effect. Closer to the corneal plane adds plus to the overall power.)
- Alternate occlusion (demonstrates the dominant eye for distance visual): This method uses a "cover test" method to determine the distance dominant eye. Simply have the patient view the distance acuity chart while occluding the eyes in an alternating format. Ask the patient which eye appreciates the sharpest quality of vision while alternating the occluder. The eye with the sharpest vision is the dominant eye. After determining the distance dominant eye in this method, proceed to the "plus lens" method to determine the level of "blur tolerance" at distance and near.
- "Camera to eye" or "targeting eye" method (defines distance dominant eye): Place the final distance correction into a trial frame. Have the patient take a camera and put it to the eye he or she would normally use to take pictures. This is the dominant distance eye. If a patient is active in sports that require firearms, archery, and so forth, ask the patient which eye he or she would usually use for targeting. Again, this would be the dominant distance eye. After the dominant eye is determined, proceed with the introduction of plus lenses over the near eye to determine the tolerance for blur.
- Refractive variance: Generally, the more myopic (or least hyperopic) eye will accept less plus at the near point. Therefore, the more myopic eye should be biased for the distance correction.

There are many lens designs available, each having a different level of complexity in fitting and ability to satisfy the visual and environmental needs of the patient. The designs include monovision, modified monovision, simultaneous view bifocals, and translating bifocals (Table 16-16).

When refining a monovision correction, the near eye should be able to achieve a distance visual acuity of approximately 20/40 to 20/50 vision (Table 16-17).

Reference

1. Mandell RB, Moore CF. A bitoric lens guide that really is simple. *Contact Lens Spectrum.* 1988;4(11):83-85.

Unless otherwise noted, all text, tables, and figures are adapted or reprinted with permission from Daniels K. Contact Lenses. *Thorofare, NJ: SLACK Incorporated; 1999.*

Table 16-16.

Contact Lens Options for Presbyopes

✓ = below average ✓✓ = average ✓✓✓ = above average

Factor	Monovision	Modified Monovision	Translating Bifocal	Simultaneous Design	Modified Bivision
Visual demand at distance	✓✓	✓✓✓	✓✓✓	✓✓	✓✓✓
Visual demand at intermediate	✓	✓✓	✓	✓✓✓	✓✓✓
Visual demands at nearpoint	✓✓	✓✓	✓✓✓	✓✓	✓✓✓
Add power	< +1.75	< +2.50	< +2.50	< +1.75	< +2.50
Pupil dependency	None	Minimal	Variable	Variable	Variable
Pupil size limitations (mm)	No limitation	> 3	3 to 4	3 to 4	3 to 4
Expense	Low to moderate	Average to moderate	High	Variable	High

All modalities are available in rigid lens materials in various designs. Hydrogel lenses are available in the various designs with a more limited, but expanding, availability.

Reprinted with permission from Daniels K. Contact Lenses. *Thorofare, NJ: SLACK Incorporated; 1999.*

Table 16-17.

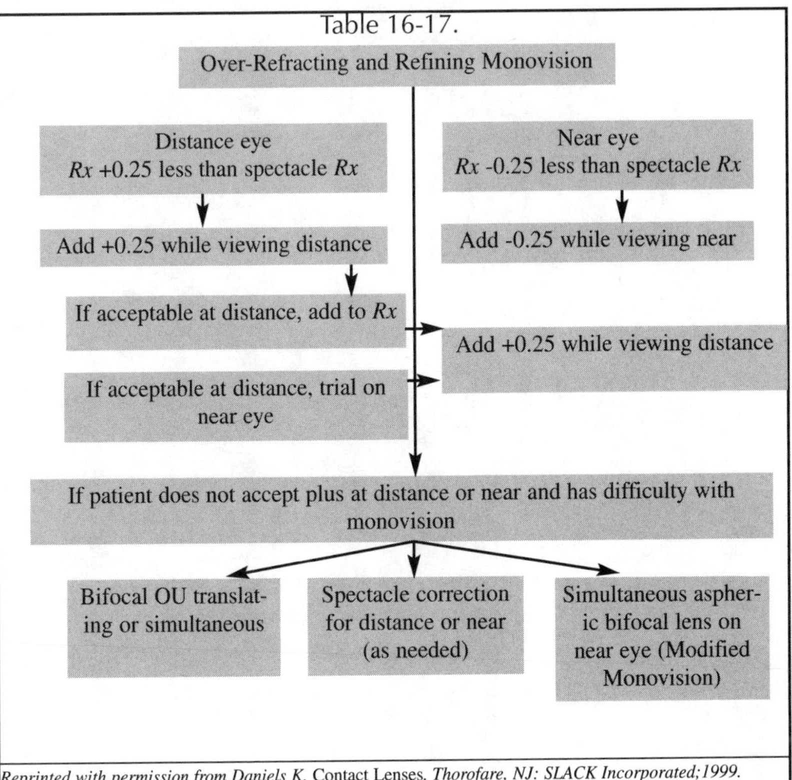

Reprinted with permission from Daniels K. Contact Lenses. *Thorofare, NJ: SLACK Incorporated;1999.*

Chapter 17

Ophthalmic Medications and Pharmacology

Prescription Writing (Table 17-1)

Table 17-1.
Common Abbreviations Used in Prescription Writing

ac	before meals
bid	twice a day
c, cum	with
caps	capsule
Coll., Collyr	eyewash
d.	day
disp.	dispense
gt (t)	drop(s)
h	hour
hs	at bedtime
no., #	number
OD	right eye
Oh	every hour
OS	left eye
OU	both eyes
p.c.	after meals
po	by mouth
prn	as needed
q	every
qh	every hour
qid	four times a day
qs	as much as needed
q2h	every 2 hours
Rx	prescribe
s, sine	without
sig	instructions
sol	solution

(continued)

Table 17-1. (continued)

Common Abbreviations Used in Prescription Writing

susp	suspension
tab	tablet
tid	three times a day
ung	ointment
ut dict	as directed
i	one
ii	two
iii	three

Reprinted with permission from Duvall B, Kershner RM. Ophthalmic Medications and Pharmacology. *Thorofare, NJ: SLACK Incorporated; 1998.*

Autonomic Drugs

- The autonomic nervous system consists of two branches: the sympathetic and parasympathetic. The actions of these two systems generally oppose one another.
- The sympathetic system is responsible for the excited state of the body. Pupillary dilation occurs as a result of sympathetic stimulation (Table 17-2).
- The parasympathetic system is responsible for the body's resting state. Pupillary constriction and accommodation are a result of parasympathetic activity (Table 17-3).
- Neurotransmitters are chemical messengers of the nervous system. Certain pharmaceuticals work by stimulating, mimicking, or inhibiting these messengers. This helps manipulate the autonomic functions.

Diagnostic Pharmaceuticals

- Mydriatics dilate the pupil (Figures 17-1 and 17-2).
- Cycloplegics dilate the pupil and suspend accommodation (Figures 17-3 and 17-4).
- Tropicamide is the drug of choice for routine dilation. It is often combined with phenylephrine or hydroxyamphetamine for added effect.
- Cyclopentolate is the drug of choice for routine cycloplegia.
- Topical ophthalmic dyes should be instilled only after evaluation of the cornea and anterior chamber, as they can alter the clinical picture.

Table 17-2.

Clinical Use of Ophthalmic Adrenergic Agents

Clinical Use of Ophthalmic Adrenergic Agents
Mydriatics (dilate the pupil):
phenylephrine
hydroxyamphetamine
cocaine
Antiglaucoma agents (decrease aqueous formation):
apraclonidine
betaxolol
levobunolol
metipranolol
timolol
Antiglaucoma agents (increase aqueous outflow):
epinephrine
dipivefrin
Vasoconstrictors (whiten the eye):
phenylephrine
naphazoline
oxymetazoline
tetrahydrozoline
Dilation reversal:
dapiprazole HCl

Reprinted with permission from Duvall B, Kershner RM. Ophthalmic Medications and Pharmacology. *Thorofare, NJ: SLACK Incorporated; 1998.*

Table 17-3.

Clinical Use of Ophthalmic Cholingeric Agents

Clinical Use of Ophthalmic Cholingeric Agents
Miotics (constrict the pupil):
pilocarpine
carbachol
physostigmine
echothiophate
Cycloplegics (paralyze accommodation):
atropine
scopolamine
homatropine
cyclopentolate
tropicamide
Diagnosis of myasthenia gravis:
edrophonium

(continued)

Table 17-3. (continued) **Clinical Use of Ophthalmic Cholingeric Agents**
Paralysis of extraocular and lid muscles: botulinum A toxin

Reprinted with permission from Duvall B, Kershner RM. Ophthalmic Medications and Pharmacology. *Thorofare, NJ: SLACK Incorporated; 1998.*

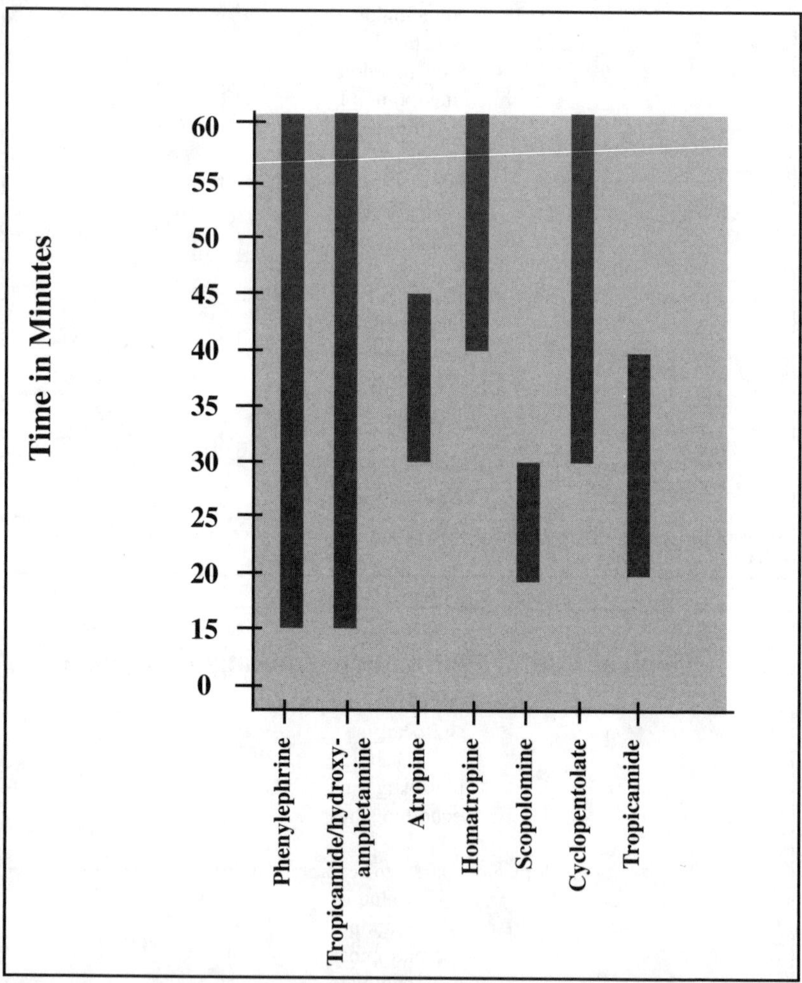

Figure 17-1. Time to maximum mydriasis (reprinted with permission from Duvall B, Kershner RM. *Ophthalmic Medications and Pharmacology*. Thorofare, NJ: SLACK Incorporated; 1998).

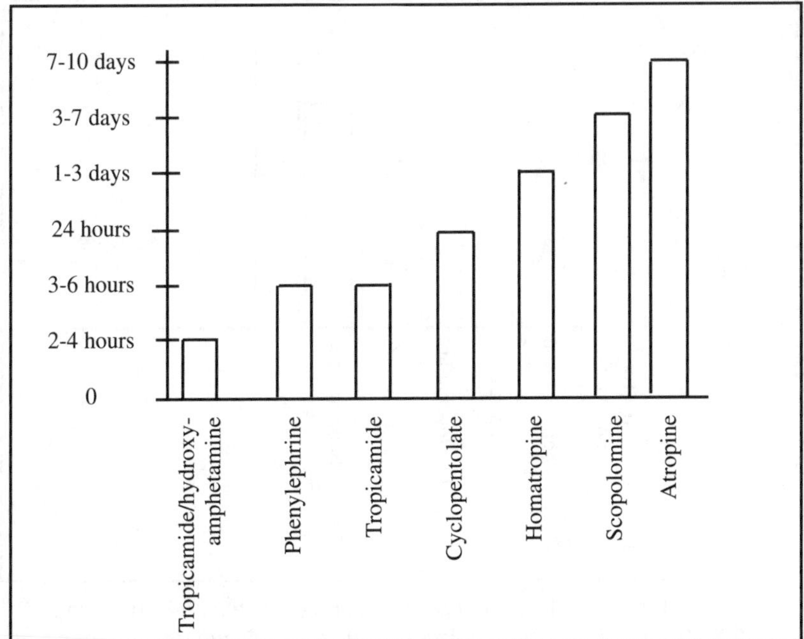

Figure 17-2. Time to mydriasis recovery (reprinted with permission from Duvall B, Kershner RM. *Ophthalmic Medications and Pharmacology*. Thorofare, NJ: SLACK Incorporated; 1998).

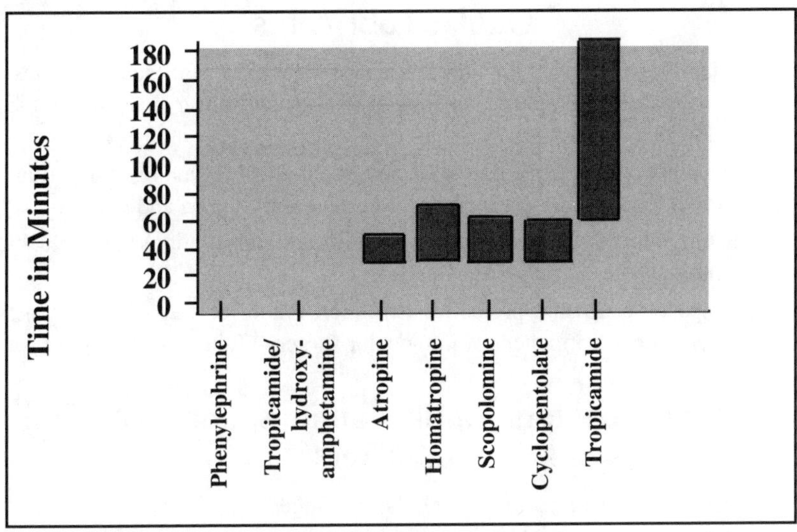

Figure 17-3. Time to maximum cycloplegia (reprinted with permission from Duvall B, Kershner RM. *Ophthalmic Medications and Pharmacology*. Thorofare, NJ: SLACK Incorporated; 1998).

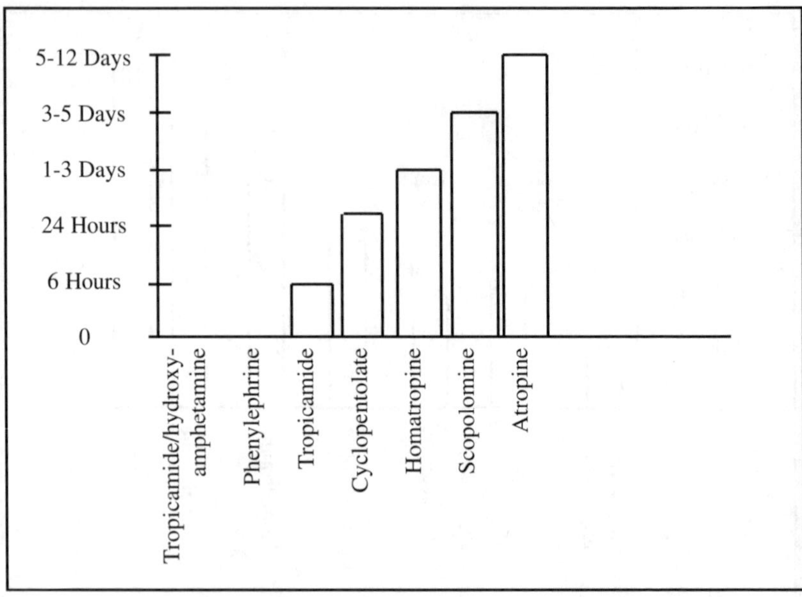

Figure 17-4. Time to cycloplegic recovery (reprinted with permission from Duvall B, Kershner RM. *Ophthalmic Medications and Pharmacology*. Thorofare, NJ: SLACK Incorporated; 1998).

Ocular Lubricants

- Ocular lubricants are the initial therapeutic choice for ocular dryness. Preservative-free preparations should be used whenever possible (Tables 17-4 through 17-7).
- Topical hyperosmotics are used to decrease corneal edema resulting from a variety of conditions and are helpful in increasing vision and comfort.
- Mucomimetic, irrigating (Table 17-8), and coupling solutions have valuable but limited roles in ophthalmic care.
- The space-occupying, protective, and inert nature of viscoelastics makes them a critical component of intraocular surgery (Table 17-9).

Vasoconstrictors, Antihistamines, and Mast Cell Stabilizers

- When administered topically, ocular decongestants (or vasoconstrictors) constrict the superficial conjunctival blood vessels and thus reduce congestion and redness (Table 17-10).

Table 17-4.

Partial List of Nonpreserved Artificial Tears (Brand Names)

Bion Tears
Celluvisc
Dry Eye Therapy
Hypotears PF
Ocucoat
Refresh

Reprinted with permission from Duvall B, Kershner RM. Ophthalmic Medications and Pharmacology. *Thorofare, NJ: SLACK Incorporated; 1998.*

Table 17-5.

Selected Preserved Artificial Tears (Brand Names)

Absorbotear
AKWA Tears
Hypotears
Ultratears
Zacril
Liquifilm Tears
Genteal
Nutra-Tears
Tears Naturale II
Vit-A-Drops

Reprinted with permission from Duvall B, Kershner RM. Ophthalmic Medications and Pharmacology. *Thorofare, NJ: SLACK Incorporated; 1998.*

Table 17-6.

Selected Lubricating Agents in Order of Increasing Viscosity (Brand Names)

Dry Eye Therapy
Hypotears
Refresh
Tears Plus
Tears Naturale
Bion Tears
Ocucoat
Celluvisc

Reprinted with permission from Duvall B, Kershner RM. Ophthalmic Medications and Pharmacology. *Thorofare, NJ: SLACK Incorporated; 1998.*

Table 17-7.

Ophthalmic Lubricating Ointments (Brand Names)

Preserved

Dura Tears Naturale
Hypotears
Duralube
Lacrilube SOP

Nonpreserved

AKWA Tears
Lacrilube NP
Lipo-Tears
Duolube

Reprinted with permission from Duvall B, Kershner RM. Ophthalmic Medications and Pharmacology. *Thorofare, NJ: SLACK Incorporated; 1998.*

Table 17-8.

Selected Extraocular Irrigating Solutions (Brand Names)

AK-Rinse
Blinx
Collyrium Eye Wash
Dacriose
Eye Stream
Eye Wash

Reprinted with permission from Duvall B, Kershner RM. Ophthalmic Medications and Pharmacology. *Thorofare, NJ: SLACK Incorporated; 1998.*

Table 17-9.

Viscoelastics (Brand Names)

Healon
Healon GV
Ocucoat
ProVisc
Viscoat
Vitraz

Reprinted with permission from Duvall B, Kershner RM. Ophthalmic Medications and Pharmacology. *Thorofare, NJ: SLACK Incorporated; 1998.*

Table 17-10.
Selected Decongestants (Brand Names)

Selected Decongestants (Brand Names)
Naphazoline
Allerest
Clear Eyes
Naphcon
Vaso Clear
Opcon
Oxymetazoline
Ocuclear
Visine LR
Phenylephrine
Prefrin
Relief
Tetrahydrozoline
Murine Plus
Visine
Collyrium Fresh

Reprinted with permission from Duvall B, Kershner RM. Ophthalmic Medications and Pharmacology. *Thorofare, NJ: SLACK Incorporated; 1998.*

- Ocular antihistamine and decongestant combinations have some value in treating mild allergic conjunctivitis (Table 17-11). They are inexpensive and easily obtained over the counter. However, they are often ineffective.
- Any product containing a decongestant should be used sparingly. Frequent use can result in increased redness and dryness.
- Mast cell stabilizers are useful in treating chronic ocular allergic symptoms. Preventative in nature, they must be used religiously, and their effect is often noticed only after days of treatment.

Corticosteroids

- Corticosteroids are very potent inhibitors of inflammation but can cause serious side effects (Tables 17-12 through 17-14).
- Patients on corticosteroid therapy must be monitored closely. Long-term, chronic use of these drugs is not advised.
- Topical corticosteroids rarely cause adverse systemic effects, although ocular effects (such as elevated intraocular pressure) can occur frequently.
- Caution should be exercised when corticosteroids are to be used in the presence of recurrent, chronic, or acute infection.

Table 17-11.

Selected Decongestant Combinations (Brand Names)

Decongestant/Antihistamine
Naphcon-A
Vasocon-A
Opcon-A
Ocuhist
Albalon-A
Decongestant/Astringent
Zinc Frin
Vaso Clear-A
Visine AC

Reprinted with permission from Duvall B, Kershner RM. Ophthalmic Medications and Pharmacology. *Thorofare, NJ: SLACK Incorporated; 1998.*

Table 17-12.

Selected Uses for Corticosteroids in Ophthalmic Practice

Chemical burns
Allergic conjunctivitis
Immune graft reaction
Stromal Herpes simplex keratitis
Sterile corneal infiltration
Interstitial keratitis
Uveitis
Scleritis/episcleritis
Retinitis
Optic neuritis
Temporal arteritis
Orbital pseudotumor
Graves' ophthalmopathy

Reprinted with permission from Duvall B, Kershner RM. Ophthalmic Medications and Pharmacology. *Thorofare, NJ: SLACK Incorporated; 1998.*

Table 17-13.

Relative Anti-Inflammatory Potency of Selected Corticosteroids

Drug	Relative Strength
Betamethasone	25
Dexamethasone	25
Methylprednisone	5
Triamcinolone	5
Prednisone	4

(continued)

Table 17-13. (continued)
Relative Anti-Inflammatory Potency of Selected Corticosteroids

Drug	Relative Strength
Prednisolone	4
Hydrocortisone	1

Reprinted with permission from Duvall B, Kershner RM. Ophthalmic Medications and Pharmacology. *Thorofare, NJ: SLACK Incorporated; 1998.*

Table 17-14.
Selected Corticosteroids

Generic	Brand Name(s)
Prednisolone	Pred Forte, Econopred Plus, Pred Mild, Econopred, Ak-Pred, Inflamase Forte, Inflamase
Fluorometholone	Fluor-op, FML SOP, FML Forte, Flarex, Eflone
Dexamethasone	Ak-Dex, Baldex, Decadron, Dexotic, Maxidex
Rimexolone	Vexol
Medrysone	HMS

Nonsteroidal Anti-Inflammatory Drugs (NSAIDs)

- NSAIDs are generally less potent anti-inflammatory agents than the corticosteroids and have fewer adverse effects. This makes them a better alternative in many cases, especially where chronic use is indicated.
- Oral NSAIDs are readily available and are effective in reducing pain, fever, and inflammation arising from a variety of causes (Table 17-15).
- Topical NSAIDs work very well in reducing pain associated with corneal injuries, such as an abrasion or keratorefractive surgery (Table 17-16).

Anti-Infectives (Tables 17-17 through 17-20)

- Most common ocular infections can be treated topically, although systemic treatment may be indicated for lid, orbital, and posterior segment involvement.

Table 17-15.
Selected Oral NSAIDs

Drug	Brand Name
Aspirin	Bayer, Bufferin
Acetaminophen (non-NSAID)	Tylenol
Diclofenac	Voltaren
Diflusinal	Dolobid
Flurbiprofen	Ansaid
Ibuprofen	Advil, Motrin, Nuprin
Indomethacin	Indocin
Ketoprofen	Orudis
Ketorolac	Toradol
Naproxen	Anaprox, Naprosyn, Aleve
Piroxicam	Feldene
Sulindac	Clinoril
Tolmetin	Tolectin

Reprinted with permission from Duvall B, Kershner RM. Ophthalmic Medications and Pharmacology. *Thorofare, NJ: SLACK Incorporated; 1998.*

Table 17-16.
Topical NSAIDs

Generic	Brand Name
Flurbiprofen	Ocufen
Suprofen	Profenal
Diclofenac	Voltaren
Detorolac	Acular

Table 17-17.
Selected Combination Antibiotic Ointments (Brand Names)

Polymixin B/Neomycin/Bacitracin
Neotal
Nertracin
Triple Antibiotic
Ak-Spore
Neosporin

Polymixin/Bacitracin
Ak-Poly-Bac
Polysporin

Polymixin/Neomycin
Statrol

(continued)

Table 17-17. (continued)

Selected Combination Antibiotic Solutions (Brand Names)

Polymixin B/Neomycin
Statrol

Polymixin B/Neomycin/Gramicidin
Ak-Spore
Neosporin
Neotracin

Polymixin B/Trimethoprim
Polytrim

Reprinted with permission from Duvall B, Kershner RM. Ophthalmic Medications and Pharmacology. *Thorofare, NJ: SLACK Incorporated; 1998.*

Table 17-18.

Selected Antibiotic/Steroid Ointments (Brand Names)

Chloromphanicol/Polymixin B/hydrocortisone
Clormycetin Hydrocorts
Ophthocort

Bacitracin/Neomycin/Polymixin B/hydrocortisone
Cortisporin
Coracin

Prednisolone Acetate/Gentamycin
Pred G SOP

Neomycin/Dexamethasone
Neodecadron

Tobramycin/Dexamethasone
Tobradex

Neomycin/Polymixin B/Dexamethasone
Ak-Trol
Dexacidin
Maxitrol

Selected Antibiotic/Steroid Solutions and Suspensions (Brand Names)

Neomycin/Hydrocortisone
Cortisporin
Bactiocort

Oxytetracycline/hydrocortisone
Terra-cortric

(continued)

Table 17-18. (continued)
Selected Antibiotic/Steroid Solutions and Suspensions (Brand Names)

Neomycin/hydrocortisone
Ak-Neo-Cort

Rhomycin/Prednisolone Acetate
Poly Pred

Gentamycin/Prednisolone Acetate
Pred-G

Neomycin/Dexamethasone Sodium Phosphate
Ak-Neo-Dex
Neo Decadron

Tobramycin/Dexamethasone
Dexacidin
Ak-Trol
Maxitrol
Dexasporin

Chloramphenicol/Hydrocortisone
Chloromycetin Hydrocortisone

Reprinted with permission from Duvall B, Kershner RM. Ophthalmic Medications and Pharmacology. *Thorofare, NJ: SLACK Incorporated; 1998.*

Table 17-19.
Selected Steroid/Sulfonamide Solutions and Suspensions

Combination	**Trade Name**
Sulfacetamide/fluoromethalone	FML-S
Sulfacetamide/prednisolone acetate	Blephamide
	Sulfacort
	Isopto Cetapred
	Ak-cide
	Ophtha P/S
	Metimyd
	Or-Toptic M
	Predsulfair
	Sulphrin
Sulfacetamide/prednisolone phosphate	Vasocidin
	Optimyd
Steroid/Sulfonimide Ointments	
Sulfacetamide/prednisolone acetate	Blephamide SOP
	Cetapred
	Ak-cide
	Predsulfair

(continued)

Table 17-19. (continued)

Steroid/Sulfonimide Ointments

Sulfacetamide/prednisolone acetate	Metimyd Vasocidin

Reprinted with permission from Duvall B, Kershner RM. Ophthalmic Medications and Pharmacology. *Thorofare, NJ: SLACK Incorporated; 1998.*

Table 17-20.

Antiviral Therapy

Generic	Brand Name(s)
Idoxuridine	Herplex, Stoxil
Vidarabine	Vira-A
Trifluridine	Viroptic
Gancyclovir	Cytovene (oral, IV), Vitrasert (Cytovene implant)
Foscarnet	Foscavir (IV)

- A "shotgun" approach to treating ocular infection is not recommended. Therapy should be directed specifically at the causative organism. Cultures and drug sensitivities should be obtained when necessary (see Chapter 10).
- Anti-infectives must be used responsibly. Over use can result in the development of resistant organisms. Highly potent agents, such as fluoroquinolones, should be reserved for more serious infections so as to avoid resistance and maintain effectiveness.
- Infections that do not resolve after an appropriate length of therapy may be the result of targeting the wrong organism, using an improper agent, or the development of resistance. Consider, also, a possible allergic or toxic response to the medication.

Anti-Glaucoma Therapy (Tables 17-21 and 17-22)

- The theory behind glaucoma management is to decrease the intraocular pressure to a point where further optic nerve damage and visual field loss ceases. This is done pharmacologically by decreasing aqueous production or increasing outflow.
- Although laser and filtering surgery has advanced (see Table 18-5), retiring many traditional drugs, pharmacologic management is still the primary step in the treatment of glaucoma.
- Beta blockers have long been the drug of choice in glaucoma management. However, newer medications, such as topical anhydrase inhibitors and prostaglandin analogues, may challenge this position with increased efficacy and safety.

Table 17-21.

Commonly Used Medications for Treating Open-Angle Glaucoma

Class	Generic	Brand	Manufacturer	Dosage
Miotics	Pilocarpine	Multiple		0.5-6% drops—two times/day
	Pilocarpine gel	Pilopine	Alcon Laboratories, Fort Worth, Tex	4%—once daily
	Carbachol	Isopto Carbachol	Alcon Laboratories, Fort Worth, Tex	0.75-3% drops—two to three times/day
	Echothiophate	Phospholine iodide	Wyeth-Ayerst Laboratories, Philadelphia, Pa	0.03-0.25% drops—one to two times/day
Prostaglandins	Latanoprost	Xalatan	Pharmacia & Upjohn Co, Bridgewater, NJ	0.005% drops—once daily
Combined alpha and beta adrenergic agonists	Epinephrine	Multiple		1-2% drops—two times/day
	Dipivefrin	Propine	Allergan, Inc, Irvine, Calif	0.1% drops—two times/day
Pure alpha-2 adrenergic agonists	Apraclonidine	Iopidine	Alcon Laboratories, Fort Worth, Tex	0.5% drops—two to three times/day
	Brimonidine	Alphagen	Allergan, Inc, Irvine, Calif	0.5% drops—two to three times/day
Non-selective beta adrenergic blockers	Timolol*	Timoptic	Merck & Co, Inc, West Point, Pa	0.25-0.5% drops—one to two times/day
		Betimol	Ciba Vision, Atlanta, Ga	
	Timolol gel	Timoptic-XE	Merck & Co, Inc, West Point, Pa	0.25-0.5%—once daily
	Levobunolol	Betagan	Allergan, Inc, Irvine, Calif	0.25-0.5% drops—one to two times/day
	Metipranolol	OptiPranolol	Bausch & Lomb, Inc, Tampa, Fla	0.3% drops—two times/day
	Carteolol	Ocupress	Otsuka America Pharmaceutical, Rockville, Md	1% drops—two times/day

(contin-

Table 17-21. (continued)

Commonly Used Medications for Treating Open-Angle Glaucoma

Class	Generic	Brand	Manufacturer	Dosage
Selective beta-1 adrenergic blockers	Betaxol	Betoptic	Alcon Laboratories, Fort Worth, Tex	0.5% drops—two times/day
	Betaxolol suspension	Betoptic-S	Alcon Laboratories, Fort Worth, Tex	0.25% drops—two times/day
Carbonic anhydrase inhibitors	Dorzolamide*	Trusopt	Merck & Co, Inc, West Point, Pa	2% drops—two to three times/day
	Brinzolamide	Azopt	Alcon Laboratories, Fort Worth, Tex	1% drops—two to three times/day
	Acetazolamide	Diamox	Lederle Laboratories, Pearl River, NY	125, 250 mg pills, 500 mg capsule—one to four times/day
	Methazolamide	Neptazane	Lederle Laboratories, Pearl River, NY	25, 50 mg pills—one to three times/day

*Cosopt, a combination product containing timolol and dorzolamide, is also available (Merck & Co, Inc, West Point, Pa).

Reprinted with permission from Duvall S, Lens A, Werner EB. Cataract and Glaucoma for Eyecare Paraprofessionals. *Thorofare, NJ: SLACK Incorporated; 1999.*

Table 17-22.

Side Effects of Commonly Used Glaucoma Medications

Class	Side Effects	Comments
Miotics	Small pupil, blurred vision, dim vision, night blindness, headache, increased myopia, increased cataract, tearing, red eyes, increased ocular inflammation, retinal detachment, abdominal cramps, diarrhea, sweating, urinary retention.	Systemic side effects more likely in smaller individuals. Echothiophate is considerably more potent than pilocarpine or carbachol.
Prostaglandins	Increased iris pigmentation, burning, irritation, allergy, increased ocular inflammation, red eyes.	Latanoprost acts by increasing uveoscleral outflow.
Combined alpha and beta adrenergic agonists	Red eyes, irritation, allergy, dilated pupil, blurred vision, pigment deposits in conjunctiva and tear ducts, increased blood pressure, rapid or irregular heartbeat, heart attack, headaches, anxiety, insomnia.	Dipivefrin usually has fewer side effects than epinephrine, but fewer than 50% of patients can tolerate either long-term.
Pure alpha 2 adrenergic agonists	Red eyes, irritation, allergy, dry eyes, dry mouth, decreased blood pressure.	Brimonidine may be better tolerated long-term than apraclonidine.
Non-selective and selective adrenergic blockers	Burning, allergy, corneal erosions, decreased corneal sensitivity, slow heartbeat, heart failure, low blood pressure, fainting, depression, loss of libido, fatigue, shortness of breath, asthma, decreased exercise tolerance, sudden death.	Betaxolol (a selective beta blocker) has fewer side effects than the nonselective agents but is less effective in lowering intraocular pressure.
Carbonic anhydrase inhibitors	Red eyes, irritation, allergy, tingling in fingers and toes, weakness, fatigue, depression, loss of appetite, weight loss, alteration of sense of taste, loss of libido, Stevens-Johnson syndrome, kidney stones, increased urination, acidosis, anemia, bone marrow suppression.	Dorzolamide, the topical eyedrop, has less risk of side effects than the oral agents acetazolamide or methazolamide. Carbonic anhydrase inhibitors should not be used by patients who are allergic to sulfa drugs.

Reprinted with permission from Duvall S, Lens A, Werner EB. Cataract and Glaucoma for Eyecare Paraprofessionals. *Thorofare, NJ: SLACK Incorporated; 1999.*

- Glaucoma therapy involves treating the patient, not just the disease. Factors relating to patient compliance, lifestyle, and systemic health, as well as the expense of therapy must always be considered when determining the appropriate course of action.

Notes

- In addition to the drug, pharmaceutical preparations have added ingredients to control pH, tonicity, viscosity, and microbial contamination.
- Pharmaceutical breakdown occurs as a result of extreme temperature, moisture, and light. Store pharmaceuticals to avoid these factors.
- Preservatives are used to control microbial contamination. They can, however, cause corneal toxicity in some patients.
- Anterior segment conditions are normally treated topically. In addition to being more effective, topical medications also avoid the increased risks and side effects of systemic administration.
- Always list all medications that a patient is taking in order to avoid possible interactions and side effects.
- Listen carefully to a patient's symptoms. They can often be drug-related.
- Eye exams are recommended for all patients on prednisone and chloroquine.
- Many topically used drugs can have effects on other organ systems.

Unless otherwise noted, all text, tables, and figures are adapted or reprinted with permission from Duvall B, Kershner RM. Ophthalmic Medications and Pharmacology. *Thorofare, NJ: SLACK Incorporated; 1998.*

CHAPTER 18

Overview of Ocular Surgery and Surgical Counseling

Surgery of the Skin and Lids (Table 18-1)

Table 18-1.
Surgery of the Skin and Lids

I. Removal of Growths

Procedure: Biopsy/removal (excision)
Description: Growth is removed in part or entirety and sent to pathology lab for evaluation
Anesthetic: Local
Notes: If growth is frozen or cauterized, there is no tissue for biopsy

Procedure: Cautery
Description: Uses high temperature to burn the tumor
Anesthetic: Local
Notes: Usually used after a biopsy has been performed or when the doctor has determined that the growth is not extensive

Procedure: Chemotherapy
Description: Cancer-fighting drugs used systemically or applied locally to the tumor
Anesthetic: None
Notes: Often used if the patient is unable or unwilling to undergo surgery; after the surgical removal of a tumor, to treat cancerous cells that might be left behind

Procedure: Cryotherapy
Description: Cryoprobe is placed on the tumor to freeze it
Anesthetic: Local
Notes: Usually used after a biopsy has been performed or when the doctor has determined that the growth is not extensive

(continued)

Table 18-1. (continued)

Surgery of the Skin and Lids

Procedure: Frozen section
Description: Suspected malignant growth is removed, sent to the lab, quick-frozen, and examined while the patient is still on the table
Anesthetic: Local or general
Notes: Tissue is removed until pathology reports that margins are clear

Procedure: Laser
Description: Directed at the tumor to break down the tumor or vaporize the cancer cells
Anesthetic: Topical or local
Notes: Often used if the patient is unable or unwilling to undergo surgery; after the surgical removal of a tumor, used to treat cancerous cells that might be left behind

Procedure: Micrographic (Mohs') surgery
Description: Suspected malignant growth is removed in layers and evaluated microscopically while the patient is still on the table
Anesthetic: Local or general
Notes: Preserves more normal tissue

Procedure: Radiation
Description: X-ray beams are aimed at the tumor to either kill the cancer cells or prevent the cells from spreading
Anesthetic: None
Notes: Often used if the patient is unable or unwilling to undergo surgery; after the surgical removal of a tumor, used to treat cancerous cells that might be left behind

II. Reconstructive Surgery
Procedure: Blepharoplasty
Description: Removal of excess skin (and sometimes orbital fat) from the eyelids
Anesthetic: Local
Notes: Surgery is considered functional if the vision is impaired by the condition; if the vision is not impaired, the surgery is designated as cosmetic

Procedure: Brow lift (direct approach)
Description: An incision is made down to the subcutaneous layer, and the brow is raised to the correct position
Anesthetic: Local
Notes: May be performed in conjunction with a blepharoplasty and/or ptosis repair if needed; may leave a scar just above the brows

Procedure: Brow lift (endoscopic)
Description: The skin is lifted off from the forehead down to the brow area, releasing muscles as needed; the brow is then pulled into the correct position
Anesthetic: Local
Notes: Scar hidden in hairline

(continued)

Table 18-1. (continued)

Surgery of the Skin and Lids

Procedure: Cryotherapy (of eyelashes)
Description: The tip of the probe is held in position for about 30 to 45 seconds to freeze the hair follicle
Anesthetic: Local
Notes: Used to treat a larger area of lashes

Procedure: Ectropion repair
Description: A wedge of skin is removed from the lid (cautery is used to control the bleeding) and the edges of the wound are sewn together
Anesthetic: Local
Notes: Purpose is to pull the eyelid against the globe

Procedure: Electrolysis (of eyelashes)
Description: A fine wire tip is applied to the hair follicle, and a weak electric current is used to destroy the hair follicle
Anesthetic: Local
Notes: Generally used if only a few lashes need to be treated

Procedure: Entropion repair (Quickert suture)
Description: A suture is passed from the inside of the eyelid into the conjunctiva and through the eyelid below the eyelash line
Anesthetic: Local
Notes: Purpose is to turn the eyelid away from the globe

Procedure: Entropion repair (tarsal strip)
Description: A designated amount of lid margin and conjunctiva are removed, and the tarsal strip is pulled laterally and secured with sutures
Anesthetic: Local
Notes: Purpose is to turn the eyelid away from the globe (this more complex procedure has the best chance for a lasting result)

Procedure: Flap
Description: Uses skin adjacent to the wound to cover the wound
Anesthetic: Local
Notes: The adjacent skin is moved over but not completely excised, bringing along its own blood supply

Procedure: Graft
Description: Tissue from one part of the body is removed and used to repair the wound
Anesthetic: Local
Notes: Graft may be obtained from excess skin of the upper eyelid, the inner arm, behind the ear, or above the collar bone

(continued)

Table 18-1. (continued)

Surgery of the Skin and Lids

Procedure: Ptosis repair
Description: The levator muscle is sutured to the tarsus; a sling procedure to connect the eyelid to the frontalis muscle may be used when the levator muscle has little or no functional ability of its own
Anesthetic: Local
Notes: Can be performed alone or with a blepharoplasty if indicated

Procedure: Tarsorrhaphy
Description: Upper and lower lids are stitched together
Anesthetic: Local
Notes: Done to protect the cornea from exposure

Surgery of the Tear System (Table 18-2)

Table 18-2.

Surgery of the Tear System

Procedure: Dacryocystorhinostomy (DCR)
Description: A large opening is made beneath the tear sac in the bone of the nose, which opens the lacrimal sac directly into the nose, giving the tears a place to drain
Anesthetic: Local or general
Notes: A silicone tube may also be inserted through the puncta into the tear system and tied in the nose

Procedure: Irrigation
Description: Washing out of the lacrimal passageway; cannula (lacrimal needle) is inserted into the canaliculus, and saline is flushed into the system
Anesthetic: Topical
Notes: If the lacrimal system is open, the patient will be aware of the saline running into the back of the throat; if there is a blockage, the saline will run down the face

Procedure: Tear duct intubation
Description: A silicone tube is passed through the puncta, through the canaliculus, into the tear sac, and into the nose
Anesthetic: Local or general
Notes: The tube usually remains in the eye for 6 months or longer

Procedure: Tear duct probing
Description: A fine metal wire is passed through the punctum, through the canaliculus, into the tear sac, down the nasolacrimal duct, and into the nose to relieve a blocked nasolacrimal system
Anesthetic: Local or general
Notes: May be combined with irrigation

Corneal Surgery (Tables 18-3 and 18-4)

Table 18-3.
Corneal Surgery

Procedure: Astigmatic keratotomy (AK)
Description: Corrects astigmatism via arcuate incisions in the peripheral cornea
Anesthetic: Topical
Notes: The incisions stretch the cornea while they heal, causing the central portion of the cornea to change shape

Procedure: Corneal transplant (lamellar keratoplasty [LKP])
Description: Only the cloudy layers of cornea are removed; the donor button is then inserted on top of the remaining host tissue and sutured in place
Anesthetic: Local or general
Notes: Usually entails a long recovery period

Procedure: Corneal transplant (penetrating keratoplasty [PKP])
Description: The full thickness of the cornea is replaced with donor corneal tissue
Anesthetic: Local or general
Notes: Usually entails a long recovery period

Procedure: Laser assisted in situ keratomileusis (LASIK)
Description: A thin section of cornea (corneal cap) is removed or made into a flap, and the excimer laser is used to reshape the corneal stroma, then the corneal cap is placed back on the eye
Anesthetic: Topical
Notes: Performed for moderate and high amounts of refractive error

Procedure: Photorefractive keratectomy (PRK)
Description: Removal of tissue from the cornea via excimer laser to correct a refractive condition
Anesthetic: Topical
Notes: The amount of tissue that is removed is guided by a computer and controlled by the eye surgeon; the location and length of time of the laser pulses will determine how much correction will be made

Procedure: Phototherapeutic keratectomy (PTK)
Description: Removal of tissue from the cornea via excimer laser to correct a medical eye condition
Anesthetic: Topical
Notes: Used to treat conditions such as recurrent erosion or superficial corneal scarring

Procedure: Radial keratotomy (RK)
Description: Corrects myopia via radial incisions in the peripheral cornea
Anesthetic: Topical
Notes: The incisions stretch the cornea while they heal, causing the central portion of the cornea to change shape

Table 18-4.
Comparison Between RK and PRK

	RK	PRK
Range of treatment	Low to moderate amounts of myopia	Can correct higher amounts of myopia
Location of treatment	Performed on the peripheral cornea, not invading the optical zone	Performed on the central cornea
Postoperative recovery	The eye is structurally weaker and results are less predictable	There is no weakening of the cornea and the laser allows more predictable and reproducible results
Postoperative pain	Mild pain up to 24 hours	Moderate pain up to 3 days
Postoperative eyedrops	Usually 1 week	Up to 6 months
Success rate of achieving 20/40 vision or better	About the same	About the same
Enhancement rate	Much higher than PRK	Much lower than RK
Risk of severe vision loss	About the same (quite low)	About the same (quite low)
Contact lens wear after surgery	More problematic with RK	Generally successful
Long-term effects	Possible hyperopia	Possible regression to myopia
Cost of procedure	Less expensive than PRK	Generally more expensive than RK

Reprinted with permission from Pickett K. Overview of Ocular Surgery and Surgical Counseling. *Thorofare, NJ: SLACK Incorporated; 1999.*

Glaucoma Surgery (Table 18-5)

Table 18-5.
Glaucoma Surgery

Procedure: Argon laser trabeculoplasty
Description: Creates burns in the trabecular meshwork, which stretch the drainage holes in the meshwork, allowing the fluid to drain more easily
Anesthetic: Topical
Notes: Questionable lasting effect

Procedure: Cyclocryo
Description: A freezing probe is externally applied to the sclera at the location of the ciliary body to reduce aqueous production
Anesthetic: Local or general
Notes: Infrequently used; done when other methods have failed

Procedure: Filtering implants (valve)
Description: A tube (called a seton) is inserted with the open end extending into the anterior chamber; a plate or ring is sutured to the sclera and covered by a flap of Tenon's capsule and conjunctiva
Anesthetic: Local or general
Notes: The tube opens when the intraocular pressure reaches a certain level, allowing aqueous to flow out of the eye; the plate should prevent the bleb from failing even if scarring occurs

Procedure: Laser microendoscope cycloablation
Description: Laser is applied to the ciliary body to decrease the amount of fluid in the eye
Anesthetic: Local or general
Notes: May be done alone or may be combined with cataract surgery

Procedure: Surgical trabeculectomy
Description: A surgical opening is made in the sclera and covered by conjunctiva, forming a bubble or "bleb" into which aqueous drains
Anesthetic: Local or general
Notes: This is the most commonly performed glaucoma surgery today

Procedure: YAG laser iridotomy
Description: Used to create a hole in the iris that allows the aqueous to drain out of the eye even if the iris blocks the angle structure
Anesthetic: Topical
Notes: Used to treat angle-closure glaucoma; argon laser may also be used to perform iridotomy

Cataract Surgery (Table 18-6)

Table 18-6.
Cataract Surgery

Procedure: Extracapsular extraction
Description: The cataract is essentially delivered whole; cortex may be removed manually with a needle or with an irrigating/aspirating (I/A) unit; an intraocular lens implant is inserted
Anesthetic: Local or general
Notes: Wound must be sutured shut

Procedure: Phacoemulsification
Description: Uses ultrasonic vibration to emulsify the cataract; a foldable intraocular lens implant is inserted
Anesthetic: Local or general
Notes: A smaller incision may be used; sutures frequently unnecessary

Strabismus Surgery (Table 18-7)

Table 18-7.
Strabismus Surgery

Procedure: Adjustable suture
Description: During the initial recession or resection, the suture is tied in a slip knot, which the physician later manipulates to bring the eye(s) into correct alignment
Anesthetic: Local or general
Notes: A topical anesthetic may be used during the adjustment procedure

Procedure: Muscle recession
Description: The muscle is detached at the insertion and resutured to the sclera behind the insertion point
Anesthetic: Local or general
Notes: Done to loosen a muscle

Procedure: Muscle resection
Description: The muscle is detached at the insertion, trimmed slightly shorter, and resutured to the sclera at the insertion point
Anesthetic: Local or general
Notes: Done to tighten a muscle

Retinal Surgery and Enucleation (Table 18-8)

Table 18-8.
Retinal Surgery and Enucleation

Procedure: Cryotherapy
Description: Freezing forms a scar around the detachment or tear to keep it from enlarging
Anesthetic: Local
Notes: Usually used for small tears

Procedure: Enucleation
Description: Surgical removal of the globe; a synthetic implant is placed into the socket to provide volume
Anesthetic: General
Notes: A prosthesis is fit after healing is complete

Procedure: Retinal laser procedures
Description: Laser-applied photocoagulation or photovaporization
Anesthetic: Topical or local
Notes: Hemorrhage from diabetic retinopathy and hypertension, abnormal blood vessel growth from diabetic retinopathy and macular degeneration, and retinal tears are common laser treated retinal conditions

Procedure: Scleral buckle
Description: Cryotherapy or laser photocoagulation is performed around each break; the scleral buckle is then sutured to the sclera, pushing the sclera and choroid inward; gas or water may be injected into the eye to flatten the retina against the sclera and to add volume to the eye
Anesthetic: Local or general
Notes: Used for larger tears or detachments

Notes

- The patient is the primary focus of the eyecare team.
- A well-informed operative patient is more likely to have a successful surgical outcome.
- The best possible patient handling is achieved when the patient's physical and emotional needs are considered.
- The patient has the right to refuse treatment.
- Proper documentation is an important aspect of surgery scheduling.
- Keeping the patient well informed may help alleviate some of the anxiety associated with surgery.

- Good communication between the physician and surgery scheduler can aid the scheduler in performing the job.
- The main goal of the scheduling system is to assist the physician in providing the best care for the patient.

Unless otherwise noted, all text, tables, and figures are adapted or reprinted with permission from Pickett K. Overview of Ocular Surgery and Surgical Counseling. *Thorofare, NJ: SLACK Incorporated; 1999.*

CHAPTER 19

Refractive Surgery

Preoperative Examination of the Refractive Surgery Patient (Table 19-1)

- Understand a patient's motivation for refractive eye surgery.
- Be realistic about a patient's expectations and results.
- Eye diseases and diabetes are contraindications to surgery.
- Take time to educate, inform, and counsel on the procedures, risks, side effects, and potential complications.

The Refractive Surgical Patient

- Careful selection of patients to receive refractive surgery is essential.
- Staff members need to know the particulars of refractive surgeries performed at their practice (Table 19-2).
- Careful preoperative counseling, including informed consent, is essential to the successful refractive surgery practice.
- Postoperative care must be meticulous. (For postoperative history questions, see Table 19-3. For postoperative slit lamp evaluation, see Table 14-12, sections VII and VIII.)

Radial and Astigmatic Keratotomy

- The three most common incisional refractive procedures are radial keratotomy (RK), astigmatic keratotomy (AK), and automated lamellar keratoplasty (ALK).
- RK, which is performed for low to moderate myopia, is a procedure in which microscopic incisions are carefully placed in a radial pattern on the cornea. These incisions flatten the cornea, causing the light rays coming through the eye to focus closer to the retina.

Table 19-1.

Preoperative Examination of the Refractive Surgery Patient

Preliminaries

- Soft contact lenses must be removed for a period of no less than 1 week prior and rigid contact lenses no less than 3 weeks prior to the examination.
- It is more effective to examine the patient more than once.
- A successful interaction between the physician and the team can ensure a good working relationship with each and every patient. If this cannot be achieved for a given patient, then it is always better judgment to not proceed with any surgery.

The History

- Age
- Occupation
- Extracurricular activities, hobbies
- Social situation (Married? Children?)
- Why do you desire a surgical alternative to eyeglasses and contact lenses?
- Medications (including over-the-counter medications, birth control pills, etc)
- Any known drug allergies
- Allergies to contactants
- Women—pregnant?
- Experience with the healing process (Does the patient tend to form keloids?)
- Ocular disease or injury
- Family ocular history

The Examination

- Uncorrected visual acuity measured one eye at a time
- Corrected visual acuity measured one eye at a time
- Best-corrected binocular and monocular visual acuity (best to use cycloplegic refractometry, including objective retinoscopy and subjective refractometry)
- Determine eye dominance
- Record previous refraction, contact lens and/or eyeglass correction, and prescription stability over time. Has the prescription recently been changed? How old are the present glasses?
- Pupillary testing with special attention to pupil diameter in normal illumination and in the dark
- Iris color
- Confrontation fields
- Ocular motility testing
- Gross external examination to note any eyelid abnormalities or tear function problems
- Slit lamp examination with special attention to the cornea
- Dilated anterior segment and funduscopic examination
- Keratometry
- Computer-assisted video keratography
- Corneal pachymetry
- Intraocular pressure

Table 19-2.

Types of Refractive Surgery

Procedure	Purpose
Radial keratotomy (RK)	Reduce myopia
Astigmatic keratotomy (AK)	Reduce astigmatism
Photorefractive keratectomy (PRK)	Reduce myopia and astigmatism
Laser assisted in-situ keratomileusis (LASIK)	Reduce myopia
Automated lamellar keratoplasty (ALK)	Reduce myopia or hyperopia
Phakic intraocular lens (IOL) implant	Reduce myopia—may be used in the future for hyperopia

Reprinted with permission from Gayton JL, Kershner RM. Refractive Surgery for Eyecare Paraprofessionals. *Thorofare, NJ: SLACK Incorporated; 1997.*

Table 19-3.

Postoperative Refractive Surgery History Questions

- Is your eye uncomfortable in any way? Scratchy feeling?
- Have you had any pain?
- Has there been much redness?
- Has there been any discharge? Tearing?
- How is your vision? Does it fluctuate from one day to the next? How? Does it fluctuate during the day? Describe this. Is it more clear when you get up in the morning, or does it progressively clear as the day goes by? Do you see equally well at distance as you do up close?
- Have you experienced any double vision? Distortion?
- Are you light sensitive? Have problems with glare? See halos around lights?
- Tell me how you are using your medications.
- *If appropriate*: Has the contact lens stayed on your eye?

Reprinted with permission from Ledford JK. The Complete Guide to Ocular History Taking. *Thorofare, NJ: SLACK Incorporated; 1999.*

- AK corrects astigmatism with arc-shaped incisions in the cornea or limbus. The incisions are placed across the steep meridian, usually in pairs on either side. This relaxes the cornea and thus flattens it.
- ALK uses a machine to slice sections off the front of the cornea to correct high myopia and hyperopia. It is also used to create a flap for the LASIK procedure.
- Incisional refractive procedures change the eye's refractive error by altering the shape of the cornea.
- The refractive outcome can be modified positively or negatively by postoperative treatment.

- Over- and under-correction are the most common complications of refractive surgery.

Cataracts and Astigmatism

- Cataract surgery has become the most accurate refractive surgery procedure.
- In order to achieve an optimum postoperative refraction, meticulous attention must be devoted to the preoperative work-up.
- Several options exist if a significant refractive error persists after cataract extraction, including incisional refractive surgery.

Post-Corneal Transplantation Refractive Error

- Intraoperative control of refractive error in corneal transplant cases is limited to the suture closure.
- After corneal graft surgery, the most useful tools for management of refractive error is refractometry and corneal topography.
- If selective suture removal does not alter the postoperative refractive error sufficiently, incisional refractive surgery may be considered.
- RK and AK are performed very cautiously in corneal graft patients because of the stress to the donor button.
- Normal side effects in an eye undergoing RK or AK can mimic the signs and symptoms of graft rejection. Patient education and meticulous slit lamp examination are crucial.

Excimer Laser Photorefractive Keratectomy

- Excimer laser photorefractive keratectomy (PRK) removes layers of corneal tissue to flatten the cornea, reducing myopia and astigmatism.
- PRK is generally for individuals with mild to moderate nearsightedness (-1.00 to –7.00 diopters and less than 1.25 diopters of astigmatism).
- There is a period of healing that can last 3 months or longer.

Automated Lamellar Keratoplasty and Laser Assisted In Situ Keratomileusis

- In ALK, a keratome is moved over the surface of the cornea in a controlled fashion to excise the cap. This cap of epithelium and stromal tissue can be either folded back (hinge technique) or removed entirely (free cap technique). The keratome can then be used for a second pass over the cornea to remove a predetermined amount of tissue for a given degree of flattening. The procedure is designed to correct myopia.

- Although the ALK technique is effective for excising the corneal cap, it is less predictable when removing subsequent amounts of tissue. PRK, however, is extremely accurate in ablating or removing a given amount of tissue.
- LASIK uses the cutting keratome to create a flap of central cornea ALK under which laser PRK can be performed.
- In LASIK, the photorefractive ablation occurs within the stroma rather than on the surface of the cornea.
- LASIK is a method for providing greater corrections of myopia than is possible with PRK alone.

Intraocular Contact Lenses and Intraocular Lens Implants

- Removal of the human crystalline lens and replacement with an intraocular lens implant (pseudophakia) can simultaneously correct myopia and hyperopia in either the cataract or noncataract patient.
- Intraocular lens implantation in the phakic patient (intraocular contact lens, or ICL) can correct most forms of refractive error and has the added benefit of being reversible. It does not require removal of the natural lens.

Unless otherwise noted, all text, tables, and figures are adapted or reprinted with permission from Gayton JL, Kershner RM. Refractive Surgery for Eyecare Paraprofessionals. *Thorofare, NJ: SLACK Incorporated; 1997.*

CHAPTER 20

The Ophthalmic Surgical Assistant

Ophthalmic Diagnostic Testing: An Overview

- Diagnostic testing provides crucial information required in the preoperative decision-making process, intraoperative course, and postoperative management (Table 20-1).
- Diagnostic testing may be used to document the need for surgery.

Anesthesia (Table 20-2) and Pharmacology

- Local anesthetics should not be mixed too far in advance of a surgical procedure as they may deteriorate, compromising their anesthetic effectiveness. Patient discomfort could result, discounting the advantages of performing the procedure under local anesthesia.
- Medication labels and expiration dates should always be checked during preparation and immediately before administration of any drug.
- An important part of preoperative preparation is confirmation of the patient's identity and operative eye before the administration of any drops or ointments.

Note: For information regarding other medications used in conjunction with ophthalmic surgery, see the following:

- Anti-infectives, Tables 17-17 through 17-20
- Corticosteroids, Tables 17-12 through 17-14
- Dilating and constricting drugs, Tables 17-2 through 17-3 and Figures 7-1 through 7-4
- Nonsteroidal anti-inflammatories (NSAIDs), Table 17-16
- Viscoelastics, Table 17-9

Table 20-1.

Preoperative Tests

Type of Surgeries	Diagnostic Tests Performed
Oculoplastic surgery	Photography, external measurements (exophthalmometry), visual field testing, optional: Schirmer testing
Extraocular muscle surgery	Photography, muscle balance
Corneal surgery	Corneal topography, optional: pachymetry, keratometry, specular microscopy
Refractive surgery	Corneal topography, pachymetry, keratometry, refractometry
Glaucoma surgery	Visual field testing, photography of disc
Cataract surgery	A-scan biometry and calculation, refractometry, keratometry, optional: specular microscopy, B-scan ultrasound, PAM, BAT, and contrast sensitivity
Retinal and vitreous surgery	B-scan ultrasound

Reprinted with permission from Boess-Lott R, Stecik S. The Ophthalmic Surgical Assistant. *Thorofare, NJ: SLACK Incorporated; 1999.*

Table 20-2.

Anesthesia in Ophthalmic Surgery

Type	Generic	Notes
Topical	Proparacaine Tetracaine Cocaine	
Local	Lidocaine Marcaine	Local anesthetics are commonly combined with epinephrine to reduce bleeding and prolong anesthesia and with hyaluronidase to increase diffusion and enhance effectiveness. Facial nerve blocks: • Van Lint block—injected directly into the orbicularis muscles of the lid • O'Brien block—injected into VII N • Atkinson block—injected into stylomastoid foramen for a complete motor block of facial muscles on that side *(continued)*

Table 20-2. (continued)
Anesthesia in Ophthalmic Surgery

Type	Generic	Notes
		Retrobulbar injection: injected into base of lids or behind globe; produces temporary paralysis of EOMs Peribulbar injection: injected into floor of socket or roof of orbit; infiltrates soft tissue Intracameral: lidocaine administered through a corneal stab incision; anesthetizes the iris
General		Used to obtain control over the intraoperative situation, for long procedures, and where patient is unable to cooperate under local anesthesia Further discussion is beyond the scope of this text

Disinfection and Sterilization Techniques (Tables 20-3 through 20-5)

- The goal of disinfection is to reduce the sources of infection. Using chemical solutions is the most common method.
- Sterilization is the complete destruction of all microorganisms. Instruments are either sterile or nonsterile. There is nothing in between.
- To ensure successful sterilization, ophthalmic surgical instruments must be wiped clean and irrigated thoroughly after use to remove any residual blood or tissue products.
- The two most common methods of sterilization are pressurized steam (autoclaving) or gas (ethylene oxide or EO_2).
- Infection control programs must be followed by all personnel in hospitals and operating rooms.

Preoperative Scrubbing, Gowning, and Gloving Procedures

- Preoperative hand scrubbing, gowning, and gloving protocols should be established and regularly reviewed by the individual facility's policy and procedure.

Table 20-3.

Common Methods of Sterilization

Method: Steam (autoclave) sterilization
Mode of action: Moist heat under pressure; microorganisms are destroyed by breaking down protein within the cells
Use: In general, less sterilization time is required if pressure and temperature settings are higher; 15 lbs of pressure at 250°F (121°C) requires 15 to 30 minutes exposure time for effective sterilization
Comments: The most frequently used form of sterilizing instruments

Method: Flash sterilization
Mode of action: High speed sterilization in a conventional autoclave
Use: 270°F (132°C) under 28 to 32 lbs of pressure; flat surface items can be sterilized for 3 minutes; any cannulated item must be sterilized for 10 minutes
Comments: Should only be used when there is not enough time to sterilize by other methods and an individual item is needed immediately

Method: Plasma sterilization
Mode of action: Low-temperature hydrogen peroxide gas plasma is used to achieve fast low-temperature, low-moisture sterilization
Comments: One of the most technologically advanced procedures in sterilization

Method: Chemical or cold sterilization
Mode of action: Various chemicals are used to kill organisms (Table 20-4)
Use: Minimum time for chemical sterilization is 20 minutes
Comments: Add a rust inhibitor to the germicidal chemical solution to prevent instruments from rusting; pad the bottom of the pan to protect instruments

Method: Gaseous chemical sterilization (ethylene oxide discussed here)
Mode of action: Gas used under specific temperatures and humidity to kill organisms
Use: Exposure times range from 1.5 to 2 hours with a temperature range of 50° to 60° and a humidity range of 40% to 80%
Comments: The least taxing on fragile microsurgical instrumentation; proper time for cooling and aeration must be allowed prior to handling or use
Advantages: Usable on materials that cannot tolerate other sterilization methods; the least damaging to fragile instruments; excellent penetration; very effective against all microbes and spores
Disadvantages: Expensive; requires special equipment; takes longer to achieve adequate sterilization; the compounds used are toxic and highly flammable

Table 20-4.
Major Categories of Chemical Disinfectants

Disinfectant	Advantages	Disadvantages	Uses
Alcohol (ethyl or isopropyl)	Fungicidal Bactericidal Tuberculocidal Active against viruses Nonstaining Fast acting	Nonsporicidal Ineffective on evaporation Cannot be used on instruments with cement mountings (dissolves cement) Inadequate for AIDS virus	Housekeeping disinfectant Used on semicritical instruments after 0.2% sodium nitrate is added Disinfects thermometers Skin antiseptic
Halogens (chlorine or iodophors)	*Chlorine* Highly active as free chlorine in slightly acidic solution Effective against hepatitis, gram positive and gram negative viruses and bacteria Low cost, toxicity, and irritancy	Cannot be used on instruments (corrosive to metals) Nonsporicidal Inactivated by organic matter Difficult to combine with detergent for single cleaning formula	Disinfects renal dialysis equipment Widely used for disinfection for toilets, lavatories, bathtubs Bleach for laundry Sanitizer for dishwashing Disinfection of hydrotherapy tanks
	Iodophors Bactericidal Pseudomonacidal Fungicidal Tuberculocidal Virucidal Versatile Rapid action Nonirritating if no iodine allergy exists and is fully rinsed	Harmful to rubber and some plastics May burn tissue Inactivated by organic matter Corrosive to metals unless combined with rust inhibitor May stain some fabrics, plastics, and other synthetic materials	Instrument disinfection after 0.2% sodium nitrate is added Thermometers (tincture of iodine or iodophors) Disinfecting some kitchen or nursery equipment
Phenols	Bactericidal Pseudomonacidal Fungicidal Lipid virucidal Remains active after prolonged drying	Leaves a film on surfaces (build up must eventually be removed) May cause skin irritation and depigmentation with long periods of use	Housekeeping disinfectant Used as instrument disinfectant if instruments are not designed for skin or mucous membrane contact

(continued)

Table 20-4. (continued)

Major Categories of Chemical Disinfectants

Disinfectant	Advantages	Disadvantages	Uses
		Nonsporicidal Inactivated by organic matter Corrosive to rubber and some plastics	
Quaternary ammonium compounds	Germicidal Detergent properties Cationic surface active compounds Wetting agents Effective against *M. tuberculosis* and gram negative bacteria	Nonsporicidal Absorbed and/or neutralized by cotton wool Ineffective as skin antiseptic Incompatible with soap Decreased action in the presence of organic matter	Housekeeping programs for walls, floors, and furnishings Should never be used for disinfecting instruments
Aldehydes	*Glutaraldehyde* Bactericidal Pseudomonacidal Fungicidal Tuberculocidal Virucidal in alcohol Active in the presence of organic matter Compatible with metal, rubber, and plastic materials	Unstable (effective life 2 to 30 weeks) Some glutaraldehydes may cause chemical burns on skin and mucous membranes Contamination is possible during wrapping and drying process Alkaline glutaraldehyde will corrode and stain high carbon metals Destroys proteins Will damage lenses after long periods of use	Respiratory therapy and anesthesia equipment Certain items that cannot be steam or gas sterilized Widely used for semicritical instruments
	Formaldehydes (37% in water, 80% in 70% isopropyl alcohol) Bactericidal Pseudomonacidal Fungicidal	Toxic to tissue (must be thoroughly rinsed from instruments) Highly corrosive Vapor has limited uses as sterilant	Can be used for cold sterilization of instruments after adding 0.2% sodium nitrate Sometimes used to clean hemodialysis water systems

(continued)

Table 20-4. (continued)

Major Categories of Chemical Disinfectants

Disinfectant	Advantages	Disadvantages	Uses
	Tuberculocidal Virucidal	High risk when cleaning hemodialysis systems: toxic to patients and personnel Absorbed by porous materials	

Data from Brooks G. Medical Microbiology. *19th ed. Norwalk, Conn: Appleton & Lange; 1991 & Soule B.* The Apic Curriculum for Infection Control Practice. *Dubuque; 1983.*

Table 20-5.

Recommendations for Packaging[1]

- The type of sterilization method used determines proper packaging for sterilization.
- Packaging materials should be durable to prevent tearing and puncture (by staples or clips) and should provide an effective barrier against microorganisms.
- The two common methods of wrapping articles for sterilization are envelopes and peel packs.
- Packages are sealed with a heat sealer or heat/gas-sensitive indicator tape.
- Single-use items are not meant to be resterilized.
- Allow for adequate penetration and release of gas and moisture for gas sterilization.
- Allow adequate air removal and steam penetration for steam sterilization.
- Muslin-wrapped items should be double-wrapped immediately.
- Manufacturers of packaging materials other than muslin must show data that indicate their products are equivalent to the muslin time temperature profile when steam sterilization is used.
- Polypropylene film (1 to 3 mm thickness) is the only plastic acceptable for steam sterilization.
- Nylon is not acceptable packaging for gas sterilization.
- Per hospital or ambulatory surgery center (ASC), any sterilized package should be marked or labeled with a lot control number that identifies the date of sterilization, sterilization used, and the date of expiration.
- Pack sizes should be no larger than 12 in x 12 in, no heavier than 12 lbs, and no denser than 7-2/10 lbs per cubic foot.

- After scrubbing, sterile gowns and gloves should be worn. This produces an effective barrier that will minimize the passage of microorganisms between sterile and nonsterile areas.
- The front of the gown, from the chest to the level of the sterile field, is considered sterile.

- Nonsterile areas are the neckline, shoulders, back, and under the arms and sleeve cuffs.
- Any item that is not known to be sterile must be considered nonsterile.

Surgical Hand Scrub Procedures

Nail polish may chip, crack, or harbor organisms and should be removed before handwashing. Acrylic or artificial nails may also harbor organisms and fungi and should not be worn by scrub personnel. The skin is a major source of contamination in the operating room (OR) environment. AORN states that the purpose of the surgical hand scrub is to:

- Remove debris and transient microorganisms from the nails, hands, and forearms
- Reduce the resident microbial count to a minimum
- Inhibit rapid rebound growth of microorganisms[2]

Therefore, all personnel should be in surgical attire before beginning the surgical hand scrub[2]: all jewelry removed or secured to a two-piece scrub suit consisting of pants and shirt (tucked in), head covering, mask, and shoe covering.

A surgical hand scrub agent, as approved by the facility's infection control committee, should be used for all surgical hand scrubs.[2] According to AORN it should:

- Significantly reduce microorganisms on intact skin
- Contain a nonirritating antimicrobial preparation
- Have a broad spectrum
- Be fast acting and/or have a residual effect[2]

Many operating rooms have sinks with elbow, knee, or foot controls. The surgical hand scrub procedure is standardized according to the institution's policy and procedure.[2]

How-To: Surgical Hand Scrub[2]

AORN has published the following guidelines that should include, but not be limited to, the following:

- Thoroughly moistened hands and forearms should be washed using an approved surgical scrub agent and rinsed before beginning the surgical scrub procedure.
- Areas underneath the nails should be cleaned under running water using a nail cleaner as designated by the facility.
- An antimicrobial agent should be applied with friction to the wet hands and forearms.
- The fingers, hands, and arms should be visualized as having four sides; each side must be scrubbed effectively.

(continued)

How-To: Surgical Hand Scrub[2] (continued)

- Hands should be held higher than the elbows and away from the surgical attire to prevent contamination and to allow water to run from the cleanest area down the arm.
- The brush or sponge used should be discarded appropriately.
- Care should be taken to avoid splashing water onto surgical attire as a sterile gown cannot be placed over damp surgical attire. This would result in contamination of the gown by soak-through moisture.

Gloving

How-To: Gloving

Closed Gloving Technique:

- Slide hands into the sleeves of the gown until the cuffs can be grasped between the fingers and thumbs. The hands do not protrude beyond the gown.
- Lay the gloves on the table with the gown-covered hand. Place the glove thumb-down on the sleeve, with the fingers pointing toward the shoulder.
- Grasp the cuff of the glove by the thumb and forefinger inside the sleeve and pull down completely over the gown cuff.
- For the opposite hand, simply pick up the remaining glove with the gloved hand and follow the same procedure.
- Inspect gloves for any holes or tears.

Open Gloving Technique:

- Pick up the sterile glove by the inside cuff with one hand. Take care not to touch the glove wrapper with bare hands.
- Slide the glove onto the opposite hand with the cuff down. Then, using the partially gloved hand, slide the fingers into the outer side of the opposite glove cuff.
- Inspect gloves for any holes or tears.

Gloving Another:

- Widely open the sterile glove for the surgeon or additional scrub person to insert his or her hand into, pulling the glove over the cuff of the gown.
- Inspect gloves for any holes or tears.

Common Errors in Aseptic Technique

- Mask that covers only the mouth and not the nose.
- Masks that are not tied securely.
- Hair protruding from surgical caps.
- Long fingernails.
- Allowing run-off from the hands instead of the elbows during the surgical scrub.
- Short scrub time and lack of systematic scrub routine (must adhere to institutional policy).
- Splashing water onto scrub clothing. This contaminates sterile clothing donned in the OR.
- Using wet towels to dry scrubbed areas.
- Allowing towels to touch nonsterile clothing.
- Contaminating sterile clothing by brushing against nonsterile objects in the OR.
- Holding gloved hands against the body while waiting.

Operative Setup

- Since most ophthalmic surgical procedures are performed on a conscious patient, the ophthalmic assistant (OA) should tell the patient what is being done and what to expect, even during the skin prep stage.
- The surgical team is comprised of scrubbed and circulating personnel. Personnel who scrub their hands, arms, and change into sterile gowns and gloves are scrubbed. Those who coordinate the room activities, interact with the patient, and provide support and supplies to the scrubbed personnel are circulators.
- It is the responsibility of every individual on the ophthalmic surgical team to monitor and preserve asepsis and to initiate corrective action when a sterile field has been violated.

Basic Instrumentation (Table 20-6)

- Ophthalmic microsurgical instruments are an investment on the part of the ophthalmologist, hospital, or ASC.
- All microsurgical instruments should be inspected under the microscope.
- Scissors with bent tips, forceps with misaligned jaws, and instruments with surface breaks should be removed from the surgical set for repair and/or replacement.
- Sterilizing an instrument is not the same as cleaning it. Used instruments must be thoroughly wiped and flushed clean with demineralized/sterile water.

Table 20-6.
Basic Instrumentation

Instrument Type	Function	Description
Forceps	Used to grasp tissue, suture, tubing	May be toothed or smooth; teeth vary in size (0.12 to 0.5 mm); curved, bent, or straight
Scissors	Used to cut tissue, suture	Blunt or sharp; curved or straight; locking or non-locking
Needleholders	Used to hold suture needles	Micro or large; locking or nonlocking
Hooks	Used to identify muscles, grasp IOL loops	Straight or smooth; hooked
Probes/dilators	Used in lacrimal surgery to open obstructed canals	Vary in size and diameter
Clamps	Used in lid surgery to isolate sections or lesions for excision; create hemostasis	Vary in size and plate diameter
Calipers	Used to measure distances	In ruler or compass form
Cannulas	Used to deliver fluids and substances	Straight, curved; varying surface finishes and gauges
Speculum	Used to separate/hold eyelids	Wire or adjustable; varying size

Reprinted with permission from Boess-Lott R, Stecik S. The Ophthalmic Surgical Assistant. *Thorofare, NJ: SLACK Incorporated; 1999.*

- Never use saline for rinsing instruments because the salt content will adhere to the surface and result in instrument corrosion, increasing rust, or deterioration of the metal.
- Dried blood, tissue, and saline disrupt the integrity of the sterilization process.
- OR personnel who handle instruments should know the name and purpose of each instrument, as well as how to maintain it.

Oculoplastics (Tables 20-7 through 20-10)

Table 20-7.
Lid Surgery Set

BSS irigator	Muscle hook #1
Towel clamp	Muscle hook #2
Mosquito forceps, straight (2)	Fixation hook, sharp
Mosquito forceps, curved (2)	Chalazion curette #1
Utility scissors	Chalazion curette #2
Miniature blade #69	Chalazion curette #3
Blade handle	Chalazion curette #4
Westcott scissors, blunt	Fixation forceps
Stitch scissors	Conjunctiva forceps
Ptosis forceps	Tissue forceps
Needleholder, delicate	Fixation forceps, angled
Kalt needle holder	Suturing forceps
Lid plate	Tying forceps, curved
Caliper	Chalazion forceps, round
Lid retractor #1	Chalazion forceps, oval
Lid retractor #2	Lid forceps
Lid retractor #3	

Reprinted with permission from Boess-Lott R, Stecik S. The Ophthalmic Surgical Assistant. *Thorofare, NJ: SLACK Incorporated; 1999.*

Table 20-8.
Lacrimal Surgery Set

BSS irigator	Lacrimal chisel, straight
Towel clamp (2)	Lacrimal chisel, curved
Mosquito forceps, straight	Pigtail probe
Mosquito forceps, curved	Retrieving hook
Kerrison rongeur	Intubation set
Nasal speculum	Lacrimal probe set
Bone rongeur	Dressing forceps
Mallet	Tissue forceps
Miniature blade #65	Utility forceps
Blade handle	Suturing forceps
Self retaining retractor	Rake retractor (2)
Lacrimal cannula, straight	Stevens scissors
Lacrimal cannula, curved	Utility scissors
Lacrimal dilator	Needleholder
Periosteal elevator	Stitch scissors

Reprinted with permission from Boess-Lott R, Stecik S. The Ophthalmic Surgical Assistant. *Thorofare, NJ: SLACK Incorporated; 1999.*

Table 20-9.
Enucleation Surgery Set

Speculum	Tenotomy scissors
Tissue forceps	Enucleation scissors
Mosquito forceps	Muscle hook

Reprinted with permission from Boess-Lott R, Stecik S. The Ophthalmic Surgical Assistant. *Thorofare, NJ: SLACK Incorporated; 1999.*

Table 20-10.
Oculoplastic Surgery Set

Lester-Burch eye speculum	Tissue forceps, standard 1x2, straight
Schepens orbital retractor	Francis chalazion forceps
Desmares lid retractor #2	Hartmann mosquito forceps
Jaeger lid plate, stainless steel	Castroviejo needleholder, straight with lock
Wright fascia needle	Kalt needleholder, delicate
Knapp retractor, four-prong, blunt	Freer periosteal elevator
Meyerhoefer curette #3	West lacrimal chisel, straight
Bunge evisceration spoon, large	Wilder lacrimal dilator #2
Fixation hook, double, sharp, large	Bowman lacrimal probe #3-4
Graefe muscle hook	Pigtail probe with suture holes
Stainless steel rule	Bard-Parker handle
Stevens scissors, standard, straight	Bard-Parker blade #11
Enucleation scissors, medium, curved	Bard-Parker blade #15

Reprinted with permission from Boess-Lott R, Stecik S. The Ophthalmic Surgical Assistant. *Thorofare, NJ: SLACK Incorporated; 1999.*

Extraocular Muscles (Table 20-11)

Table 20-11.
Muscle Surgery Set

BSS irigator	Jameson muscle hook, small
Serrefine (2)	Jameson muscle hook, large
Towel clamp	Tenotomy hook
Mosquito forceps, straight (2)	Muscle hook #1
Mosquito forceps, curved (2)	Muscle hook #2
Utility scissors	Muscle hook #3
Speculum	Stainless steel rule
Tenotomy scissors, straight	Dressing forceps
Tenotomy scissors, curved	Conjunctiva forceps
Stitch scissors	Fixation forceps
Westcott scissors, blunt	Tissue forceps

(continued)

Table 20-11. (continued)

Muscle Surgery Set

B-P handle #3 and blade #11	Suturing forceps, 0.3 mm
Beaver handle and blade #6900	Muscle forceps, child
Caliper	Muscle forceps, adult
Lid retractor #1	Needle holder, delicate
Lid retractor #2	Needle holder, standard

Reprinted with permission from Boess-Lott R, Stecik S. The Ophthalmic Surgical Assistant. *Thorofare, NJ: SLACK Incorporated; 1999.*

Cornea (Table 20-12)

Table 20-12.

Corneal Transplant Set

BSS irigator	Superior rectus forceps
Towel clamp (2)	Fixation forceps, 0.3 mm
Mosquito forceps (2)	Colibri forceps, 0.12 mm
Wire speculum	Corneal forceps, 0.12 mm
Serrefine	Tying forceps, curved
Transplant scissors, left	Tying forceps, straight
Transplant scissors, right	Double corneal fixation forceps
Vannas scissors	Suture placement marker
Stitch scissors	Paton spatula
Trephine blade, 7.5 mm	Air injection cannula, 30 gauge
Trephine blade, 8.0 mm	Viscoelastic injection cannula, 26 gauge
Trephine handle, 7.5 mm	Viscoelastic aspiration cannula, 22 gauge
Trephine handle, 8.0 mm	Needleholder, micro
Fixation ring set	Needleholder, standard
Intraoperative keratometer	Donor button punch

Reprinted with permission from Boess-Lott R, Stecik S. The Ophthalmic Surgical Assistant. *Thorofare, NJ: SLACK Incorporated; 1999.*

Refractive Surgery (Tables 20-13 through 20-15)

Table 20-13.
Radial Keratotomy Set

Wire speculum, solid	Visual axis marker
Diamond micrometer, double edge	Optic zone marker
Blade gauge	Radial marker, 6 lines
Marking pen	Radial marker, 8 lines
Thornton fixing ring	Incision spreading forceps
Fixation forceps, straight	Incision depth gauge
Fixation forceps, angled	Irrigating cannula, 27 gauge

Reprinted with permission from Boess-Lott R, Stecik S. The Ophthalmic Surgical Assistant. *Thorofare, NJ: SLACK Incorporated; 1999.*

Table 20-14.
Astigmatic Keratotomy Set

Wire speculum, solid	Axis marker
Diamond micrometer, double edge	T-incision marker
Blade gauge	Optic zone marker
Marking pen	Thornton corneal marker
Thornton fixing ring	Arcuate incision marker
Fixation forceps, double	Irrigating cannula, 27 gauge
Fixation forceps, 0.12 mm	Incision spreading forceps
Visual axis marker	Incision depth gauge
Degree gauge	

Reprinted with permission from Boess-Lott R, Stecik S. The Ophthalmic Surgical Assistant. *Thorofare, NJ: SLACK Incorporated; 1999.*

Table 20-15.
Instrumentation for Laser Refractive Surgery

PRK Surgical Tray	
Leiberman speculum	Katena fixation ring
Fukasaku hockey knife	Optic zone marker, 7 mm
Paton spatula	McPherson tying forceps
LASIK Surgical Tray	
Leiberman speculum	Marking pen
Corneal marker	Microkeratome instrumentation
Spatula	McPherson tying forceps

Glaucoma (Table 20-16)

Table 20-16.
Glaucoma Surgery Set

BSS irrigator	Colibri forceps, 0.12 mm
Towel clamp (2)	Caliper
Mosquito forceps (2)	Suturing forceps, 0.12 mm
Wire speculum	Tying forceps, straight
Utility forceps	Tying forceps, angled
Sclerotome blade	Trabeculotomy probe, right
Blade handle	Trabeculotomy probe, left
Super sharp blade	Air injection cannula, 27 gauge
Blade handle	Corneoscleral punch
Westcott scissors	Cyclodialysis spatula
Stitch scissors	Needleholder, micro
Vannas scissors	Needleholder, standard
Iris scissors	Diamond step knife
Dressing forceps	Tonometer
Bishop-Harmon forceps	

Reprinted with permission from Boess-Lott R, Stecik S. The Ophthalmic Surgical Assistant. *Thorofare, NJ: SLACK Incorporated; 1999.*

Cataract (Tables 20-17 and 20-18)

Table 20-17.
Planned Extracapsular Cataract Extraction (ECCE) Set

BSS irrigator	Kelman-McPherson forceps
Towel clip	Utrata capsulorrhexis forceps
Mosquito forceps	IOL forceps
Serrefine (2)	IOL manipulator
Wire speculum	Kuglen iris hook
Super sharp blade	Cyclodialysis spatula
Blade handle	Needleholder, micro
Corneal section scissors, right	Needleholder, standard
Corneal section scissors, left	Lens loop and probe
Westcott scissors, blunt	Thornton limbal ruler
Stitch scissors	*Kansas nucleus trisector
Capsulotomy scissors	*Kansas nucleus bisector
Iris scissors	*Kansas vectis, solid
Caliper	*Kansas nucleus loop
Conjunctiva forceps	*Keener nucleus divider
Superior rectus forceps	*Loop for nucleus divider *(continued)*

Table 20-17. (continued)

Planned Extracapsular Cataract Extraction (ECCE) Set

Colibri forceps, 0.12 mm	*Kansas nucleus fragment forceps
Diamond step knife	Viscoelastic aspirating cannula, 22 gauge
Intraoperative keratometer	Air injection cannula, 30 gauge
Tissue forceps	Viscoelastic injection cannula, 26 gauge
Suturing forceps, 0.12 mm	Cystotome
Tying forceps, straight	Capsule polisher
Tying forceps, angled	I/A cannula

**Additional instruments for manual small incision*

Reprinted with permission from Boess-Lott R, Stecik S. The Ophthalmic Surgical Assistant. *Thorofare, NJ: SLACK Incorporated; 1999.*

Table 20-18.

ECCE (Phacoemulsification) Surgery Set

Wire speculum	Suturing forceps, 0.12 mm
Diamond knife, trifacet	Superior rectus forceps
Keratome blade	Conjunctiva forceps
Round blade	Tying forceps, straight
Incision enlarging blade, 4.0 mm	Tying forceps, curved
Incision enlarging blade, 5.2 mm	Utrata capsulorrhexis forceps
Sideport incision blade	Kelman-McPherson forceps
Blade handle (4)	IOL forceps
BSS irrigator	Intraoperative keratometer
Colibri forceps, 0.12 mm	*Soft IOL holding forceps
Mosquito forceps, straight	Needleholder, standard
Mosquito forceps, curved	Needleholder, micro
Towel clamp	Viscoelastic aspirating cannula, 22 gauge
Capsulotomy scissors	Anterior chamber cannula, 30 gauge
Nucleus rotator	Cystotome
IOL manipulator	Hydrodissection cannula, right
Internal caliper	Hydrodissection cannula, left
Westcott scissors, blunt	Capsule polisher
	Viscoelastic injection cannula, 26 gauge

**For foldable IOLs.*

Reprinted with permission from Boess-Lott R, Stecik S. The Ophthalmic Surgical Assistant. *Thorofare, NJ: SLACK Incorporated; 1999.*

Retina and Vitreous (Table 20-19)

Table 20-19.
Vitreoretinal Surgery Set

Eye speculum, large	Caliper
Baby towel clamp 2 1/4 in (2)	Scleral marker
Serrefine (4)	Scleral depressor
Towel clamp 3 1/2 in (2)	Sleeve spreading forceps
Mosquito forceps (2)	Conjunctiva forceps 1.2 mm (2)
Baby mosquito forceps (2)	Utility forceps, smooth
Eye scissors, straight	Utility forceps, serrated
Eye scissors, curved	Suturing forceps 0.12 mm
Stevens scissors	Fixation forceps 1 x 2
Westcott scissors, right	Tying forceps, straight (2)
Vannas scissors	Colibri forceps 0.12 mm
Blade handle (2), K-Blade #64	Needleholder, straight
Orbital retractor	Needleholder, curved
Stiletto blade (20 gauge) and handle	Intraocular scissors, angled
Muscle hook, large	Intraocular forceps, serrated
Retinal detachment hook (2)	Intraocular forceps with platform

Reprinted with permission from Boess-Lott R, Stecik S. The Ophthalmic Surgical Assistant. *Thorofare, NJ: SLACK Incorporated; 1999.*

Notes

- Proper patient education is an asset in preoperative and postoperative compliance.
- Informed consent procedures have a medicolegal impact on the ophthalmic surgical candidate.
- The typical informed consent consists of an explanation of the procedure, anesthesia, risks, and complications.

References

1. Jackson-Williams B. *Ophthalmic Surgical Assisting*. 2nd ed. Thorofare, NJ: SLACK Incorporated; 1993.

2. *Standards and Recommended Practices.* Denver, Colo: Association of Operating Room Nurses Inc; 1996.

Unless otherwise noted, all text, tables, and figures are adapted or reprinted with permission from Boess-Lott R, Stecik S. The Ophthalmic Surgical Assistant. *Thorofare, NJ: SLACK Incorporated; 1999.*

CHAPTER 21

Office and Career Management

Records Management

The primary purpose for keeping medical records is to fully document the patient's visit and progress. It also represents security in case of an audit from a government or private peer review organization.

It is important to remember that the contents of the chart itself are medical/legal documents and thus must be handled appropriately.

How-To: Correct Patient Records

- Never use White Out (Bic Corporation, Millford, Conn) or a similar product; never erase anything.
- If a change needs to be made, strike a single line through the inaccuracy, and write the correction clearly next to it.
- Place your initials next to the correction.

Occasionally, a patient may leave the practice and need his or her medical records. Records release forms are legal documents authorizing the transfer of patient records to another physician or to the patient. It is important to remember that the medical charts and records belong to the patient as his or her sole property and may not be transferred without the owner's consent. It is wise to document the receipt and issuance of patient records in the patient's chart before photocopying, faxing, or otherwise transferring the record. The patient's record request should be signed by the patient, power of attorney, or legal guardian.

Other communication in regard to the patient's medical records is also considered a legality. Giving anyone information in a patient's chart over the telephone or through fax communication may breach patient confidentiality. The person and reason for the request should be very carefully screened before divulging any information.

For information on office forms, see Table 21-1.

Table 21-1.
Common Office Forms

Form	Description	Notes
Authorization for payment	Assigns payments received from third-party source to doctor providing the service	Payment comes directly to physician, rather than going to the patient
Authorization for responsibility	Documents who is responsible for payment	Usually the patient; may be a power of attorney, guardian, or family member
Informed consent	Denotes patient acceptance of the risks, benefits, and actions to be performed	Usually for surgical procedures; may be written or video taped
Initial patient registration	Demographic and medical information	Filled out at first visit; includes referring source
Interval visit registration	Update form for demographics, medical, and benefits	Usually shorter; filled out at subsequent visits
Records release	Authorization to release records to patient or physician	Must be signed by patient or legal guardian
Waiver of liability	Patient assumes financial responsibility for a procedure that may not be covered by a third-party payer	Usually for surgical procedures; may be a service

Patient Management

The way that patient care is delivered can make or break a practice. It does not matter how successful your marketing program is at bringing patients to your door. If they are not treated well, receiving a high level of care, not only will they find someone else to take care of their eyes... they will tell everyone they know to do the same.

When calling your patient from the reception room, eye contact and a smile are always in order. If your patient needs a hand for steadiness, offer it. (As a general rule, geriatric patients like the caring touch that is offered. Patients who are in their more active stages in life usually do not.) Health care professionals have a unique opportunity to make a positive difference in a person's day. Treat your patients with dignity and care. Your warm touch or smile may be the only one your patient gets that day.

Patients who become irate feel either insulted or hurt in some way. (It might even have been something that happened before they arrived at your office.) It may fall to you to smooth those ruffled feathers. Listening is one of the best ways to do that. Not just hearing, but really listening to your patient. Try to listen objectively, not defensively. The patient's concern is rarely a personal attack. Pay particular attention to the last thing your patient says. It is usually the issue that is the greatest concern to him or her.

If the patient is verbally upset and around other patients, it is best to direct him or her to a quiet out-of-the way spot where others will not be disturbed. On rare occasion, a patient will become verbally abusive. If this happens, simply excuse yourself from the patient's presence and let the doctor or office manager handle the situation.

Create an environment that is free of potential hazards to your patients as they move around in the office. Lanes need to be well lit when entering and exiting the room. If your examination chair has a foot platform, fold it up out of the patient's way as he or she gets in or out of the chair. Warn patients in advance if they are going to be seated on a chair that has wheels. If you are assisting blind or low vision patients, have them rest their hand on your elbow or shoulder while you walk in front of them, describing any uneven flooring or turns they will have to maneuver.

Wipe all areas of patient contact with alcohol or some other solution that is approved by OSHA standards. Have patients sit back if an adjustment is necessary in the positioning of equipment in which their chin is resting. If you have a patient with a contagious disease (such as chicken pox, etc) isolate him or her from the rest of your staff and patients.

Health care professionals are mandated reporters of suspected abuse in many states. What this means is that we are required by law to report (or cause reports to be made) to the proper officials if we suspect that abuse has occurred. The person reporting does not have to prove the abuse has taken place. Because the law to report abuse mandates health care providers, we are also protected by the law. We cannot be sued for reporting suspected abuse even if we are wrong. Check the laws in your state.

Look at your patients as whole people instead of "a cataract" or some other case. This will enable you to treat them with the respect and dignity they deserve. If each patient is listened to and his or her needs are assessed and then met, you will find your job more rewarding than you ever thought possible.

Other Matters

- The patient is the most important person in the practice.
- Any gross dissatisfaction, threat to bring legal action, or incident that could possibly result in legal action should be documented and brought to the physician's attention at once.
- The Good Samaritan Law varies from state to state and is designed to protect both victims and medically trained rescuers.
- You and you alone are responsible for your success.
- Write down your long-term goals. Then list the steps you need to take to achieve your goals.
- Success is not a destination; it is a process.
- Certification tells your employer and patients the value you place on what you do.
- You are what you think.
- It is not what happens to you that is important, it is what you do with what happens to you that is important.
- The key to preventing burnout is to control stress.

Unless otherwise noted, all text, tables, and figures are adapted or reprinted with permission from Borover B, Langley T. Office and Career Management for the Eyecare Paraprofessional. *Thorofare, NJ: SLACK Incorporated; 1997.*

Index